THE DARK
ORCHESTRA

FOREWORD BY DONNY SHANKLE

JON NORTH   JAMES MCDERMOTT

The Dark Orchestra
Copyright © 2014 by Jon North & James McDermott

Design Credits

Cover design by Jordan Aguilar
Book design by Jordan Aguilar
www.JAdesign.us

Executive Producers - Christopher Smith & Kayleigh Gratton

Photo Credits

Jasha Faye – Cover Photo
Nat Arem – www.HookGrip.com: (8.1)(8.2)(8.3)(8.4)(8.5)(8.6)(8.7)(9.1)(9.2)
(10.3)(11.1)(12.1)(12.2)(12.3)(12.5)(12.6)(13.1)(Back Cover)
Maria Murray Photography: (11.4)(13.5)
California Strength: (8.8)(10.5)(10.6)(12.7)(12.8)
Caleb Ward: (11.2)
Muscle Driver USA: (13.4)(13.5)(13.6)
Joe Nissim: (About James McDermott)

Content Credits

International Weightlifting Federations – www.IWF.com: Definitions (1)(2)(3)

Editors

Patrick Regan – Head Editor
Joanna Toman
Jessica North
Juanita Smart
Kiera Taylor

Printed in the United States of America

The Troy Book Makers • Troy, New York • www.TheTroyBookmakers.com

LinguaLinx • Troy, New York • www.LinguaLinx.com

To order additional copies of this title visit www.TheAttitudeNation.com

ISBN: 978-0-692-34539-9

EDITORS NOTE

Becoming a professional athlete is a goal held by countless people around the world who aspire to be like those they idolize in their respective sports. Having a role model is important to the development of an inexperienced or rookie athlete because it helps to provide them with inspiration to act upon their dreams. Having a positive example to follow is a wonderful thing, but up and coming athletes should also realize that there is more to being a professional than just the success they see on the outside. Training is laborious, taxing not only the body, but the mind as well. This is why Jon North created his online journal (blog) The Dark Orchestra.

The Dark Orchestra opens a door to a side of the sport of Weightlifting few are privileged enough to witness. Jon uses this deep personal outlet to communicate and share his philosophies about life and being an athlete with the world outside of the concrete walls of a gym. His blog also gave him a means to escape from the daily demands of hard training and the ability to express his creativity and passion for his craft. Within this text you will have a closer view on the social aspects, psychology and deep emotions that come with being a high-level athlete. You will gain knowledge from the successes and failures that Jon has experienced on his journey in the sport - something he hopes you will take to heart so that you can be a better athlete or coach.

Within the book, the blogs serve as artistic pieces to compliment the main text and enhance your experience. They were written throughout a large part of Jon's career while he was developing his methods. Due to this some instruction on technique discussed in the blogs may contradict how he views things now in the main text. Think of the main text as the production that drew you into the concert venue all dressed up in your best formal attire. Throughout the performance your ears are filled with the beautiful notes created by the strings of violins, the hum of horns and beating of drums. The beautiful music pleasures the senses and peaks the imagination guiding you on a path of self discovery and the development of your own personal technique. Think of the blogs as interludes – brief breaks from the music of the Orchestra that still add to the overall harmony of the show.

After much debate, we made the decision to present the blogs unedited in their raw natural form. These blogs are much too personal for Jon to allow another hand to alter and to do so would ruin their messages and the context from which they were originally written. Take note of the progressive improvement in Jon's writing over the years. As he becomes a better athlete, refining his technique and finding success in the sport, his skills as a writer in both structure and content also dramatically improve.

The following have not been changed to preserve the original spirit of the blogs: grammar, punctuation, spelling and typos.

For consistency, the following have been altered from how they initially appear - positioning of dates, signatures and titles.

Throughout the text you will periodically notice QR (Quick Response) Codes. It was our intent to create a very interactive experience for you. This was especially so because Jon is very active on Social Media platforms such as YouTube. To gain access to the content the QR Codes provide, you will need to download a QR Code Reader App on your mobile device. We recommend doing that now and practicing with the QR Code to the right.

We, the editing team, have worked hard to provide you with a fun, unique experience and hope that you enjoy your journey into The Dark Orchestra. We want you to know that we are not professionals, just individuals who care about health, fitness, Weightlifting and the two authors. This was quite literally the first project of its kind that anyone involved has worked on. Along the way we learned a lot about the processes for writing, editing, and developing a book. We hope that you can forgive us should a comma or two be out of place.

Thank You,
Patrick Regan (Head Editor)

JON NORTH AND JAMES MCDERMOTT
PRESENT
THE DARK ORCHESTRA

PROGRAMME.

TO COMMENCE AT EIGHT THIRTY O'CLOCK PRECISELY.

RESERVED SEATS, 5S. | UNRESERVED SEATS, 2S. 6D | FAMILY TICKETS TO ADMIT FOUR TO THE UNRESERVED SEATS, 7S. 6D.
THE OVERTURE HAS BEEN ARRANGED FOR THREE VIOLINS, FLUTE, VIOLONCELLO, PIANOFORTE, HARMONIUM, AND DRUMS.
BY THE INTRODUCTION OF THE HARMONIUM, THE EFFECT OF A FULL ORCHESTRA IS OBTAINED.

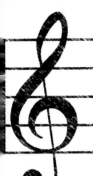

FOREWORD

BY DONNY SHANKLE

   I first met Jon North in 2009. After being introduced
at a local competition, he and his wife Jessica drove to
California Strength. Since then Jon and I have developed a
friendship which lasts today. On the platform we are intense
and passionate about weightlifting. Off the platform that
same passion we have for attacking the bar carries over into
other areas of our lives. Perhaps, this level of commitment to
weightlifting and the desire to live life to its fullest, form
the cornerstone of our friendship.

   Jon asked me to write the foreword to this book quite a
while ago. I am not sure he realized how difficult of a task
this was for me. Our language especially in training has always
been something unspoken. It is more of an intuitive feeling not
expressed through words. Our language is a language of champions.
Jon has now done a remarkable job sharing this language with you
and the etymology behind it begins with understanding passion.
As you develop your own principles and virtues through practice
which make you strong, never lose the passion you feel
from day one. Passion keeps you alive. It keeps you
believing in yourself even when you feel yourself
on the edge of the event horizon ready to tip
into what he calls the Dark Orchestra. There
are countless men who can get
you to think but few men who
can get you to feel. Jon is
one of those men. His blogs which
were the genesis to his book
are spoken to you in a way
champions speak to each
other. They are not
written in an outline
with structure by
some pedantic academic.
Instead, they are written to
you straightforward and from

the heart. They are not edited nor changed in any way from its original form. All of what Jon has written has been drawn from living life passionately. You will feel his pain as he pulls you into his darkness and rejoice with him as he pulls back the night sky and shows you his sterling spirit.

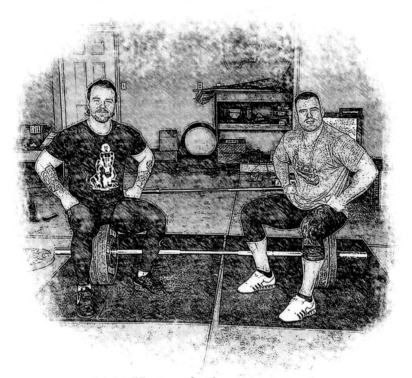

2011 National Champions in the 105KG Class (Donny) and the 94KG Class (Jon).

Ivan Abadjiev said one of the four pillars to becoming a world champion is attitude. Jon has always possessed this champion quality. He built his company on the back of it known as the Attitude Nation. It is the loadstar to his philosophy. Wherever he gets this from, I do not know for sure. But I think perhaps he finds it through the love he has for Jessica. Who can speak of the limitless strength of any man without praising his companion? Jessica has trained alongside Jon since the two of them first met. Weightlifting is a bond between them and it was after victory in competition he asked her to marry him. Sometimes we win and sometimes we fail. In weightlifting you may have to wait patiently for your next lift to retake your gold medal. Jon won something even greater than gold in Jessica. He won lasting happiness.

As you read this book, you will gain insight on how Jon teaches. He will share his own immutable style on how to train the Snatch and the Clean and Jerk to become great. All of his teachings are passed to you in the champion's language shared only in a way Jon can explain. The Superman Pull, Hit and Catch, and Horses Out of the Gate are all original ideas he has framed to make sense for you what made sense for him. How he teaches is anything but dull as you will soon find out. His style is filled with passion and of course, attitude. Alongside his teachings are blogs filled with the philosophy that guided him. Some of my favorites include Tigger, Devil In a Red Dress, Wanderlust, The Overall Man, and his personal best The Old Show. In these blogs Jon reveals more than a man who is great at weightlifting. He humbly discloses to us a man who set out on his own and as he would say, "chased the atmosphere".

Whether you love or hate him, Jon is genuine. He is a champion full of swag and grit. His accomplishments on the platform stretch from representing his country with pride on team USA to becoming the best weightlifter in the United States as a 94 kilo man. As I read his book, I was reminded of our moments in the gym. The competitive fights we shared on the platform and the laughs afterwards. The times spent at the writing table in between training sessions where both he and I worked relentlessly sharing our wins, our losses, and our lives. In a sport which will whale on you with Leviathan weights, it's important to remain strong both physically and mentally. The best way to start doing that is how Jon did and keeps doing. With attitude.

JON NORTH AND JAMES MCDERMOTT
PRESENT
THE DARK ORCHESTRA

PART I.

CHAPTER 1:
PUMPING IRON
FOR DELIVERANCE

Room 2

Thursday, November 17, 2011

The closer you got to room 2 the darker the hallway got. The
lights would flicker and the wind would whistle through the broken
door leading to the outside court yard. The same yard where I
would cry before class. The same yard I would sit in, while class
was in session. Eyes where sad, heads were down, and bad attitudes
were in full effect. Anger and sadness where the two feeling's
you got while being around room 2. The sky was not the limit for
us, therefor the sealing was lower and the options for life were
scars. In room 2 you will find zombies that never went far from the
room, lunches were eaten fast in a different part of the cafe, and
soon back to base. A place where we were catergorized, put to the
side for the other kids to play and grow like weeds. Room 2 was a
place for kids who were "special" a place for kids who had trouble
learning, a place where I called home from 1st grade to 12th grade.

5+5=11 what did I just read? What is the teacher
talking about? Why are all the kids writing?
the room is so quite from all the heads down
taking the test. I wonder why jimmy whore that
green shirt, why is the teacher reading about
planes? I can't keep my head
down; I am going to fail this
test very badly, just like all
of them. I hate school, I hate
this classroom. My mom told
me never to say hate, but
I hate this test. The
writing on the paper is
in Spanish and I can't
stop moving my feet. All
I feel is frustration and anger.
I keep staring outside the window

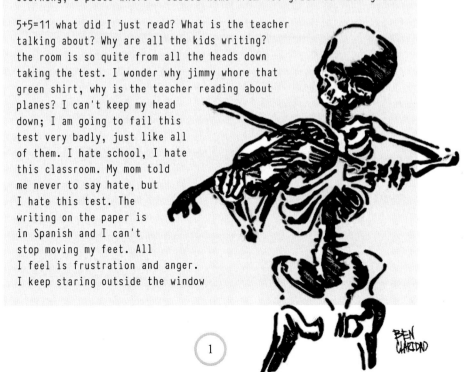

BEN
CARIDAD

1

wondering what's out there for me. What am I going to do in that big world? Kids start to turn their papers in with smiles, and I keep writing over my name bolder and bolder, over and over, with a look of defeat. I need to move, I need to get out of this school and get into the world. I am in jail; this book is my hand cuffs, this school is my prison. I want to be free, I want to lift weights, run, play football, get into a fight, be hit, hit, try new things, go to the edge and almost fall over. I want to live, I want to move on to the next room and say goodbye to 2 and see how 3 or 4 is. I want to explore, find a world of my own and live there forever.

c,d,c,f,c,d,c on my report card. I really thought this one was going to be better. I will go train in the school gym, a place that I could just sit in and feel good. A place that was always cold but warm, a place where I could feel confident in, a place that always felt like Christmas morning. The worse my report card was, the more weight I lifted, and the more I realized that I must learn how to play the game of life. Find my own way through this maze, I must be a fighter, must attack the world from a different direction than most, or I will die in room 2.

But my plan of attack was not working. College came around and I was chained deep in the dark whole of room 2 never to be seen again. I would here the kids talking about jobs, money, success, dreams, there major, there interviews and achievements. I remember wanting to be them so very bad, I wanted to have something I could do, touch, have control over, make my own, just like all of them. I was upset at myself, know one else.

Room 2 let me go when they finally kicked me out for bad grades. The jail cell opened and the outdoors light was bright, the sounds were loud like I just stepped onto a new planet for the first time. No money, no job, no life. I would sit on the outside bench watching all the people walk by me back and forth like they were in a movie being directed by a director. I was still moving my feet, having random twitches in my arms and shoulders. There was something in me that wanted out, an alien that was about to rip my stomach open and start hoping over cars.

The night was freezing when I was woken by an angel with three white stripes looking down on me. I was still on my bench when

I saw this women with wings. There were know more people, know more loud sounds, just me and this women in the cold night. She was beautifull. Take this bar sweet child, and lift it above your head with all the might in the world. Do this and you will have a purpose, lift this bar and you will be set free, lift this bar and you will find love in your life and even change the lives of others. Go ahead grab it, take it in your hands and raise it above your head like it's the world. Now go, follow the path the bar has for you, and make your mother proud, your sister proud, and yourself proud, walk and never look back.

I was lost back then but now I am found. I was confused back then but now I am smart, I was an F now I am an A, I was losing back then now I am winning, I was laughed at now I am laughing, I had 5 special attention teachers, now I teach. I was sad now happy, I failed English now I write, I had hate in me and now I love. Now I lift every day. I lift the world over my head, I lift for my family, I lift for my wife, I lift for you mom, I love you mom. Attitude Nation I salute you.

2012

Like many of you out there in the Attitude Nation, I have lived through some dark times. From an early age I struggled with drug addictions, my vices often guiding my path. Crystal Meth was my father, Cocaine my mother and Weed my sister – we were a perfect nuclear family. We laughed together living in crack houses, night clubs, and bars. I always had a desire to be engulfed in the nightlife, a drink in my hand and music vibrating through my bones.

At five-feet nine inches tall, I was a skeleton weighing in at one hundred twenty pounds – just the rigid framework of a person. By the time I had turned twenty, I had lost all of my back teeth and my hair was falling out. I battled with insomnia, and sleep became just a word, as the Crystal Meth made that next to impossible. Coupled with a lack of sleep and malnutrition; I experienced psychological effects that stemmed from my behavior such as a deep sense of insecurity and severe depression.

After coming down from my high, I would feel nervous, alone and at times afraid. It was a swift transition from the life of the party to a guy sitting in the corner crying. I felt like I was trapped in a world that I did not belong in, but had no way of escaping. A stranger in a strange land; if I wanted to find acceptance, I would have to do it with narcotics.

I was a lost soul, trying to survive and find myself on the streets of Eugene, Oregon.

♪ ♪ ♪

I consider myself to be a very shy and quiet person by nature. It takes a lot for me to get past my insecurities and break through my comfort zone. I found that I needed the drugs to be outgoing and *that guy* who was the life of the party. Once I was on them, I was able to come out of my shell and have a good time. A blizzard of white would dust the inside of my nostrils, shots would pour down my throat, and dancing would commence. I was like a man possessed out there on the dance floor. My body moved any direction it desired; I laughed for no reason and talked to strangers. I did things that would never have been possible when sober.

As the night progressed, I made my way to the places many would consider frightening. The hum of the music from the club faded as I walked down dark streets, traveling to neighborhoods where the police prowled – shining spotlights down every alleyway. Not all of the street lights worked, and the risk of being mugged…or worse was high. The projects are known for violence, vandalism, suspicious activity and drugs. My destination was a dilapidated building where I happened to be friends with people who provided me with crystal meth.

The white two-story house with plywood shutters was falling apart, like many others in the area. The grass was uncut, and the front bushes were overgrown. A flight of concrete steps led from the sidewalk to the front porch which was surprisingly clean, so as to not draw unwanted attention. Inside the house, the scene was more subdued than at the club. It was dark, quiet, and the overall atmosphere was one of sadness. The floor was lined with a stained burgundy carpet and littered with garbage. All of the tables and countertops were covered in a graveyard of cigarette butts and empty bottles. The air was thick with the scent of smoke, stale beer and mildew.

I preferred to hang out in the living room. There was a couch, a loveseat and an old tube T.V. with a DVD player setup. I liked to sit on the loveseat, which was next to a boarded up window and look at the outside world through the cracks. That was a very peaceful place for me. There I could be calm and think about life and the world. I would look out into the darkness, at the empty street thinking I was a happy person, but deep down I knew better. In many ways, I was a prisoner, and this was my cell. Whether I was willing to come to the realization or not; I knew deep down I would either have to part ways with my addictions or die.

♪ ♪ ♪

There was something peculiar about that night and as I sat in my loveseat staring out the window, I was in deep reflection of my life. I thought about stories I had heard of others in my close social circle going through rough patches in their lives involving their health and the law. Those stories made me think about how every time I too chose to feed my addictions, I gambled on my future. This game I was playing was dangerous and did not stop at just drug and alcohol abuse, but included fighting as well. Dwelling on the past, I remembered how when I was in middle and high school, I enjoyed fighting. It was something I felt I was good at because I never lost. When I was high I was bolder and more confrontational. It was only a matter of time before the repercussions of my decisions in life would come to a head in a much more violent way than I would have preferred.

I remember, it was a usual Saturday night – We pre-gamed, taking shots of vodka and other hard liquors at a friend's house and then went to a party to enjoy the rest of the evening. We ended up at a house party, but it was not your typical teenage drink and dance gathering, but instead a drug party. The crowd was a mix of older kids and adults, many of which had gang relations and were not the kind of people you would want to cross.

I was having a great time. I mingled with people that I knew and indulged in the party favors that were available. It is hard to remember the exact reason – the littlest thing can set people off in this type of environment, but I offended one of the guys at the party. These were not people I wanted to push the issue with, so after words were exchanged, I decided to leave and salvage the night elsewhere.

It all happened very quickly. Upon leaving the party, my friend and I were followed by some of the partygoers I had offended – among them was the guy I had words with and I knew I was in trouble. Three Black and two Hispanic men encircled us. One of them held my friend back while the rest attacked me. I fought hard – punching, elbowing and thrashing around, but I was not strong enough to fend them off. They wrestled me down to the ground and repeatedly punched and kicked me. I was hit numerous times in the face and kicked in my ribs and stomach. As I was spitting out blood while still trying to protect myself, and my vision began to blur from a hard shot to the nose. The last thing I remembered was watching the heel of a boot driving to my face. Then there was nothing.

I was certain at that moment that the end had finally come. I was going to die lying on the sidewalk in a pool of my blood. I woke up in a hospital room with my real family at my side. I had been nearly beaten to death and I can only imagine how terrifying the whole situation was for them. The ordeal left me with puffy black eyes, a broken nose, cuts on my face and a few broken ribs. My mother and step-father pleaded with me to change my behavior. While their pleas came from a place of concern and love, they fell on deaf ears. I was a stubborn kid who was more concerned with having fun and my social life.

Three weeks later, I was out of the hospital and back at Spencer Butte Middle School. While hanging out with my girlfriend at the time, Shannon, a car containing a few of the guys that had assaulted me pulled up in front of us. They tossed a bag of weed to Shannon and apologized to me. I had wronged their friend at the party, and while they liked me the incident was just business.

I was running with a dangerous crowd and participating in things I should not have been. My addictions were too powerful to be beaten out of me physically.

I needed something stronger to show me the way. A spiritual reawakening that would cause the walls of my reality to fall, exposing the fact that I was a prisoner of my life. Unfortunately, that would have to wait as I continued my drug use throughout my teenage years and into college.

♪ ♪ ♪

I had been slumped over the arm of the loveseat, staring off into space while pondering my past for quite some time. That evening where the nightlife had almost fully consumed my teenage-self had come and gone – now here I was a stoned sophomore at College of the Siskiyous located in Weed, California who had no intention to go to class the next day. It was now two o'clock on a Wednesday morning and I was sobering up. Not a whole lot happens at that hour and others in the house probably felt like I did, bored. Little did I know it, but the reawakening that would forever redefine my life was finally about to take place.

There was some discussion about putting in a movie when a very tall black guy with an orange afro came downstairs and into the living room. He looked at me and said "North! I got something for ya!" I had no idea who this guy was and was surprised he knew my name. He opened up the DVD case and tossed it on my lap. I picked it up to study the cover. It featured a colossal looking, muscled, half-naked man. "Pumping Iron starring Arnold Schwarzenegger." The tagline stated: "This movie has heart, soul, blood, guts, perspiration and plenty of muscles."

Pumping Iron is a documentary on the sport of Bodybuilding. The film follows famous Bodybuilders Franco Columbu, Lou Ferrigno and Arnold Schwarzenegger on their journey to the 1975 Mr. Universe and Mr. Olympia competitions. During the movie, you watch them lift weights and observe the drama that unfolds in their lives. This film is considered by many to be a rite of passage for gym goers to see before embarking on serious training. My life could have been changed by anything that popped up on that television screen. Had it been something about golf, mixed martial arts or cooking and I might be pursuing those careers right now. I often imagine how "home décor" with Jon North would have panned out.

From the moment it started I was completely enthralled. Others may watch Pumping Iron in amazement at how big and strong the Bodybuilders are, but not me. There was something else that spoke to me, something I had been searching for; my whole life. I had been gasping for air, trying to find my place in the world, but Arnold was not. I watched his every movement and was fascinated by his every word. When he spoke, people listened. When he was on stage, there was a presence about him and unbelievable confidence in his smile.

Halfway through the film, I realized what the difference was between Arnold and I. He was free and I was not. I was tired of endlessly trying to prove myself on the streets through fighting. I was sick of numbing reality with drugs and being a prisoner of my own mind. That is not what Arnold fucking did. He loved his life and was not afraid to go out and get what he wanted. I sat there on that loveseat next to the window clutching the DVD case in my hands. I was shaking, tears running down my face, but no one noticed. The other people in the room were stoned, passed out or fixated on the glow of the television. I looked around the room, my eyes bloodshot and watery. I came to the conclusion that I would never set foot in this fucking place again.

♪ ♪ ♪

The next morning, I woke up at eight o'clock after having hardly an hour of sleep. I took a long hot bath to cleanse the filth of the crack house from my skin and set out into the world. My first order of business was to join the Rockhouse Gym in Mount Shasta, California. This was not Gold's Gym or 24 Hour Fitness. It was an old school facility with mismatched plates everywhere and posters from the sixties and seventies on the wall. I bought a membership, signed the papers for my twenty-four hour access card and walked out on the weight room floor.

Rockhouse Gym had all sorts of equipment available. There were machines, dumbbells, and treadmills everywhere. I was a little lost on where I should start, so I spent a few minutes just exploring. I stared at the posters on the wall that depicted men like Arnold posing for the camera. Eventually, my eyes fell upon an EZ Curl bar lying on the floor next to one of the benches. I picked it up and looked at a poster that showed a bunch of arm exercises. Arnold had big arms, so that seemed to be a good place to begin. That was the first time I had ever touched a barbell, and I enjoyed the way the weight felt in my hands.

I started doing curls. At ten my biceps started burning. At fifteen, they were on fire and I was sweating profusely. At twenty, my hands, forearms, and biceps felt like they were going to explode! At twenty-five I dropped the barbell. I was breathing heavy and blood was flooding through my arms. That was the pump I heard Arnold talking about in the movie and it felt incredible. The high I felt from that pump was better than any I had ever experienced when on drugs. I was hooked and I wanted more. I picked up the bar again for set two. This would be the beginning of a much more positive and fruitful era in my life.

♪ ♪ ♪

I can be an extreme person. When I set out to do something, I go all in. That was part of the problem in my partying days – it was my only outlet to channel all of my energy into. Bodybuilding became a new, but positive addiction for me to focus my attention on. I went out and bought magazines and protein powder and I practically lived at the Rockhouse Gym. I started eating cleaner instead of getting high and working out instead of fighting. Eventually, these changes in my lifestyle also re-ignited passions from my childhood such as Football. As a young kid, I was very athletic and loved to play Football. The prospect of joining the College of the Siskiyous Football team made me work even harder in the gym.

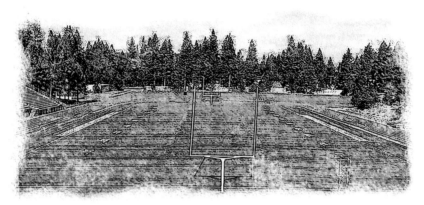

College of the Siskiyous Football Field.

I was blessed with genetics that allow me to put on muscle quickly. Between working out and the protein shakes I was drinking, my weight increased significantly. That, coupled with my prior knowledge of playing Football and athletic abilities, made it easy for me to land a spot on the team. We were the Eagles, and Eagle Football is huge in Mount Shasta, California. I now had a purpose in life and goals that I was committed to busting my ass to achieve.

It was on the Eagle Football team that I met my good friend Rob Chicano. We shared a mutual love for Bodybuilding and he became my very first training partner. He pushed me to work even harder in the gym and I would push him right back. After hard workouts we would have a posedown *right there* in the Rockhouse gym.

With our shirts off, we would try to mimic Arnold's poses and make intense faces. Just as in competitions, we would rub oil all over ourselves. I would say "hey bro, can you get my back" because that was the one spot I could not reach. We even went as far as to shoot a training video of us hitting big sets and yelling a lot just like Ronnie Coleman and Jay Cutler – two Bodybuilders who were famous at the time for their intense battles on the stage. Unfortunately, that video has been lost over the years.

♪ ♪ ♪

I have never been a good student. I often struggled with my grades and it usually created a lot of problems. Playing Football required that I had an overall passing average. If I did not do well in my classes, I risked losing my spot on the team. However, this time my poor academic abilities ended up being a blessing in disguise adding more beauty to my life than I ever could have imagined. Her name is Jessica.

The first time I saw Jessica West we were both taking a summer painting class. She was a straight A – student, and she sat at the front of the classroom. She was taking this class to learn something new and thought it would be fun. I, on the other hand, was only in the room because I needed to maintain a C- average and sat in the back of the room. Jessica was too beautiful for me to stay encamped all the way back there. Over the course of the semester I slowly migrated to the front searching for excuses to joke and talk with her. She is the only reason I did well in the class. I made sure never to be late, showing up bright eyed and bushy tailed every day.

I find it very fitting that I met her in an art class, because when I look at her it is as if I am looking at a masterfully done painting. I remember the world would move in slow motion around her as she would walk into the room and took her seat next to mine. Jessica is tall and slender with long dark hair. Her infectious smile melted my heart. Last, but not least, she has eyes that saw through me piercing the tough guy persona I tried to portray. As I look back on it now, it's kind of crazy to think that if I had been a better student, I might never have met her. I only chose that class because I thought it would be an easy passing grade, but I ended up just seats away from the future love of my life.

Eventually, over the course of the semester, she buckled to my charm, and we have been together ever since.

♪ ♪ ♪

A coach is like a good friend, someone who is practically a member of the family. They are someone who believes in you and the things you have set out to accomplish. A person who gives a damn about you so much that they will fight through hell for you. They guide you when you are lost and share knowledge so you can be successful. Coach Tim Frisbie became that person to me during my time at College of the Siskiyous. He is a man that I greatly admire.

While I played, Coach "Friz" was the Offensive Line coach and head strength & conditioning coach to the Football team. Simply put he was and still **IS** Eagle Football. He is extremely well respected at the University as well as its surrounding communities. Coach Friz is one of those men who is a backbone of their community. A stalwart man who is quiet, but straight to the point when he tells you what is on his mind. Everyone looked to him for advice because you knew you could trust him to either have the answer or point you in the right direction.

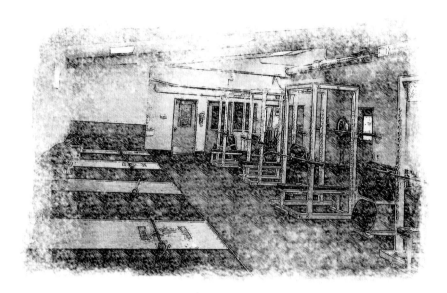

Coach Friz's Weight Room.

I spent three years training with Coach Friz who has a very time-tested style of molding athletes into unstoppable machines. The foundations of his method were respect and communication. He knew that the bonding of a team in the weight room is what leads it to success – we not only needed to be strong, but in sync with one another. Coach Friz had very strict rules in his weight room. We were not allowed to listen to music or wear iPods because those things would hinder our team communication. Wearing cut-off shirts, weight belts and disrespecting fellow teammates were also forbidden.

Coach Friz's instructions were very concise. If you did not know what was going on it meant you were not listening. Failure to listen or breaking the rules meant you had to run the bear tail. The bear trail is a 1.7 mile route that takes you around the campus perimeter and through the woods. Many students like to walk it to take pictures of nature or exercise. We ran it for punishment.

It was under Coach Friz that I was first exposed to the Weightlifting movements of the Snatch and the Clean & Jerk. We used these lifts often when training for the explosive power and strength needed out on the Football field. Cleaning heavy weight was one of my favorite things to do in the weight room. I probably looked forward to it even more than playing Football. In addition to learning those lifts, quite possibly the most valuable thing he taught me was how to squat low. When I say low, I mean low as in your ass is touching your ankles at the very bottom of the squat.

♪ ♪ ♪

After ridding my life of drugs, training hard in the gym and playing Football for three years, I was ready to graduate with my associate's degree. Everyone I knew was utterly shocked that I was not only going to be graduating from junior college, but also continuing my education. As the word spread, I had friends and family coming in from all over the country just to watch me walk across the stage and receive my diploma. Knowing my track record, everyone felt the need to come and witness this miracle for themselves. They all believed in me of course, but to this day even I do not know how I pulled it off. It was not until I was asked what gown size I needed that it dawned on me what was happening. I suppose anyone can get lucky if you take enough P.E. credits.

♪ ♪ ♪

Graduation day was terrifying because it left me with a new question: "What do I do now?" I had my Associates Degree in my hand, but nowhere to go with it. The lanterns on the path ahead had not yet been lit and I did not know how to make fire. After the ceremony, Coach Friz helped me answer the question.

Coach pulled me into his office and sat me down for a serious talk. Like any good coach, he had excellent eyes. He saw something in me that others, even myself, had overlooked. He saw potential. Coach asked: "Do you know about the sport of Weightlifting?"

He was an avid supporter of Weightlifting and thought that I would have a future in the sport. He knew people at Sacramento State College and pulled some strings to get me an interview. He took me under his wing and even helped Jessica and I to move out there. Over the years, he had given me all the help and support he could. Then he pushed me out of the Eagle's nest and said **"Fly you S.O.B.!"**

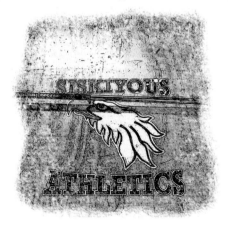

Siskiyous Athletics Weightlifting Platform.

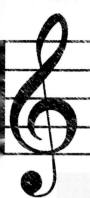

CHAPTER 2

REDEFINE THE POSSIBLE

24 Hour Fitness

Wednesday, September 26, 2012

A family of hard workers, hard workers and professional mess-a-rounders. Great people who made the job even greater, and finalizing it with the crown of "best job I have ever had". It was a job I will never forget, a job that to this day makes me smile from great memories. It was a job that made me excited and alive while I drove to work, a job that I looked forward to every morning. It was a second home that brought me comfort, stability, and a meaning to my life. A band of brothers is what my co-workers were, brothers in arms who I couldn't wait to mess with and sell more than. 24 Hour Fitness was a fucken blast, and also the start of the most hated man in USA weightlifting, Jon North.

Walking into work at 24 hour fitness you would think the busy bees and bright lights never shut off for closing. It was an ongoing coffee break without the break. I looked out to a sea of money through the window my desk sat by everyday, a desk crushed next to many other desks like bunk beds full of sales people... wait no, sales friends, while people and cars past by. Grumpy elf is what we called him, grumpy in a good way I should add, a funny "ok ok boss man I will get back to work and stop playing table football" way. I should also add even though I got yelled at for messing around with the triangle piece of folded paper, grumpy elf was the one playing with me! I think it's because I was winning that made him snap out of

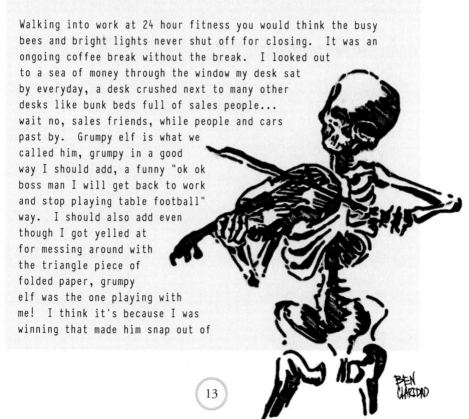

BEN
CARIDAD

fun time and back into work time. The best boss, leader, friend, and all around person that I have ever met, Greg Husten. Thank you Greg for hiring me and taking me under your wing when I needed one so very badly. Thank you for everything you have taught me in sales and in life. I looked up to you then, and I still do now.

Greg Husten aka the boss man

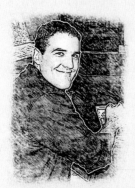

Charles Shipman, yes you might know this name; he is a weightlifter, and my best friend. Charles's first day at 24 was my second day, and we hit it off right away. Beat boxing and free-styling was not unusual. Actually, we sold more memberships after a good rap battle. Nice cloths, gelled hair, coffee in hand, and the world at our feet. We were membership salesmen and we were damn good at what we did. Well..... Charles was, I was too busy watching Shankle videos on my phone at a time before I ever met Donny, or became part of the Cal Strength Mafia. Wow..... just thinking about the 24 hour fitness days seems like a lifetime ago, but then again I can remember everything so clearly. I was a firecracker back then, keep in mind this was right when I first became a weightlifter. If you think I am crazy and wild now, then you should of seen "Jumping Jonathan North" back then.

Charles Shipman

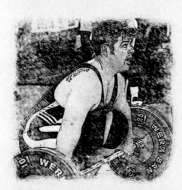

It was never about the commission, it was about beating Charles and Greg in sales. When a client walked in it was all business, the gym changed into a white house meeting. All three of us concentrating on our sale in front of us, but always with one eye cocked to the side seeing how Greg, Charles and any other rookie (not apart of the cool crew) was doing. Either high fives at the end or throwing of a pen or clip board. Sales

was a lot like weightlifting, a bitch. But at often times a
high that kept you coming back for more. I have smoked meth,
and done my fare share of coke back in my party days, and I
will be the first person to tell you that making a big lift or
landing a membership sale is the exact same high. Having my
boss Greg tell me "good job" made my day, and only made me want
to sell more. I loved Greg's style of leading, very much the
same style as my coach Glenn Pendlay. They let me breath, they
lead from behind, and they both let me create my own style of
training or selling. A leader who leads from behind has always
pushed me more, and made me want to achieve the goal at hand,
not only for myself but for them as well. Working with Greg and
Charles was a lot like training with my weightlifting teammates
now; there is very little difference the more I think about
it. A lifestyle full of goals and hard work, intertwined with a
healthy dose of laughter and fun, which in my opinion is the key
for success in anything.

A statue of a strong buff man holding the world over his head some
how climbed itself onto Greg's desk. I think it was a sales award
he won, and a well deserved one at that. Greg was magic when it
came to selling. Greg is not the type to go showing off, but one
morning the statue was just there, sitting on his desk for all
to see. Lol, just writing this blog is hard because I am already
laughing so hard from the image I see in my head. I see Greg
sitting there, typing at his desk with his long chin stuck out as
he types so relaxed and confidently. I walk in a few minutes late
like I have been known for still to this day. He does not stop
typing, but his eyes look over to the side giving me the "your
late look". I sit down at my desk scrambling to begin my work day
trying to show him that I have a "busy" day ahead, even though we
both know that's a lie. He finally stopped typing, and this time
his whole head turned with his eyes along for the ride, he said,
"glad you could join us today Jon boy". It was so hard to keep
a straight face with Charles at his desk quietly laughing at the
situation. Before I even gave him an excuse or told him, "sorry
it want happen again" line, I looked at his overly big and bright
statue and without thinking replied, "hey look, statue looks like
me". LOL!!!!!! I slightly laughed while looking back and forth
from the statue to Greg, waiting to see his reaction. But there
was none, he just stared at me for a good minute until he slowly

turned back to his computer screen and began typing again. I looked over to see Charles's reaction, and yes, Charles was almost on the floor laughing.

Ever since that morning anytime anybody would walk by Greg's desk, he would say very loudly and cartoon like "Ooooo yea, statue looks like you". And then he would come back into himself and under his breath say, "God dude, get over it," The best part about this was that the people Greg joked with never said anything about the statue, or even knew about the inside joke in the first place! The poor guy would just walk away scratching his head. LOL!!!!! I am dying laughing, and if you don't think this is funny that I am sorry, I guess you just had to be there, or I am not writing this correctly. At the end of the day Greg would crack a small smile and tell a joke, letting you know that deep down he was just messing around.

After a year went by we all got broken up and went our own ways, but we all still stay in touch, and are very good friends to this day.

24 Hour Fitness 2016   Charles Shipman 2016
Greg Husten 2016   Pre pay 2016   Two Week Pass 2016

"Redefine the Possible" is the mantra that drives the day to day pursuits of all who attend California State University, Sacramento. Coach Friz, opened the door here and I was now on a mission – to join the Weightlifting club. My Football career was over after numerous concussions, but I still wanted to be involved in sports. I had always enjoyed performing the Snatch and the Clean & Jerk while training in the College of the Siskiyous weight room and Coach Friz thought Weightlifting would be perfect for me to showcase my athletic abilities.

It was hot and sunny on my first day and I was already in my workout clothing – I was sweating quite a bit. I was told to report to the Eli and Edy Broad Field House, at one-thirty in the afternoon to meet Kathy and Paul Bowling.

♪ ♪ ♪

The weight room was stunning and everything was very polished. Down the center of the room there were several rows of squat racks and each rack had it's own wooden Weightlifting platform with the college logo printed in the middle and a barbell with a stack of rubber plates. I arrived early for my meeting to make sure that everything went right when I finally met Kathy and Paul, who were both already veterans in the sport of Weightlifting.

Kathy was a kindergarten teacher in the Sacramento City Unified School District. Already an alumni of Sac State, she was currently enrolled to gain a master's degree in Education. She is a Collegiate Nationals Gold medalist in the 69KG weight class, and a World Team Trial 1st place winner. She also holds numerous Silver and Bronze medals at the American Open and Senior National events in the 63KG weight class.

Paul or "P-Funk" as he is lovingly called is equally as decorated. He holds a Bachelors in Science Degree in Kinesiology from California State University, Sacramento. Like Kathy, he is a Marine Corps veteran where he also served as a computer technician. Lifting in the 105KG weight class, he won the 2003 American Open and Arnold Classic events. Paul is also a national level Weightlifting coach through the USAW (USA Weightlifting).

Together Kathy and Paul ran the Sacramento Olympic Weightlifting club. In the eyes of the college the "team" was unofficial – more of a recreational club since they did not offer Weightlifting as a sport. However, the name was listed as an official Barbell Club through the USAW at the time.

♪ ♪ ♪

As I walked around the gym, I noticed a poster hanging high on the wall in front of one the first platforms. It was a National Championships promo poster and on it was Jeff Wittmer the top 94KG American Weightlifter. He was holding up his hands, yelling triumphantly after winning the 2006 Senior Nationals. I could not take my eyes off of it. I could see how much this victory meant to him. I imagined all the hard work he had put in leading up to that very moment. It must have felt incredible.

Jeff Wittmer is one of the greatest American Weightlifters ever to live. His resume is awe-inspiring. He was a three-time Collegiate National Champion, a three-time Collegiate All-American team member, a five-time Junior National Champion, and a two-time Senior National Champion in the 94KG weight class. He won that title back to back in 2006 and 2007. He was also on world teams and an unstoppable force in the sport.

I broke my gaze from the poster as I noticed Kathy and Paul had entered the gym. I nervously approached and introduced myself. They were delighted to meet me finally and excited I was interested in joining the Weightlifting club. Kathy was a small yet powerful looking, beautiful woman. Paul was a big man who almost crushed my hand when he shook it.

We sat down on some benches and spoke a little bit about my background in sports and weight training. I had some experience lifting at College of the Siskiyous, but I wanted to learn more. After a few minutes, Kathy asked me "What are your goals?" My hand immediately shot into the air and I pointed at the Jeff Wittmer poster across the room. "I want to beat him and win Nationals," I replied. I was dead serious and they were pleased with my enthusiasm.

♪ ♪ ♪

A lot of schools out there are not fortunate enough to have a club for Weightlifters to join or at least they did not back then. I treated the club as if it were my old Eagle Football team. I gave it everything so that both it and I could succeed. Every day I was learning about equipment, competition, rules, and technique. Under the Bowlings, I learned a more traditional American type of Weightlifting. It was very similar to what was taught through the USAW.

While training at Sac State, I really connected with fellow club member Ben Claridad. Ben is a very well-known Weightlifter right now, but back then he was my first training partner in the sport. I will never forget our first practice session and seeing this gorilla of a man with huge arms throwing around heavy weights like toys. When I saw that I knew I was right where I needed to be. To those of us in the club, Ben was the captain. It was not his official title, but since he was the best athlete, we all looked up to him and sought his guidance.

He was one of the first athletes to welcome me into the sport. He took me under his massive wings and showed me how to be a Weightlifter – little things like using chalk and the shoes I needed to buy. He looked out for me just like a coach would and it made me feel very much a part of their training family. Ben and I share the belief that Weightlifting is art – a form of self-expression through physical performance. Not only does he express himself on the competition stage, but Ben is also an excellent artist.

While I enjoyed my experience with the Sac State club, it lasted for only a brief few months. They met twice per week and the college had restrictions on when the gym would be open. I realized that I needed more than that if I was to become a National Champion. As fate would have it, I crossed paths with my next coach Jackie Mah on campus.

Jackie Mah is a phenomenal coach with well over a decade's worth of experience. As an athlete, she was a Collegiate Champion in the 76KG weight class. She won the American Open with back to back victories in 1995 and 1996 in the 83KG weight class. Jackie also has over ten top place finishes throughout her career. As an added bonus, Coach Mah also has a Masters Degree in Physical Therapy.

At the time Jackie was a coach at the Hassle Free Barbell club down the street and also helped out at the Sac State club from time to time. She has a keen knack for discovering individuals with potential and she saw a lot of it in me. She saw my hunger to excel in the sport and that I was a caged animal that needed to be let loose on the platform. Training for one hour twice a week was just not enough. During one of her visits to the college, she asked Jessica, Ben and I to go train with her at the Hassle Free gym. I felt like I was being invited to an exclusive event like something right out of the movie Fight Club. She instructed us to meet her at ten o' clock the next morning where she would introduce us to the Head Coach, Paul Doherty.

♪ ♪ ♪

The Hassle Free Barbell Club is one of a kind. It is without a question one of the United States most prestigious Weightlifting facilities. It is run by brothers Paul and Kevin Doherty in two separate locations. Kevin runs a gym located on the campus of Lincoln High School in San Francisco, California. Paul's gym can be found at Sacramento High School. Together they train hundreds of athletes including young children.

Kevin and Paul are both outstanding coaches and between the two of them they have trained countless Junior and Senior National Champions, American Open Gold Medalists, and world team members. Athletes such as Ian Wilson, D'Angelo Osorio, and Donovan Ford all came from, and to my knowledge still train at Hassle Free. They are top level international coaches, and I'm blessed that I had the opportunity to train in their facility.

It was Paul's gym that would come to be my home and when I first saw it my jaw hit the floor. It was one of the most intense atmospheres I had ever experienced in sports. As I walked around the gym, there were children of all ages training. I saw Fifth graders all the way up to collegiate athletes putting their heads down and doing serious work. To say I was motivated would be an understatement. These kids were maxing out, hitting lifts and I wanted to be right there with them.

I remember Jackie Mah looked at me and smiled as I stood there wide-eyed and said "I told you so." Ben walked passed me, giving me a light punch on the shoulder and said "You're going to love this place Jon." Both of them had thought this would be a better fit for me and they were right. The Sac State club was great and I learned a lot, but it ultimately felt like I was just dabbling in Weightlifting. It was all about fundamentals, the basics and only a few times a week. It was a tease. Hassle Free on the other hand, was the real deal. I learned a lot about myself training there. I figured out how much I had in the tank and if I did indeed want to be a Weightlifter. The answer was an irrefutable **"YES!"**

I trained at the gym for three weeks with no official coach since Paul was a very busy man and traveling a lot. I used this time to find myself as an athlete in the sport – I performed only the Snatch and Clean & Jerk every workout. It was a lot of volume and countless repetitions, but it helped me learn how to move my body like a Weightlifter. Within a few weeks Jackie officially became my coach and under her tutelage I began my climb up the rankings of the USAW.

♪♪♪

This all felt like a very magical time in my life. I was living in an apartment with Jessica in Sacramento and both of us were attending the university. While I pursued my Weightlifting dreams daily, I also held one of the best jobs I have ever had. I was a "Sales Counselor" at the 24 Hour Fitness in Carmichael, California. I was in charge of selling new memberships to potential clients. I met and became great friends with my manager Greg Husten and co-worker Charles Shipman. It is a time I truly cherish when I look back on those days.

24 Hour Fitness is a health club franchise chain. They have over four hundred clubs all over the country, and you can find them everywhere in California. Since there were bills to pay and I needed money for local meets, it just made sense to work in a field that was related to Weightlifting. Jessica was working at Gold's Gym and I had filled out applications there and other fitness clubs in the area.

My first day on the job was Charles's second. We hit it off right away and became good friends. I would tell him all about Hassle Free and the type of training I was doing. His response was to look at me confused and say "Oh like deadlifts and stuff like that?" I was still new in the sport myself, so I concluded that it would be easier just to show him. I said, "Just be at Sacramento High at six tonight."

He showed up that night to train with myself and guys like Donovan Ford, David Garcia, and Ben Claridad. You would think that going from a fitness center to a hardcore Weightlifting gym would be unnerving, but Charles loved it. He was able to squat quite low and had incredible flexibility. It allowed him to take to the Snatch quickly, and I was so proud of him when he Snatched 80KG. Here was another soldier, recruited in the quest for more kilos and he was a natural.

Greg Husten was the head of sales and he helped introduce me to the working world. He reinforced the value of being on time, taught me how to act like a professional and talk to people. I can honestly say that I learned more from him than I ever did taking classes in school. These were real skills like how to manage money, make sales and be sure that the customer is happy.

Charles and Greg were caring people that would give you the shirt off their backs. We were like a family and it was a place I could go for support. I found out quickly that Weightlifting can be a frustrating sport and having a place like 24 Hour Fitness and guys like Greg and Charles kept me positive and on a good track. When you come from where I have been, it is paramount to have role models and a healthy atmosphere to be around. It was not a job to me, but a home with a family I loved.

♪♪♪

When I arrived at Sac State and said I wanted to win Nationals I was dead serious. I want to be clear that Kathy and Paul were excellent coaches. They taught me a lot, but wanted me to go slower than I was comfortable with. They wanted me to focus mainly on the fundamentals and train for a year or two building a foundation before I competed. Great advice for most, but I needed to get my feet wet. I could not handle going slow and I wanted to dive head first into the sport.

Jackie Mah took my goals to heart and let my competitive side run wild. We made smaller goals that would eventually lead up to my big one. First, I needed to win a spot on the podium at a local meet. Second, would be to qualify for the American Open and finally qualify for Nationals. The help Jackie provided me on my journey up through the rankings was invaluable. She helped give me momentum to start making a name for myself in the Weightlifting community.

Within a year, I found myself in the warm up room at the 2007 American Open. The meet was held from November 30th to December 2nd in Birmingham, Alabama. I had accomplished my first two goals by battling in the trenches at local meets and was ready to lift on one of the biggest stages our country has to offer. I was going to be lifting in the 94KG weight class with such athletes as Phil Sabatini, Greg Everett, and Jeff Wittmer. By this time I had already grown to become a huge fan of Wittmer's and I admit to being a little starstruck when I saw him warming up.

Wittmer was lifting weights that were far beyond my capability at the time. He would not be my opponent that weekend – I would end up engaging in an epic battle with Greg Everett instead for fun.

I was proudly representing the Hassle Free Barbell Club and since it was the American Open, I wore a very patriotic singlet. It was metallic red with white and blue stripes running down the side. Greg was lifting for Team Southern California.

I had already become known in the Weightlifting community as "Jumping" Jonathan North. I would stand back about ten feet from the barbell staring out at the crowd. To psych myself up I would jump up and down, turning my hips side to side and swing my arms. It made me feel like I was on the sideline at a Football game, waiting for the coach to put me in.

My first lift on the big stage was a successful one. I easily completed a 112KG Snatch and declared 117KG to be my next lift. Greg hit 115KG and then I finished my second attempt at 117KG. I was pumped to make this weight – I was keeping up with these guys and upon completing that lift I yelled "Yeah! Come on let's get this!" Greg ended up missing his second attempt at 120KG due to a press out. Here was my chance to beat him in the Snatch event. I walked out on the stage with 122KG on the barbell. I needed to make this and I stomped my feet, let out a loud grunt and ripped it off the floor. I nailed it, yelling loudly in as I stood, waited for the down signal and then **SLAMMED** that bar as hard as I could. I had made all of my attempts in the Snatch. I ran backstage yelling to find Jessica and Jackie.

Calm and collected, Greg went to the same weight and made it with ease. Damnit! We were all tied up and it was all going to come down to the Clean & Jerk event. Greg opened with 140KG, and I followed with 150KG. For his second lift, Greg hit 145KG and I hit 154KG in mine to clinch the win in our mini battle. Greg ended up missing his final attempt of 150KG and I missed at 158KG. I finished in 8th place overall with a 276KG total with Greg right behind me with a 268KG total. It was an honor to be able to share the stage with him and everyone else who competed that day. One year into the sport and I completed five out of my six lifting attempts. The whole experience, while fun and exciting, only left me hungry for more.

♪ ♪ ♪

My life was pretty close to perfect. I had been drug-free for a few years and nothing could pull me back to that world. I was at Hassle Free every day training as close to full time as I could. I was even allowed to start coaching by helping out with the Football and youth Weightlifting teams. When I was not at the gym, I was spending time with my family at 24 Hour Fitness. Achieving my goals one lift at a time, I honestly felt I was unstoppable.

I was so wrong. Over the course of a week the fabric of the life I had created started to unravel and I would lose almost everything. To be honest, school was never my priority – I had no desire to sit behind a desk. Between Hassle Free, 24 Hour Fitness and Jessica; something had to give – and it was my class work. I should not have been surprised when Sacramento State kicked me out for my bad grades. What really shook me was what happened next.

Jessica and I were training one night at Hassle Free; each on our own platform going through lifts. Some punk college kid, who I did not remember seeing before, decided he was going to take over Jessica's platform. All of the other lifting areas were in use and instead of trying to work in somewhere else; he was bullying my fucking girlfriend. She asked him several times to please leave. When he ignored her, I got involved.

I asked him politely to move, but he still refused. I could feel my blood beginning to boil and I repeated my request. He told us to fuck off and I saw red. Being rude to me is one thing – being rude to Jessica is a whole different story. As the guy was telling us off, all these different emotions started to fill my head. With every word he spoke, the kid inside me who used to get in fights outside of parties gradually awoke. Each time he opened his mouth it was as if I was back there getting kicked in the ribs over and over. When he finished his sentence, I had no choice. I had to knock his ass out.

The gym went silent. The sound of barbells bouncing on the platforms vanished and I felt terrible. I was still riled up and needed air so I stormed out of the gym with Jessica behind me. I prayed that this whole thing would blow over, but Jackie and Paul eventually learned about the incident. They were furious with me and I felt like I had let them down. I was able to stay for a day, but word spread to the school's principal. When they learned about what I had done, I was banned from the facility and surrounding properties.

Knocking that guy out, was one of the dumbest things I had ever done in my life. But looking back on it, I was fortunate. That is because that one punch would lead me to Shankle...

♪ ♪ ♪

My mother had always been my biggest supporter. She encouraged me to play sports and forced me to play outside when I was young. She fed me well made sure I was in good health. I always had a safety net with my mom and it was not until I decided to give up on school that it was taken away. My mother is an old school conservative parent. She did not approve of me being kicked out of school for bad grades. To her dismay, I was content with not going back. Instead, I wanted to focus on Weightlifting full time.

She did not know anything about the sport and that led her to be worried and doubtful. She questioned whether I was making the right choice since I would not have anything to fall back on if it did not work out. At the time I did not understand, but now I see that she had my best interest in mind. If I was going to quit school – she was no longer going to support me financially.

To make my financial situation worse, about two months after being banned from Hassle Free, I decided to leave my job at 24 Hour Fitness. I loved the job and my family there, but the company had decided to transfer everyone to different facilities. I was now in a new place, and it was not the home that I cared about so much. **THAT** building and **THOSE** people were what made everything seem magical.

When I was transferred to the new place it was death. I hated everything about it. We were not a family anymore. Our team that had a rhythm and a certain way of doing things was gone forever. We had been a well-oiled money making machine, signing people up for memberships, but at the same time having fun, playing pranks and drinking coffee. It was already a very depressing and emotional time for me when that was taken away.

I was not happy about the change, but I needed the money. I was going to try and make things work and to supplement my income – I attempted to personal train clients. Now I had different views on exercise – some of which contradicted what was taught at the club. I would experiment by having member's squat low or perform Clean complexes with just the barbell. I was told by management to stop or I would be fired. They said I needed to take a certification and learn their way of teaching if I wanted to gain clients. I decided to be open-minded and give it a shot.

At the certification things did not go well. I finally lost it when they were instructing us on the Front Squat. I believe in squatting low – below parallel with the crease of my hips well below my knees. These people were now telling me that was wrong and that clients should squat to exactly parallel. I had my arms extended straight in front of me like Frankenstein and a barbell across my shoulders while I sat down into a squat. There was a mirror next to me, and I turned my head to take a look at my movement. An incredible amount of disgust overcame me.

In that moment, I was not Mel Gibson from Braveheart. Instead, I had laid down my sword and was doing something I did not agree with. There was no way I was going to teach this farce to paying members at the club. As I began to walk out of the class full of fifty brainwashed future club trainers, I was stopped. The instructor said that if I walked out I would fail the certification. I said, "that's okay I quit this cert" and stormed out.

I was frustrated with how this new place was run. Not long after, more problems quickly surfaced because the new gym was not as lenient about me taking time off to do meets. Weightlifting was still the mission. Although I was down at the moment, I was still going to work hard to become a National Champion. It came to a head when an important meet popped up that would help bump me up in the rankings.

I tried to use my vacation time and anything else I could think of to take that day off. I just needed that **ONE DAY** and all would be okay. The new boss would not allow it. He did not care that I had goals or something that I was passionate about. This new place only cared about having someone there to sell, sell, and sell. The most important thing in the world to me other than Jessica was Weightlifting. I was not about to let them take it away from me. When they said "no," I said, "I quit." I walked out that day and did that fucking meet.

♪ ♪ ♪

It all just came crashing down. Sac State was gone. Hassle Free was gone. 24 Hour Fitness was gone. I had no school, no income and worst of all no club. It was a very weird and uncertain time for Jessica and me. I felt lost again. I questioned what I was doing and wondered if I should just go back home and regroup at my mother's house. Jessica worked at Gold's Gym and still attended school, but with such little income we could no longer afford our apartment.

We moved out and started living out of our Dodge Neon which I had just bought it from Charles Shipman a few months prior. I would lay in the back seat feeling dazed and confused. It was as if I had been beaten within an inch of my life again. I laid there asking myself "what happened?" Everything was going so well. Hassle Free, Jackie Mah, Ben Claridad, Sac State, 24 Hour Fitness and then poof! It was all gone in the blink of an eye.

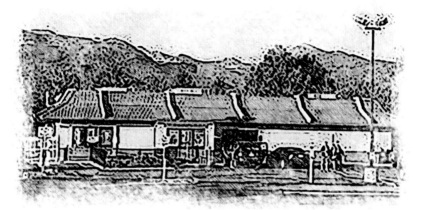

The McDonalds I Worked at to Save Money for Meets.

Together Jessica and I tried to turn things around. She still had her job and I picked up part-time work at a local McDonalds. We both barely made any money; certainly not enough to pay for an apartment in Sacramento, but it was enough for food. I would deposit bottles to scrape up extra money for gas and pay for meals from the dollar menu. All of this went on for a period of five months, but even though it was difficult, I was still committed to Weightlifting.

Jessica and I were a couple of Weightlifting nomads traveling from meet to meet. The two of us were lucky that California, being an extremely active state in the sport, hosted a lot of competitions. We were in a new city every weekend fighting to move up in the rankings. I was qualifying for the big meets of the American Open and Nationals, but I was not winning them. Instead of knowing me for lifting big weights, people knew me for my on stage antics, attitude and my extreme personality. I was hated for it. People would try to ban me from local meets or have me thrown out, but I was persistent. I kept on fighting regardless of their damn dirty looks or disapproving comments because that is who I am.

♪ ♪ ♪

Homeless, living out of my car and hated by my peers; I continued to push forward. First, I needed to find a place where I could train specifically for Weightlifting. I called all the gyms in the area and the only one that had the type of equipment I needed, bumper plates and a platform, was a Powerhouse gym about an hour drive away. The commute would be difficult, but I needed to figure out a way to keep training.

Powerhouse gym is a franchise chain that can be found all over California. This one in particular had all the usual Bodybuilding equipment, but was also keen on Strongman training. In their Strongman room they had two Weightlifting platforms and the plates I needed. The only problem was they did not have any barbells I could use for Weightlifting. I needed a bar that could spin so I would not hurt my wrist and could take the impact of being repeatedly dropped without breaking. Finding one would prove to be a difficult task because, back then, we did not have all the outlets available to buy gym equipment like we do today.

I hit the phones again this time calling gyms and other facilities asking if they had a barbell for sale. After a few days of calling around, I found the one strength and conditioning facility that had a suitable barbell they were willing to sell. I drove to their place and the guy liked me so much he allowed me to make payments on it. I think I am probably the only person in history to have had a payment plan on a barbell!

All Jessica and I had was the car, a barbell and each other. The Neon was in the Powerhouse parking lot every day and I went to work with that bar. To help pay for the bar, gas and gym membership, I picked up another job working nights at a T.G.I. Friday opening doors. We made this situation work for us the best we could and giving up was not an option. Although I was banned from Hassle Free, I still had some contact with Jackie Mah. From time to time I would go and train at her home gym in her garage. It was not something I was able to do often, and Jessica took on the rest of the coaching duties – such as programming, technique analysis and helping me at meets – while I trained at Powerhouse Gym.

The Neon would break down all the time. I would call Greg Husten to pick us up and help me put gas in it. That is how close of a family we were at 24 Hour Fitness. We were not employees, we were fucking brothers. What ex-manager would drive around Sacramento to help out an ex-employee? His support let Jessica and I breathe a little easier when something like the car stalling would come up. I do not think I could ever thank him enough.

Throughout all this chaos of making payments on barbells, the car breaking down and battling at Weightlifting meets, I began to notice something. We were homeless, living in our car, both working multiple jobs to survive – but we were together, and that is what ultimately mattered. We felt free to live every day as a new adventure. We were happy.

♪ ♪ ♪

While training at Powerhouse, I met a guy named Matt. He was a Bodybuilder and owned a local business called the Nutrishop. He knew about my situation and since we hit it off at the gym, he decided to help me out. He offered me a job at his store. That allowed me to quit working at McDonalds and spend more time at the gym.

The coolest part about the whole situation was that I knew **NOTHING** about supplements. Matt knew this and yet still decided to hire me. He liked my personality and passion for Weightlifting and thought it would bring good energy to his store. I was ecstatic and hopeful, I felt like I would be able to plant my feet back on the ground and make even greater progress in Weightlifting.

I must say though that I felt like I did nothing while I worked at the Nutrishop. We would sit and watch Weightlifting videos and drink protein shakes for the majority of our shifts. I had random little tasks to complete like sweeping the floors, taking out the garbage and organizing the inventory. None of that was very time-consuming and afterwards I would just hang out. We ate lunch together and talked about training.

If life has taught me anything, it is that good things do not last forever. Matt's plan was that eventually I would progress toward selling supplements to customers, but I had trouble retaining information about them. I would read countless articles, but I just could not grasp it. I felt like I was in school again and to be honest, I had no interest in learning about any of it. Matt and I spoke and he kindly let me go.

I understand his decision and I am okay with it. Matt helped me out for a while the best he could and let me be a part of his business. I am very grateful for that. The good times may not last forever, but the kindness of strangers is probably one of the most beautiful things one can experience.

Dodge Neon

Monday, January 20, 2014

What the fuck has happened? Shadows come alive on my wall from the fan turning above my head. Spin and click, wobble and move.....this fan creates life in my midnight room. Elephants juggle beach balls on their nose. Boo! Jokers with white face paint laugh with palms wide open, making my eyes close for a slight second....before reopening. The change of wind from my slightly cracked window turns the circus show on my wall to a more scenic adventure. Mountains of high, surrounding roads of long, as yellow lines flash as the AC blows. Windows down and sun hitting the right side of my face....I can feel it now laying on my mattress in place. Gas station stops while YouTube plays on my phone, a fast look at Steiner winning gold before my gas pump clicked with aggression. I seem to always feel a click away from one day making it big, lifting big and achieving elephant size dreams. A dollar in my pocket, as gas money came from bottles of exchange. My white dodge neon cried as the door opened, the smell of worn breaks made my eyes water, cover your nose sweetie, this car is going under. My body weak.... my mind strong......my pockets broke as my attention moves on.

"Welcome to T.G.I.Fridays," I would say. A big smile on my face that soon turned grey......my eyes shut as life prostitution

becomes sound. Selling my dreams to a door at 2 AM became
steady and bound. My life seemed fucked, this was fact. The
cold air whistling through my bedroom window reminded me of this
time way back. Opening doors for others as mine stayed shut.
Weightlifting videos played on repeat.......as my dirty clothes
stunk like piss. My bedroom wall became filled with moving parts,
all that somehow were magically put together for me to write this
diary I call this blog. The Orchestra plays a story of long.

"I got 5 sweetie,!" I would yell from the broken apartment on
the bad side of Sac. Loud bass pumping against all four walls as
cars outside sat on blocks and windows laced with locks. Shots
at night kept us up, as noodle of top filled our cups. "I got
5!," I would yell from the bedroom closet. Scattered clothes
laid out like someone opened a cargo plane door. My wife's eyes
opened like the door at Fridays as a giant leap and a hug fell
onto my arms, we spun around the room until we became weak, sweat
dripped from our foreheads from the hunt that we called pocket
searching. So hungry......so broke......finding money in some
month old jeans made for an overwhelming lump in our throats.
Joy was an understatement.....as McDonald's dollar menu made for
an early thanksgiving feast. Our bikes took us over the bridge
to dinner we pedaled.....this meal will make us lift bigger
weight than ever......and once Fridays pays me our training will
spike like no other. We even had some left over change to buy a
monster energy drink that we shared together......training that
day was like no other.

Survival not to survive......but survival to stay alive......
Weightlifting.

Random fucking jobs we would work, almost taking turns being
the pimp. Waiting for my wife outside the mall at 1 AM made my
mind fucking spin. What the flying fuck were we doing in this
town? Is weightlifting worth all this waiting around? Training
was great, but the life style fucking sucked. I felt like a
prostitute waiting to get fucked. My wife entered the neon of
broke, smell still so bad I would rather go back to blowing coke.
She cried as her boss was a dick....I guess this mother fucker
was yelling at her once again. This dick......my anger ran high,
as my motivation to win the Weightlifting National title became

overwhelmingly dyer. I would do anything to get us out of this
shit hole life! I banged the steering wheel as spit came flying
out of my dry hungry mouth. A lock on our door...........this
is where our lives hit the floor. Two months late on the rent
meant living on the car floor. Team USA to be on the moon, for
my national title packed up and moved to Mars. The shadows on my
wall were now dancing devils.....skeletons of some sort as they
played their fiddles.....I was fucked......

I let my wife down and my family. This weightlifting journey
left me in a pile of shit. Now homeless and empty with no food
or place to shit. Random bathrooms for washing, for even thinking
about training became daunting. So mad at the world road rage
became worse. Middle fingers never went down almost as a curse.
This led to me punching an athlete at Sac high, I guess the kid
was 18 years old......how was I supposed to know. Parting with
Doherty and Jackie Mah.....was one of the hardest things this
journey had to offer. To this day I feel bad......to this day I
feel awful. Now homeless and broke, no place to train, considered
reckless and wild in my weightlifting family I became.

Months dragged on, working at the Nutrishop taking out the
garbage and cleaning labels I was. Jon fucking North......
before Jon Fucken North. Chatter of training talked all around
me, as people never once noticed me. College drop out living
in a dodge neon.......bum of society....scum of the Earth. I
swept those floors solid 'til my arms fell off. I kept thinking
about my wife being yelled at by her dick boss at the mall. I
was angry but steady, I was sad but fierce. I was down but not
out.....I was defeated but not dead. The one thing that kept me
going was Weightlifting.....training.....competing. You think
we stopped? Fuck you. Once I picked up the bar at Sac State with
Ben Claridad I never put it down. Do you hear me world! Do you
hear me society! Fuck you! You might have punched me in the fucken
face.....you might have kicked me when I was down......but I am
still MOTHER FUCKEN HERE YOU MOTHER FUCKER! I still trained. On
the bus I road to the Power House Gym in Sacramento. With the
money we made I paid that monthly fucken bill, I slammed bars
still! Loafs of bread we would steal....only to eat for training
to one day hopefully become.........champions.

His hat laid low, blue and beat up. His jeans tight and his legs
out to the side, in a stance that looked like the Eiffel Tower.
Not lifting at this local meet he stood, way in the back of the
room. My piss smelled clothes and my change chattering pockets
approached. My body skinny and my dreams big. I asked him a
question about training.

Donny Shankle Replied.............

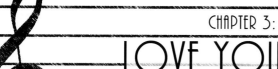

CHAPTER 3

LOVE YOUR LIFE
OR CHANGE IT

Don

Thursday, February 9, 2012

That day I ordered a number one like I usually do. Instead of the drink I got a strawberry shake, and instead of the double-double I had to upgrade to a tripple- tripple. I couldn't let Donny see me with a small meal. I wanted my first impression to be good; I wanted him to like me. My fingers were like drum sticks against the white table as my head kept turning side to side, trying to see if I could see the man himself walking towards the building. Saying I was nervous doesn't explain how nervous I really was. Not just the fact that I was about to eat lunch and train with my role model I have never met before, but the fact that I was in an unknown city by myself, just gave my college councilor my drop out forum, and just told 24 hour fitness I quit. So there I sat at the front door of my new life, hoping someone would open the door and take me in. I put everything on red, and then closed my eyes as the ball rang around the wood wheel.

I ordered Donny the same thing I got. My dad taught me well, I bought.... respect is everything. I was raised watching the Godfather's and listening to lecture's from my father on how to go about social situations. Hours among hours of "what to do" and "why to do it". The man was brilliant and still is. I keep trying to convince him to write a book, trust me.... it would sell. This man's life is a book; Dave North is a genius with people. With just one look and a touch

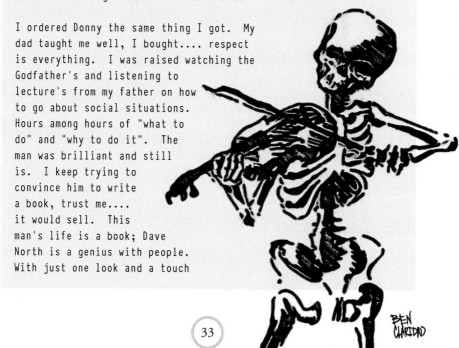

BEN CARIDAD

33

of the shoulder, he would make you melt in his hands, and he
knows it. My parents are divorced, and let's just say that my
mom and dad don't talk. But the best way I can explain my dad
is something my mom says about him. She says "that man could
have been President of the United states". When she says that it
gives me goose bumps. Pulling strings is an understatement with
him. He would give me a lecture as a child and then perform it
without anyone knowing what he was doing. It would work every
time, to this day I am still baffled at what his mind can do. I
will never forget the smell of his work suits and the presence he
carried with him. He always made the coffee drive through people
smile, and please stomp your shoes outside before getting in his
baby (aka) Lexus. Being the vice-president of Nextel on the whole
west coast....well let's just say he ran things like a boss! As a
young man I emulated him. He was after all, my father. One day
I realized that my father was not me, and I am not my father. As
my father chose the direction to take his life, I chose my own
direction. So I became jumping Jonathan North, a soldier of the
Attitude Nation, nothing more, nothing less. It feels great just
being myself. I still use many of my dad's teachings every day,
and I am lucky to have a dad that let me into his mind and help
me through many of my problems. Thank you Dad for everything you
have taught me, without it who knows where I would be today. If
we ever talk again, I would tell him to please write a book. I
beg you. I Love you dad, I always will.

As I sat there with all these random thoughts racing through my
head, I then wondered if Donny knew that I am his biggest fan. I
would sit front row at every meet he lifted in, and cheer like
the Cowboys were playing in the Super bowl again. His YouTube
videos were my motivation, and California Strength was the Harvard
of weightlifting. Hopefully I get in, and maybe someday I will
graduate with my Olympics rings.... if I play my cards right and
train hard.

He walked in like he owned the building, better yet... the city.
I stood up and shook his hand, and then we sat and ate in almost
complete silence. He didn't talk a lot, so I didn't either.
There was an understanding at the table between us both, and after
a few minutes I knew this was going to be my new home.

We trained hard that day. I met the Don (Dave Spitz) and that
went well. I will never forget what Donny said to me in the
middle of practice. He said, "I am going to break you down boy".
And O boy did he. I was about to drive back home to Sacramento
when the Don changed my life with just one line. "Come back
tomorrow and train again". I drove home with a smile ear to ear
the whole hour and half home. No music, just a replay in my mind
of everything that happened. I did it, I impressed them, they
liked me, I just might be a Cal Strength soldier.

After three weeks of hell, and hours and hours of driving there
and back, the Don had a sit down with me. The little ball hit
red. Babe call the Uhal place, we are moving. The End

                    Shankle-Don-Cal strength-Dave North 2012

Sometimes you have to take a few steps back before you can continue moving forward again. That is precisely what was happening to me. If I wanted to be successful, I needed go through all the struggles of the journey and be tough enough to overcome them. However, I did not falter and find the drugs of my past for comfort. Jessica and my passion for Weightlifting made me stronger so that I did not need to go back to those places.

I had a new drug now that was much more satisfying to the mind and other senses. It was the smell of the gym, the chalk on my hands and the shoes on my feet. The unforgiving steel firmly in my hands of a loaded barbell was what made my pupils dilate. That bar, anchored to the floor with three red plates on either side, laughing at me because I dared to challenge it.

The passion I have for this sport is what helped me keep going when life tempted me to go back home. It helped me regain my momentum again and to claw my way up the rankings. I kept coming back every single day to put in the hard work I needed to succeed. If I did not do that, I never would have found California Strength.

♪ ♪ ♪

My training continued at Powerhouse Gym, and I attended as many local meets as possible. Jessica and I would drive down the night before and sleep in the car parked outside the venue. I would go even if I was not able to afford the entry fee. Just being there made me feel like I was a part of the community, and I had the opportunity to watch my favorite lifters in action. To say I was a fan would be an understatement.

Weightlifting meets can be very subdued. It can be almost like you are watching golf instead of the greatest sport in the world. I never understood this; the guys are lifting weights heavy enough to crush them to death, but the crowd shows little emotion. I yelled and cheered as loud as I could when my favorite lifters took the stage.

There was no one that I screamed louder for than Donny Shankle. Donny is a Marine Corps veteran who served in the Iraq War. He is a five-time National Champion in the 105KG weight class. He has been on multiple world teams and is the only American Weightlifter in thirty years to defeat a foreign defending World Champion in a competition. At the 2007 Arnold Classic, Donny was awarded the "Most Inspirational Lifter" award, something that he most certainly was to me.

♪ ♪ ♪

Donny lifted for a non-profit company called American Weightlifting, aka: California Strength, located in Benicia, California. It was founded by David Spitz, who at the time wanted a serious place to train and wanted to provide something that would help the sport grow in this country. Weightlifters that were recruited for the team included Donny, Max Aita, and James Moser. Dave needed a coach that could help him achieve both his goal of winning the 2008 Olympics <u>and</u> making American Weightlifting the premier facility in California. To do that, he brought world renowned Weightlifting coach Ivan Abadjiev to America. Two Bulgarian lifters, Martin Pashov, and Nikolay Hristov also came to join the team.

Ivan Abadjiev is the most famous coach in Weightlifting history. A native of Bulgaria, Ivan earned a Silver medal at the 1957 Tehran World Championships. When his career as an athlete ended, he embarked on coaching. He was nicknamed "the Butcher" for the extreme level of commitment and discipline he expected of his athletes. Under his tutelage, the Bulgarian Weightlifting Federation became one of the most successful teams in the sport consistently winning major world titles. His greatest student was Naim Suleymanoglu, who over the course of his career won three Olympic gold medals, 7 World, and 6 European Championships and broke countless world records.

Ivan is also known for his methods and philosophies of training. He is the father of the "Bulgarian Method." Under this system of training his athletes only used five exercises in their training regime which included the Snatch, Power Snatch, Clean & Jerk, Power Clean and Front Squat. These exercises were performed using only single repetitions and to a maximum weight multiple times a day. It is incredibly difficult and demanding on the body. Currently, it is not thought to be a viable method of training for clean athletes who do not take performance enhancing substances.

♪ ♪ ♪

I could never work up the nerve to talk to Donny at the local meets in California. Both he and his team had a mystical aura about them that was extremely intimidating. They were so intense and professional as they lifted such heavy weights. I was always shocked at how good they were, and I would ask Jessica "Why don't I look like that?" or "What are those sounds the bar is making?" We could never figure it out, but instead of asking, I would just cheer him on from a distance and watch videos of him lifting online. I would imagine how much fun it would be to learn from him and train together.

It was not until a competition at Rob Earwicker's gym FIT (Focused Individual Trainers) that I found the courage to speak to the Lion Killer himself. Donny was not lifting that day, but instead just watching from the back of the crowd. He was standing near the entrance way to the gym examining each competitor as they lifted. He had a very broad stance and he kept his hands tucked into his front pockets. He looked as if he was posing for a Levi's jean commercial. He wore a white tank top under a zip up jacket, military style boots and a blue hat. Those that know him well are aware of the Shankle wardrobe.

Right when you walked into that gym, **BAM!** You were greeted by the sight of Donny Fucking Shankle. Jackie Mah, who was also at the meet, knew I was a big fan. She relentlessly egged me on to go talk to him until I finally broke. Breathing heavily, hands sweating and my stomach in knots, I walked toward him. Standing to his side, I said, "Hey Donny, I'm a big fan and I just wanted to introduce myself." I extended my hand to shake his. He turned very calmly and said "Nice to meet you" before turning away to watch the meet again.

A few awkward and silent minutes went by as we stood there. I was very excited by the fact that I was sort of hanging out with Donny Shankle. I felt like I had broken the ice, the first date was over and now I wanted to ask him a question. I was like a young cub, jumping around the alpha male of the pride as he bathed in the sun looking out over his domain. I said, "Donny, I have a question. How do I get strong like you?" His head turned to look at me and he said, "God damnit son! You just gotta get stronger." "Okay," I replied.

After that, thankfully, the conversation continued. He started asking questions about me, my training and goals. "Why don't you come out and train with me for a day?" he said. I was caught off guard by his question and not sure that I heard him correctly. I was a nobody, a homeless, low-level Weightlifter and now all of a sudden Donny was inviting me to train with him. "What time do you want me there and what day?" I replied.

He gave me the gym number and told me to meet him there at nine o'clock the next Thursday. Then he just turned and walked away. No goodbye or see you later; he was just done. There I was, with Donny Shankle's card in my hand and my knees shaking. Excitement and thoughts of "What the hell just happened!?" filled my head. That was one of the most electrifying moments in my life and one that I often look back fondly upon. It was one of those moments where I finally thought I had found my path. I knew then how Charlie from "Willy Wonka & the Chocolate Factory" must have felt, I had my golden ticket.

♪ ♪ ♪

Money was still very tight, but I had to gamble and drive out there to see where this opportunity would lead. I wanted to know if I truly had what it took to be a professional. Jessica and I collected soda cans so that we would have some extra gas money to make the trip. We hit the road, and ninety minutes later were about half a block away from the gym in San Ramon, California.

We went into an In and Out Burger restaurant and called Donny. "Hey Donny, I'm here. I'm ready to go." "Hang on, I'll meet you there," he replied. A few minutes later we saw him. Donny Shankle himself was walking toward us with no shirt on in the middle of the city. I thought to myself "Holy shit, this is happening!" Donny is a walking type of guy, but we drove him back to the gym.

My heart was pounding as we walked through the doors. All I could see was a thick cloud of smoke. I learned right away that Bulgarian lifters enjoyed smoking while resting between lifts. I heard the unmistakable **CLANG!** of a barbell being hit by an athlete's thighs during the Clean and then **SLAP!** of their feet as they smack the platform when performing the Jerk. I was shocked when I saw one of the Bulgarians Hang Snatch over 182KG.

Donny introduced me to everyone on the team. It was an honor meeting Dave Spitz, who had recently retired from competition to focus on coaching and being a business owner. All of the guys there; Mark Hazarabedian, Chris Wong, Max Aita, Martin Pashov and Jim Davis were there and all very welcoming. They were overjoyed to meet us and excited to have visitors training with them that day. Everything went even better than I could have imagined. Dave laughed at how people knew me as a crazy man in the local community. Everyone busted my balls for that and my on-stage antics. From the minute, I walked into that gym, it was as if I had come home.

My personality, attitude and bar slamming was all okay here. Instead of trying to change me, these guys accepted it all.

♪ ♪ ♪

I left Powerhouse Gym and started commuting to San Ramon from Sacramento five days a week. All of this traveling would not have been possible were it not for my mother. She realized how important Weightlifting was to me and how big of an opportunity I had at Cal Strength. Once again, she started giving me money here and there so I could make the trip to train. I chugged monster energy drinks, trained three times per week and had not yet undergone the transformation into a professional. That was all about to change in a very dramatic way.

Ivan Abadjiev was no longer coaching at Cal Strength. I had just missed him by a couple months. Instead, Donny was my coach now, and he beat the shit out of me over the course of my one-month trial. He placed me on a strict Bulgarian training system, one he no doubt learned from Ivan. I would build to maximum weights for the Snatch and Clean & Jerk five times each daily. I also maxed out the Back Squat ten times per day. I had a thirty-minute break in-between exercises and then I would do it all again.

After a week, my body and mind were breaking. The tendonitis I had in my joints was debilitating. I would lay on the floor with tears streaming down my face, and my whole body shook. It felt like Donny was killing me. The drive to and from the gym was so unbearable because my legs would cramp up. I even had trouble sleeping at night. I was not gaining any strength – just felt like I was dying.

I was not paying to train at Cal Strength. They had invited me to be there and it was my choice to go every day. I had to go and show them; to show Donny that I could handle it. I needed to prove I could be a professional. One of my worst days there was about two and a half weeks into my trial. It was the third workout of the day and I fell to the floor. I was laying on my platform, grabbing my elbow which was in intense pain from maxing out the Snatch and Clean & Jerk multiple times each day.

The training made football feel like cheerleading. Donny walked to my platform and stood towering over my body with fire in his eyes. I looked up at him, the light on the ceiling casted a luminescent mane around his head. He offered no sympathy, but instead words that I'll carry with me for the rest of my life. In his deep, Cajun-accented voice he said, "I'm going to break you down boy to build you back up." In pain, I let out a whimper. "You don't want to be a champion!" He yelled. "If you can't handle it then get the fuck out of my gym!" With that, he turned and walked away. He did not have to tell me twice; I dried my face, stood up and got back to work.

♪ ♪ ♪

They had been testing me to see if I would break, but I never did. I admit that I bent a little, but I never broke during those incredibly hard training sessions. Later that month Donny took me to the 2009 National Championships which was held in Chicago, Illinois from June 4th to the 7th.

I was so fatigued from training that I could barely walk. Donny's program continued right up to the meet. The day before the event, I completed a full day maxing out all of my lifts numerous times at the venue's weight room. Next thing I knew I was sitting in a chair, moments before my first lift scared shitless.

I had been eating too much McDonalds and had put on some fat, so I was competing in the 105KG weight class. My elbows still hurt and my legs were shaking uncontrollably. I had done competitions before, but I never felt like this. Each step I took forward to the platform was agonizingly painful.

Donny submitted an opening Snatch weight of 135KG and gave me a look that suggested I better make it. I wondered how in the world I was going to do it without killing myself. My legs burned as I squatted down to address the bar and then I felt nothing. Donny's efforts with my training, to make me a mindless robot that did not think had worked. All of a sudden, the bar was over my head and the lift was done.

I rode the confidence of that lift to complete my next Snatch of 140KG. There were four other lifters attempting the same weight I was and I managed to keep up with them. I missed my last Snatch at 145KG. I only completed my opening Clean & Jerk at 172KG and then missed at 177KG twice. I concluded the day with a 312KG Total and a fourth place finish – just 8KG shy of a spot on the podium.

My body was broken, but the experience I gained was invaluable. It showed me that I could participate in a competition of this caliber and do well. I had stayed positive through that whole month trial at Cal Strength. It may surprise many, but I rarely spoke unless I was spoken to. I only did whatever the hell Donny told me to do, always with a smile on my face – he was Coach. Dave and Donny saw my passion and how hard I was willing to work. Like a dream come true, they invited me to be on their team and train full time.

♪ ♪ ♪

I want to make one thing very clear. The best thing that has ever happened to me in the sport of Weightlifting was that one-month training with Donny. Being coached by him, Weightlifting from nine in the morning to nine at night made a man out of me. I learned that if I could make it through those four weeks, I could make it through anything. I could survive. Physical strength is one thing – now I was mentally stronger.

Something that happens in that type of training is that you go numb. Your mind and body just surrender to the pain. You cast aside your thoughts, emotions and you become a zombie. You are just there with another workout in front of you. Nothing else matters because you do not care how you feel; you just lift. You go under weight that should crush you like a bug. Some lifts you make, some you miss. With that kind of training, 80% of lifts are misses and 20% are successful.

Now, when training or even life feels hard, I think about that one month and nothing seems that difficult anymore.

♪ ♪ ♪

Toward the end of my time at Powerhouse Gym, I had enrolled in Sacramento City Junior College. I was trying to re-start my academic career. I trained at Cal Strength and took classes part-time. The goal had been to do well enough to go back to Sac State. But when Dave offered me the chance to join his team, that plan went out the window. Without hesitation, I accepted and dropped out of college again. With what little money we had, Jessica and I rented a U-Haul truck and moved to San Ramon.

Dave Spitz took care of Jessica and I. He helped us find an apartment, put food in the fridge and made sure anything else we needed was available. I had the opportunity to work at California Strength. I was paid a stipend to sweep the floors, take out the garbage and trained like a professional athlete.

I was living in one of the richest towns in the nation and training with my hero Donny Shankle. I was Weightlifting for hours each day **and** making a living. It all happened so fast my head was spinning and I felt like I was in a dream.

Behind The Gym

Tuesday, January 10, 2012

Behind the gym is where I smile. Behind the gym is where Donny
and I both smile. Behind the gym is a happy place, a place where
we can finally breathe. A place where apples and oranges the
size of our fists grow on every tree. We our sheltered by lines
of shade from the trees that bend over the top of us, as if they
were ease dropping. There are cows that sit right next to us.
Green pastures as far as the eye can see. Smells that will make
your nose twitch and your eyes water. The smoke sometimes stays
motionless right in front of my eyes. Creating patters as if
there was a small Indian making smoke signals on my nose. Donny
is still talking about how he thought training went, and I am just
glad to be out of the gym, even though I can still feel the wall
shake from the weights dropping. The air I inhale is not just air,
but a cloud of relaxation that gives me peace; Intel the Indian
makes his smoke signal again. I love this fort, this getaway, this
little world Donny and I built together. I think I might make a
no girls allowed sign and have a secrete hand shake just to get
in. The pressure, the negative forums, and the training, would
all take me under like the Titanic if it wasn't for this beautiful
alley behind my gym. Shankle Just picked an apple off the tree,
asked me what I thought about Asian women, and then took a bite
with power and conviction.....this man means business.

There is a half broken old chair that sits in the alley, in my
eyes it's a golden thrown only for the man who has the most
achievements in this sport. Donny sits in the chair and I
sit on the rocky ground.... that I have to say, is always very

comfortable. Hopefully someday I can sit in that chair, while
Shankle looks up to me. I guess that's going to take more
training days, more alley getaways, more Pendlay, and more hell.
I guess I will have many more days and nights chatting with Donny
on the ground about training. Don't tell him, but when is he not
there I sometimes sit on the chair with my head held high. I
always feel like a bad ass. Hey maybe if you ever come out to Cal
Strength and visit Donny and I, you can learn the secrete hand
shake and breath the peaceful air in the ally I call home. Just
remember, Shankle gets the chair.

Behind the gym 2012

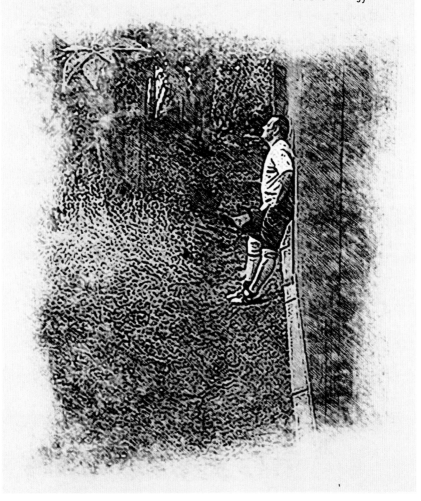

Since I had missed the Ivan Abadjiev era at California Strength – I trained with Donny under the intense Bulgarian system. That changed four months into my tenure when one of Ivan's protégés Alexander Krychev came to take the helm. Krychev was a Bulgarian Weightlifter and Ivan's very first student. His credentials included World Championships and a silver medal at the 1972 Olympic Games.

When Krychev came on as coach, it allowed Dave to focus on the business and Donny to train like an athlete. We trained together, went to local meets and more importantly started the bonding process of becoming good friends. Building a relationship with Donny was a slow and scary process for me. We were spending a lot of time together now and the last thing I wanted to do was to piss him off. He was my role model and I looked up to him a great deal.

I was also still slightly intimidated by him at the same time. Donny does not talk a lot and I, on the other hand, love to talk. I wanted to learn more about the man, where he was from and things he enjoyed. That was one big lesson I learned from Coach Friz – You have to know your fellow athletes to be an effective team. Our smoke breaks behind the Cal Strength gym provided the perfect scenario to get to know one another.

Weightlifting is a difficult sport. Our bodies would be broken down and in pain. What was needed was a quiet, peaceful place to relax – somewhere to let the mind wander. Behind Cal Strength, there are woods and cow pastures. This was our place to go and escape. There was just one old wooden chair and Donny always sat in it. He had more Gold medals than I did, so out of respect he got the chair and I had the ground. I would sit in it sometimes when he was traveling. It always felt weird, like somehow wherever he was in the world he knew I was sitting in that chair. I would hear "God Damnit Jon, that's my chair" and have to stand up for a moment.

The psychology of a cigarette is very interesting. When you have one in your hand you can be a different person. You can go behind the building to enjoy the peacefulness of the world and have a great relaxing conversation. Now take that cigarette away and that conversation would not be the same. If we had gone back behind the gym to stand in the silent woods and talk, it would have been awkward. The cigarettes provided us with an ice breaker.

♪ ♪ ♪

I never smoked in front of anyone else other than Donny. Through those cigarettes, we were able to have some of the greatest conversations in my life. We talked about training philosophies, world news and our past. I cannot comment on what Donny told me, but I shared with him aspects of my younger years that I never actually shared with anyone other than Jessica.

I remember very well one of the early days when we were still getting to know one another. Donny sat in his chair taking a drag from his cigarette and listened to me intently. I sat on the grass and tapped ash into an ashtray. I paused for a moment to look at the embers burning on the edges where I had missed. I cleared my throat and told him about my relationship with my father.

My father, David North, had been the West Coast President of Nextel. He was a successful millionaire with beautiful houses and fancy suits. When he walked into the room, he was instantly the center of attention. He is a very charismatic man, the type of guy everyone wanted to be around and listen to. My mother used to joke he could have been the President of the United States if he wanted to because of how people hung on his every word.

My relationship with him was very different from any other father-son relationship you could imagine. Early on he was just a dad. He performed the typical task of consoling me when I was scared and disciplining me when I was bad. However, as I grew older, he started to become more of a friend than father. I would tag along with him to parties and he would give me a beer. I thought it was cool to drink with my dad. I felt like we were Bonnie & Clyde – just a couple of gangsters running around together going to parties, dance clubs and raves. As I moved from middle school to high school the parties became bigger and bigger.

I lived a double life, but one that I felt was well balanced. I would have one week of white picket fences with my mother and step-father, Jim McConnell. They were strict "do your homework and go to bed at nine o'clock" parents. Then the next week I would be with my dad and his friends having a great time at happy hour. He would say "Hey Jon, get in the car" and I would be whisked away on an adventure other kids could only dream about. I would accompany him to important business meetings in the morning, watch a Football game in the afternoon, eat a fancy dinner with his friends and then hit the town at night. The thrill of sneaking into clubs was incredibly exhilarating.

My dad was a professional by day and a party animal by night. You would never have guessed it sitting next to him at a Soccer game. Together we got into the nightlife and I learned a lot of valuable lessons from it. My father's philosophy was that if I was going to do these things, I might as well do them under his supervision. He wanted me to get it out of my system while I was young, so it did not trouble me when I was older.

I would be throwing up in the toilet and he would say, "This is why you better go to college." Every night he would tell me that I better stop doing this soon. "You gotta hustle in life Jon." "You can't let the nightlife control you." We were completely immersed into our fast-paced party lifestyle and were reluctant to give it up. As father and son we went through these challenges together while at different stages in our lives.

♪ ♪ ♪

Through these experiences, I had an unexplainably close bond with my dad. I had the opportunity to get to know him in ways other kids would not ever know their own fathers. We had been through many rough times together trying to survive, running from the police or navigating rough neighborhoods. At five o'clock in the morning, he would be passed out in the back of a cab and I would lean against him to keep him from getting hurt if we hit a speed bump. I cared for him deeply. I did not just have a guy in my life who pretended to play the role of "father." I had a man who was involved in my life and aimed to make it the best one possible.

My father taught me many valuable lessons during this time. I learned how to treat people like they were human beings; equal no matter their social standing. One night we would hang out with his hardworking business friends who wore suits, ties and expensive watches. The next we were in the projects with guys who had gold grills in their mouths, bandannas on their heads and guns sticking out of their pants. My dad would be wearing a $2,000 suit – his Lexus was parked on the street, just as if everything was as normal as can be. He was not scared, because he knew them all and treated them exactly the same. He interacted with them like they mattered to him, and they did. He brought up everyone around him to his level no matter their class in society.

I remember when I was in the 5th grade he said "Son, you are going to sit down and watch these movies with me." Holding the DVD cases, I replied with "What are these Dad?" "That's the Godfather." He announced. "You are going to sit down in this chair and you are going to learn." We watched the movies and he would quiz me. Asking me questions such as "What do you do in this situation" as a scene played on the television. These were social quizzes to teach me how to think on my feet when interacting with other people.

Through these films he showed me that I should never fight for myself, but only for others. He said if he ever saw someone messing with one of my friends and I did not punch the offender in the face; I would be grounded. I would also face a similar punishment if I fought someone for messing with me directly. It all made me take an interest in that type of a mafia lifestyle. Not extreme like in the movies, but in a supportive family way. Do you need a car? Take mine. You need a place to stay? My house is your house. In a bind and need a hundred bucks? Here you go. It is why helping others in need is a big part of how I live my life today.

I want my dad to know that I love him. Over the years our relationship has been through many ups and downs, but we overcame the rocky periods and worked everything out. I cherish every second I ever spent with him. The father times and the friend times were some of the best moments of my life. All of the partying and hanging out was worth it. While I am not saying everything he did was right, I regret none of it because it made me who I am today. Anyone who might judge him negatively can go to hell because they could never understand the positives of our Bonnie & Clyde relationship. His philosophies were genius and showed me the value of working hard to find success. It was only after I stopped hanging out with him and went off to college that I lost sight of the values he taught me. When I was with my father we had control of partying, but without him there, partying had control of me.

I thank him for making me a good man. Had it not been for all those experiences, I would not be surrounded by so many beautiful people today. My path in life would have been different, and I may never have found the barbell. I might not have a passion for the sport of Weightlifting. Most importantly, I may never have met the most significant person of all, my heart and soul, the love of my life, Jessica.

CHAPTER 4

GET YOUR SHOES ON

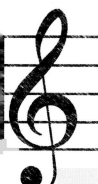

Costco

Wednesday, May 4, 2011

I am almost 100% sure that Coach Glenn Pendlay works or has worked
for the secret service, and here's why. The whole California
Strength team pulls up in two car loads into the Costco parking
lot like we are in the mafia, or better yet in the secret service.
Coach starts walking to the front door outside in the windy
parking lot. Now for some reason while Coach Glenn Pendlay
was walking toward the front door I imagined the Akon song "sexy
chick" playing. It would have fit coach perfectly! The walk, the
attitude, the weightlifting mafia behind him, shit just the whole
Glenn Pendlay way! I was thinking, "Damn that's one sexy man"!!
haha I don't know why I think that's so funny, it just is. I
think it's because he is just so damn serious it makes it that
much funnier. Its sample time baby! A couple times a week we
crash the little party of soccer moms and working dads at Costco
and eat all there samples! The first step in pulling
off this free meal between practices is getting
a cart, and pushing it around the store like we
are actually buying stuff. Coach will actually
put stuff in the cart and just slowly push it
around the store! It's like
he is a big bear trying to
fit in with the humans! haha I
am sorry but watching him making
round after round is one of the
funniest and greatest things
I have ever seen. It's
not only that, it's
the way he does it. He
will walk up looking at
the samples like it's a math
problem, look up at the little
Asian girl, look back down to

BEN
CARIDAD

49

the samples and then he will start talking to the samples lady's
about everything! "what is it" where is it from" what's it good
on" He will eat it, then he will start moving his hands around
in some sort of crazy way, gathering his flock of weightlifters
to the sample booth! "Jon have you tried this"? I will say yes
coach I have. "Well Jon then get some more!" Ok coach I will.
lol hahaha and he is dead serious, I have never seen a man so
serious in my life, and we are eating samples!!! If we walk up
to a sample table that has the food in the oven still, he will
write down when it will be done, walk around more and then yell,
"guys I think the mini hot dogs are done"!!!! "Let's go" "move
out"!!! We will all follow our great leader through the crowd of
people like little ducks down a stream. Sometimes coach will have
us spread out and attack each sample booth one at a time, then we
will switch every minute. Of course only on coach Pendlays hand
motion. It's not hard to find the leader, just look in the middle
of Costco and you will find a big man with camo pants on and a
black shirt that says "Penldlay"!!!! hahahahahaha

Light weight!!! 2012!!

I was never the greatest student during my academic career. I would sit in classrooms tapping my feet and fingers while I looked out the window. In my head I would think: "what is out there around the corner, down the road and into the next state?", "who are the people in those buildings?", "how can I be a part of the rest of the world?"

Wanderlust consumed me. I think it is one of the reasons that the Truman Show starring Jim Carrey is my favorite movie of all time. His character wanted to go to Fiji, but instead he was a prisoner of the show / the world he knew. His desire eventually became so determined that he figured out a way to escape his life. I felt just like Truman – I was restless, and I wanted to travel and learn about life; not mathematics or social studies.

California Strength allowed me to fulfill those wanderlust fantasies. I may have flunked, dropped or been kicked out of numerous schools; but this time I found the right fit for me. I was at the Harvard of Weightlifting and I intended to be the class valedictorian. Not a day went by where I was not excited to go to there.

My gym bag was not filled with papers, pencils or books, but with hard heeled shoes, tapes, and wraps. When I showed up I sat in the front row to learn from professors Krychev, Shankle, and Spitz. I took notes as I learned and listened to the old war stories of training and competition. I had the ability to travel all over the country for competitions. I met new people, saw beautiful places and made memories with Jessica. Everything was perfect and things were about to get even better. California Strength was on the cusp of a booming renaissance of Weightlifting the likes the world had never seen.

♪ ♪ ♪

Life was finally settling into an enjoyable routine of lift heavy, eat, sleep and repeat. It was a welcomed change of pace from sleeping in my car or depositing soda bottles to pay for a fast food dinner. I was living a dream I had imagined so many times before while I looked through the windshield on the way to meets. I was becoming a more polished Weightlifter with every repetition and my career was blossoming.

After a short period, Alex Krychev left the gym to pursue new projects. He was in the process of starting a supplement company called CSA Nutrition based out of Nevada and Northern California. As a high-level coach, he was also sought after by the Swedish barbell manufacturer Eleiko to open a Weightlifting academy. It was a project both he and Ivan would work on together. That left us with a void that needed to be filled. While the search for a full-time replacement started, Dave took over coaching duties.

Dave had his distinct style of coaching in contrast to Donny and Krychev. At their roots, his methods were still very Bulgarian. His workouts stuck close to the lifts, but he was extremely thorough with his explanations of little details. He taught me a lot of drills and together we worked on fine tuning my technique. Dave often gave seminars in which he taught large groups of athletes all at once and I would assist. He would direct me through his drills and that allowed me to do something crucial, not think. These movements are too fast to think about while performing. You just have to move your body or you risk committing errors. He would move me into a position and yell **"Go!"** I felt like that part of my training made my movements automatic and very smooth.

♪ ♪ ♪

At its' very core, California Strength has always been about Weightlifting. Dave had grown his business from a seed and now it was about to blossom into a very fruitful tree. He had plans to expand the training space so that half the facility could be Weightlifting and half sports performance. Because of that Dave needed to step aside from coaching so he could continue focusing on developing the business aspect of the gym. When Dave announced this, it was not the only bit of news.

Dave sat us down at a team meeting and told us he had a big surprise. Coach Glenn Pendlay was on his way from Texas. Glenn is one of the greatest Weightlifting coaches in our country's history. He had achieved the highest coaching status in the USAW as a Level 5 Coach. Glenn earned Bachelor's in

Science studying Exercise Physiology and a Masters degree in Endocrinology at Kansas State University. He was mentored in Weightlifting by famous Russian coach Alexey Medvedev. Having trained ninety National Champions and well over 20 international medalists; we could not have asked for anyone better.

Glenn would also be bringing one of his lifters with him, Caleb Ward. Caleb was already a well established Weightlifter in the junior division and now competed at a high level in the senior division. He is quite simply the most incredible athlete I have seen in my life. He was a big kid, lifting in the 105+KG weight class. As big as he was, he was the fastest, most agile person in our gym. If you search on YouTube for "Jon North vs. Caleb Ward," you can find a video us battling it out in a backflip competition. Needless to say, he won. Our already strong team just became unstoppable.

♪ ♪ ♪

My little world at Cal Strength was changing and I was both thrilled and nervous at the same time. These feelings reminded me of the first day of school. After much anticipation, the big day finally arrived and when the gym doors opened, two gargantuan men entered meaning business. Glenn is a man of very few words. He just waddled in and said "Get your shoes on."

I knew right then that I was in for some serious training. No "Hi" or "Nice to meet you." There was no pizza party to celebrate and mingle. We could exchange pleasantries later. We would have all the time in the world to laugh and learn each other's favorite movie. On that particular day, at that time, we only had time to fucking train! To tie our laces tight, grab a bar and throw something heavy over our heads!

He started coaching the second he walked into the gym. "Get your shoes on" meant let's dominate the Weightlifting world. When he spoke those words all I heard was we will make Pan American teams, win a National Championship and be number one in the country. I transcended the speeds of light and sound as my shoes slipped onto my feet. I kicked my heels together to make sure they were snug. There is no place like home – no place like California Strength. Standing on my platform, I looked at Glenn and said "I'm ready coach."

♪ ♪ ♪

In general I am a very laid back, easy going person. I have tendencies to be shy and introverted. That is the person that not many people know. Instead, on the opposite end of the spectrum, there is the Jon North you see on the platform. The guy who slams bars, kills PRs and yells **"SHANKLE!"** before every lift. It is almost like normal me is Bruce Banner and then I turn into the Incredible Hulk when it is time to lift big weights. It is the only way I could find to overcome the brutal nature of this sport.

Every Weightlifter has ways unique to them which gives them the ability to cope with grueling training. For me, survival meant bringing my mind to a place that allowed me to ignore the pain. You develop a thought process that enables you to "let go" as Donny would say and go under weights that could kill you.

"Jon North" had become a third person. People would often discuss the attitude and onstage antics with me. I would just think to myself "oh you mean that other guy." I knew of him, but we had never met. He was just someone I saw in passing or on a video someone recorded with their phone. When I looked in the mirror, I did not see the bar slamming, Shankle yelling, "Jumping" Jonathan North everyone loves or loves to hate. I saw me; a person who I was still trying to learn about.

I had found myself as an athlete, but I still did not know who I was outside of that. I was depressed if I was not Weightlifting. I would be hanging out with a guy (me) that was a stranger. Weightlifting made me confident. When I was on the platform, adrenaline would be surging through my bloodstream as I exorcized my demons. If I did not have this sport to channel my energy and draw out my addictive qualities, I would still be smoking crystal meth.

I was very fortunate to have Glenn as my coach. He may not have liked any of my antics, but he never discouraged them either. His approach was never to put shackles on his athletes. If I needed to go crazy to lift significant weights then that was okay. Everything we did was about adding more weight to that bar. We had to become stronger so we could win.

His training was strict and well thought out, but there was always wiggle room for us to breathe. If we wanted to go heavier, the answer was always yes even if it went off the programming. When I felt good on what was supposed to be a "light" day then, it was okay for me to max out. He allowed me to be an athlete while he was the coach. That is why he is one of the greatest coaches not only in this country, but the world because he was flexible. We were not a bunch of athletes he tried to "manage" or rule over. We were his stable of Weightlifting Stallions and he understood we needed to be let out into the field to run.

♪ ♪ ♪

One thing I learned from Pumping Iron was that when Bodybuilding you chase the pump. You want those muscles to fill with blood, to swell like balloons that could pop with just one more repetition. However, in Weightlifting, you chase different rabbits – atmosphere and emotion. Training in a high-energy environment is critical. You need teammates that will push you and a genius coach who guides you to find success. That is what I had at Cal Strength and it took me to the next level in competition.

Under the watchful eye of Coach Pendlay, I qualified for the 2009 American Open. The meet was held in Mobile, Alabama from the 11th to 13th of December. Lifting in the 94KG weight class, I butted heads with the legendary Phil Sabatini and my good friend Frankie Murray. Phil had been on the scene for quite some time battling against the now retired Jeff Wittmer in the 94KG class. Frankie, like me, had been working his way up the ranks.

It was a big meet for me and I was filled with all sorts of emotions that I hoped would fuel my performance. Frankie completed his opening Snatch of 132KG, and I followed him shortly with an attempt at 138KG. I was nervous and I needed an emotional edge. So I thought about one of my favorite Weightlifters of all time; Matthias Steiner.

A native of Austria, he competed in the 2008 Beijing Olympic Games in the 105+ weight class for Germany. A year prior to the Olympics, Steiner's wife sadly passed away in a fatal car accident. Mourning the loss, he battled with thoughts of quitting the sport altogether. I know from experience that it takes a lot of time in the gym to succeed and I can only imagine the level of focus needed to make it to the Olympics. The pressure must be incredible and that did not leave much time for his family. After what I can only speculate was a severe emotional battle to find the will to return to the gym, Steiner decided to keep pursuing Beijing. Not only would he keep training, but he dedicated everything to the memory of his late wife. Going into the competition, Matthias was an underdog. The famous Russian, Evgeny Chigishev or World Champion Viktors Ščerbatihs were the projected favorites to win. He stayed in the game during the Snatch opening with a 198KG Snatch, just 3KG under his all time best and 203KG on his second attempt. He needed to hit these big weights to be a contender for the podium. His Snatch session concluded when he missed 207KG. He could not hold it above his head and as it fell to the ground the bar clipped his head.

Every lift was filled with emotion. He would yell and throw his fist in the air prompting the crowd to cheer. After battling through the Snatch event, the gold medal would be decided with the Clean & Jerk. At this point, Steiner was ranked in fourth place with a total of 203KG. To stay competitive, he needed to lift 246KG. Still sapped from his final Snatch attempt, he Cleaned 246KG, but missed the Jerk.

As pressure mounted, Steiner successfully hit 248KG to guarantee himself a third place medal and the crowd erupted to help him celebrate. Ščerbatihs missed his final two attempts leaving it between Matthias and the Russian. Chigishev was on fire, setting the bar high at 250KG on his last lift. Having completed a 210KG Snatch, he was now sitting with a 460KG total compared to Steiner's 451KG.

Steiner was the last man left to lift in the session. It was his show and everything would come down to this final lift. He opted to put 258KG on the bar – Completing this lift would give him a 1KG lead over Chigishev and a Gold Medal. In this sport, a 12KG jump is unheard of, and this was a weight Steiner had never lifted. All his emotions, all the hard work throughout his journey would be tested right here.

He walked out on the stage, his coaches watching intently. Steiner setup on the bar and pulled. He was not just lifting a metal bar and rubber discs. In his hands he held a year's worth of pain and loss. The mental anguish of having to do another repetition when all he wanted to do is weep and remember the past. The Clean gave him no struggle as he brought the bar to his shoulders. As he stood so did the crowd roaring in excitement.

Matthias Steiner took a deep breath and let go of all his fears and went for the Jerk. His feet slammed down upon the platform as he moved them into a split stance. The weight effortlessly floated above his head, and his arms extended. All that was left was to bring his feet together and wait for the down signal to drop the bar. He had done the impossible. The crowd was in a frenzy yelling his name and hugging.

He did not raise his hands in the air in triumph but instead collapsed over the bar. Tears bursting from his face he slammed his hands to the platform yelling in celebration. His coach, Frank Mantek stormed the stage to congratulate his athlete. The two embraced and jumped up and down. On the podium, Matthias carried with him a photograph of his late wife so the world could see she was there with him.

♪ ♪ ♪

I wanted the crowd to be involved like they were for Steiner. After Frankie's first Snatch, I followed shortly after with 138KG. I then missed my next two attempts and my first Clean & Jerk. Phil was in the lead with a 150KG Snatch and Frankie was ahead of me completing his first Clean & Jerk.

I had missed at 170KG. To stay on Phil's heels and take the lead over Frankie, Glenn and I decided to go for 172KG. I walked out scanning the crowd and yelled **"STEINER!"** loudly. Remembering his story gave me a jolt of adrenaline and I made the lift. Frankie completed 173KG on his second attempt and Phil did the same on his third. Frankie was going to go for a much higher number to make a big jump in the rankings and I needed to make a larger jump myself to stay in the mix if he made it.

We decided to go for 176KG on my final attempt. I was still thinking about Matthias and how he must have felt. I went on stage and destroyed 176KG, slamming it down as hard as I could. Frankie then asked that 182KG be put on the bar. If he made this lift he would tie me for a total, but win on bodyweight since he was lighter at 90.84KG to my 93.30KG. He failed to complete the lift and as a result took third place. I finished the meet with a 314KG total taking a Gold Medal in the Clean & Jerk event and Silver Medal in the overall competition.

That is the power of atmosphere and emotion. Those who chase them find success.

♪ ♪ ♪

Thinking back on this time in my career, I am reminded of that television show "The Wonder Years" starring Fred Savage. The show always opened with a montage of the Arnold family's grainy 1970s style home movies. It would show them having barbecues, graduation parties and other happy moments. With Joe Cocker's "With a little help from my friends" in the background.

It felt just like that at California Strength. We were a close family who did everything together and training was our life. Everyone lived in the same apartment complex within walking distance of the gym. Before, during and after practice sessions we would lay out by the pool soaking in the California sun. Donny would eat steaks and all we would talk about was Weightlifting. It was the first time since Eagle Football I felt this level of team camaraderie and brotherly love.

Our lifestyle was made possible by the Cal Strength work-train program. Each of us made money by helping to coach other athletes and personal training. It was a revolutionary approach by the company; a program that no one else in the country was offering. American Weightlifters in general, are poor in comparison to athletes in other sports like Football or Basketball. Other countries pay their Weightlifters to train and offer significant bonuses for winning medals. In the United States, there is no government funding and if you want to succeed in this sport then you have to support yourself and work a job on the side.

California Strength was ahead of the pack in this regard and it allowed for the building of a solid professional team. Our lifters, myself included, could focus one hundred percent on the sport because it was our job. It eliminated the stresses of bills, bosses or the half-hearted pursuit of another career. Our only concerns were the gym and the barbell.

Cal Strength YouTube Channel

Friday, March 14, 2014

The gravel crunches under my feet as I take
a stroll down a once operating machine
factory I once called home, that now lays
in ruins full of old cameras and scattered
shoes. Swinging swings squeak as the the
wind swirls through the empty abandoned
park, creating a false reality of life, as
newspapers dance across the dirt, and kilo
plates fall over from the wooded blocks the
weights have gotten to know and love. A

rustic world where memories live and dreams were made. Old Cal
Strength. The original, and the place where it all started. The
longer I walk under this dark yellow sky, the deeper the Cal
Strength YouTube channel goes. Faces that bring a smile to my
face, and some a tear, as the memories are only the start, for the
surface has cracks, and deep within those cracks lie the feeling
that each person left upon me. Each person has unknowingly formed
me into the man I am today. Each video has branded me a home sick
feeling that pounds deep within my stomach. The more I write,
the more I walk, the deeper I go, the more the home sick feeling
grows, leaving me wanting to re-live each video, each laugh, each
joke, each miss, and each struggle. Adopted from what I loved
most, a shoulder to lean on, and a family to call my own. I
walk with my head down, for seeing too much makes it too hard to
continue the YouTube stroll down this graveyard of old school.
The graveyard of the very beginning.

Glenn's nicely shaved face and nervous ticks while being filmed
runs a tear down my eye as I write this blog that has already shown
itself as one of the hardest blogs to write to date. Max Aita
performing a no belt, no wraps and no hands 250kg back squat, then
afterward joking around about our little pyramid scheme, inside
joke we created after always getting approached constantly at
Costco, made my home sick feeling grow to the point of pain. Donny
Shankle telling his famous war stories on a hot summer day while we
all sat around drinking our energy drinks as if the platform was a
camp fire, and the resting chairs were our tent. Mullet jokes with

Enderton, while Spencer danced on top of the jerk blocks. Kevin
Cornell and his wise philosophy made every one's hard training day
become a little bit better, while Rob's loud skipping laugh echoed
throughout the gyms walls for all to hear.

At this point of the journey I have found myself resting on an old
white pick up truck that Max must have forgotten to drive away with
before the new school Cal Strength came through. It is no longer
white and alive, now dead and brown from the constant slashing
of the wind and dirt that never seems to let up. Sunny skies and
rolling hills have turned into forgotten paths and cow pastures
full of bones. A deserted world that once bloomed colors and
energy, now quiet and calm it sleeps. I mustered up the strength
to drag my legs down the Cal Strength channel even deeper, on the
hunt for what started everything.....the very first video.

The gravel road turned a few sharp corners as it led me down its
windy hill. The yellow sky is brighter than earlier, as black
clouds splattered throughout like spilled paint. The dirt world
is a desert waste land, but off in the distance there stands life,
tall and proud, green and alive, beautiful and fulfilling. A tree,
a single tree that my eyes followed while my feet stepped blindly.
My hands out to the side to better balance myself from my feet
stepping in all the wrong places. The wind seemed to die down, as
true silence rang throughout the waste land. A broken wall that
laid half in ruins tried desperately to stand in front of the tree.
It looked as if the wall had been defeated, as the tree stood in
victory. Was this wall once a part of the old Cal Strength? I
mumbled to myself as my hand brushed the sad wall. Sad it truly
was, I felt like at any minute the wall was going to ask me if it
could be tall and sturdy like the tree in front of it. My heart
rang out, smothering my home sick stomach, with now a stinging pain
in my heart. My other hand grabbed the bark from the tree while
my eyes stared down on the small path that ran between my legs, now
finding myself resting and relying on both objects after a long
and emotional journey. I then knew where I was. Lightning went
off and the grey clouds darkened the yellow sky. Both my hands
became free as my back hit the wall and my body slid down into the
dirt that grew so familiar. My eyes closed with a fallen tear, as
my fingers dug deep into the dirt creating a sharp pain from my
finger nails being pushed back. The tree might as well have smiled

at me and told me it has been too long. The wall had my back like it always had, and the little path that ran between both the tree and wall was the same, it was just without water running down and green grass surrounding it. My hands beneath the dirt felt a long piece of medal. My head turned to the hand that captured this treasure, and then my arm began to pick up speed moving back and forth trying to wrestle the dry dirt away to view what my hand was holding. A stubborn thing this piece of medal was, so stubborn I found myself standing up heaving with all my might. Soon after about 10 minutes of battle, the object uplifted from the graveyard of dirt, and showed itself. It was a medal chair. Bent and broken, used and then forgotten, lonely and left behind. I new I had to continue on my path down to the bottom of the deepest Cal Strength video. I must leave this memory behind me always keeping it deep down inside of me never to be forgotten. I must walk away from the once beautiful and magical place Donny and I once called our smoke break behind the gym.

I soon found myself down deep, deep where the landscape became blurry and out of focus from the small little camera Glenn used to film with. Before the beard, before the exposure, before the medals, before everything. Broken bars and broken straps that were once shinning stars of this time period. Old shoes with no laces, and echos from past lifts as screams and yells whistled with the wind. Dirt hitting empty coffee cups that made sounds of chatter about possibly putting a blog together, and the excited talk about coaching and clients, gold medal goals, and maybe one day the chance to be able to represent the Country. Dreams that were boiling like water on the stove. Videos that were mostly clips of single lifts that bloomed into multiple clips that soon became training videos. Retired YouTube views begged for more hits on the side of the gravel road like homeless bum's begging for drug money. A single number 1, was telling stories and bragging about how he was the first viewer ever, the first YouTube hit ever. He sat up high on a broken platform as he took credit for the start of the thousands and thousands hits to come. For he was the original hit, the first hit ever that created a wave of something that no one at the time ever thought possible. I broke a smile and waved at number one as I passed by, raising my head to show my respect and appreciation. I stumbled upon a blackberry that the dirt had not fully swallowed. Not the fruit, but the phone. I picked it

up and then blew the dirt off the screen to get a better look. I
knew right away that this was the phone of Dave Spitz. Keys
completely worn out from the fast typing of exciting numbers his
athletes just hit. Fast texting from the work he constantly put in
to grow the life of his baby. The owner of Cal Strength, the boss
man, the godfather, the leader, the man that made it all possible.
The man that gave me a chance when I was a young troubled kid.
The man that breathed air into my lungs and gave me a purpose.
Memories of him yelling at me while front squatting, "There is no
crying in weightlifting, Jon!" I wonder what he would yell at me
now if he saw my face. Because right now I am not weightlifting.
Maybe I will travel high up to the very top of the channel where a
world of unknown and new faces live and return his phone. Maybe
he dropped it while moving forward away from the old school waste
land. I put it in my pocket, and traveled down deeper to where
the videos became even more blurry, shaky, and innocent. I walked
deeper down to the place where I was born.

Muscle Driver and the Attitude Nation seemed a million miles
away. I started to miss my present life, but was too driven by
the good old days to stop now. Martin Pashov told stories of how
he wanted to be a soccer player in Bulgaria, but was never allowed
to because they forced him to become a weightlifter. This always
broke my heart. Anthony Grule was just a baby experiencing high
school, and Caleb Ward was still a 105 plus. Coach Glenn only
wore these gladiator sandals, or what we called, Jesus slippers.
I picked them up from the curve of an empty tire, and put them in
my bag to give to him once our paths ran into each other again. I
was close to the bottom, I could feel it in the change of the air.
The temperature started to drop dramatically, and the sky was now
pitch black. The dirt scurried past my feet as every step I took
crunched the gravel of moving rocks below me. I was far away from
Donny's and my smoke break tree, and at this point it would be
nice to have one with him from the nervous wreck I was under.

My feet met water, as a distant light house cast its light far in
the distance. The wind was heavy, but the water was glass. My
feet became bare as my hands became smooth. The dark only showed
its face for the last hour, and now the sun was rising making the
nighttime light house fade. The sun crept up my body warming my
cold heart while the dirt turned into green grass. A boat was

heading my way, but I couldn't make out who it was. It looked
like two big people from one side of the boat almost completely
tipped one way. How the boat didn't fall over was nothing but a
miracle. I was startled from the out of no where comment by Pete
standing beside me. I was startled, but more baffled on how he
got there. Pete's Asian eyes lit up as he waved the boat down as
if he was the kid in school begging to be called on. I looked
over at Pete with an excited look on my face and asked him "Who
is that Pete?" He replied with a look of confusion because of
the fact I didn't know. "That's your new coach Glenn Pendlay and
his athlete Caleb Ward!" He went on to tell me they made a long
journey from Texas to get here, and how excited they were to be
a part of the team. At this point I was waving with Pete, even
jumping up and down. I looked over to Pete while half laughing
- half yelling "Over here!" then asking "What team?" Pete looked
back at me as his face became blank and more Asian than ever.
"Team Cal Strength" Pete looked away while still keeping one
eye on me as if he was unsure I was not losing my mind. I then
realized I was home, back to the start, the very bottom of Cal
Strength's YouTube channel. I made it, my journey was a success.
I drew many tears, laughed many memories, and walked many lonely
paths, but I made it. I looked back with a smile ear to ear at
Donny sitting on the brand new chair behind the tall proud gym
wall and yelled to him with everything I had, "Donny......Coach is
here"!! Donny took a drag from his smoke while looking up into
the bright green tree and then back at me, "Good brother, now tell
em to hurry it's almost time to train brother". I waved my head
back and forth while shooing him away with my hand as if to say
that could wait 'til later, Donny. He chuckled while wiping some
moss away from his white tank top. "Max! Come fast, coach is
here!" To my surprise Max was already right next to me, beard and
glasses in full affect, and responded with just a look beyond out
to the boat. My chest became warm from my wife Jessica leaning
up against me as my arms wrapped around her body, as if we were
watching the sunset, but instead we were waiting upon two heavy
set men that were almost drowning the boat. Caleb with a barbell,
and coach with a small silver camera. Dave Spitz welcomed them
both. I then startled in excitement to show both coach and Dave
that I found their belongings on my journey to now. I held out
the blackberry phone in one hand, and the Gladiator sandals in
another, awaiting their good praises. But instead, getting funny

looks in return as I soon noticed they already had these objects
with them. I almost forgot that this interaction was only a
memory, and that the only place to go from here is forward, back
through the rolling grassy hills of San Ramon, tall tree of smoke
breaks behind the gym, back past Max's bright white Chevy truck,
brand new barbells and new shoes, and upgraded cameras to capture
all of the memories and success that happened throughout the
beginning of the Cal Strength days. All soon to one day turn back
into the waste land of forgotten times and rustic memories. At
this point view number one was not bragging on top of the broken
platform, because view number one was not alive yet.

Coach Pendlay and Dave looked at the new
and improved team with Donny off in the
distance wrapping his knees with his famous
knee wraps, and they both said at the same
time......."Well....shall we train...?".

The rest is history.

A forgotten video from the old and original
waste land

Cal Strength 2016

In our little corner of the Weightlifting world – the second Cal Strength era
was in full swing – it seemed as if all you needed to do was walk into the room
and you would be stronger. Word spread fast and more lifters wanted to join.
Our all-star team consisted of Donny Shankle, Max Aita, Kevin Cornell, Spencer
Moorman, Caleb Ward, Jessica and me. We traveled the country with our fearless
leader Glenn Pendlay leading the way.

And we were breaking new ground. At the time, it was not a regular
practice to film your lifts, write blogs or speak on podcasts. Information was
not freely shared so if you needed coaching or critiques you had to find a
coach and a gym. Cal Strength changed all that with an explosion of YouTube
training videos.

It all started one day when Glenn walked into the gym with his shoddy camera
and filmed just one lift, not even an entire training session, and then he put it on
YouTube. It was purely just for fun and to show some people around the area what
we were doing. He had no intention of shooting any more videos after that, but
much to everyone's surprise, a few days later the video had 2,000 views.

I find it funny today, but Glenn, Dave, myself and the other athletes thought there was something wrong with YouTube when we saw so many views. Glenn was sitting in his chair in the weight room looking at his laptop. Around him were all these big strong Weightlifters scratching their heads trying to figure out how to fix the damn thing – surely 2,000 people could not have watched our video so quickly. Finally, Dave emailed the company for help, and they responded that everything was fine. "You are just popular," they replied. We were astonished that so many people took an interest in watching us train. A light bulb must have flashed over Dave's head, and we started shooting more videos.

Dave began making full use of the internet to share and promote our craft. He and Glenn filmed all of our big lifts and then put them together to make training videos. They became so extremely talented at producing these videos that they began to branch out from big lifts. Cal Strength started releasing instructional videos on technique that were met with fantastic feedback from the national community. The goal was to spread the word on the gym and educate people all over the world on how to lift. It would bring a lot of attention to our incredible sport.

♪ ♪ ♪

It was almost as if we had our very own reality television show. The madness of training was now available to the world. People could tune in and see if Donny was going to hit a big lift or my crazy antics. It granted the wish of everyone who wished they could be a fly on our wall. Anyone could type our name into the search bar and see us warming up, working up to big lifts and the emotion that follows after missing. These are things every lifter could relate to and now they could soak it all up whenever they desired.

One of my favorite recorded encounters can be found by searching for "Jon North vs. Spencer Moorman at Cali Strength." I think this video depicts the training and atmosphere we had in the gym very well. Our ultimate goal as athletes was winning competitions. Often Glenn would stoke the fire of our competitive natures by adding a twist to max out days. That twist usually involved cash prizes for the lifters who were the most consistent. He judged this by the number of missed lifts.

Spencer and I had to complete seven repetitions of the Snatch and Clean & Jerk at 90% our current best totals. Whoever successfully lifted all fourteen attempts with no misses would win $100. I brought my "A" game with me and tried to use every trick I had to get into Spencer's head. I attempted to cast doubt in his mind to make him overthink the situation. I would tell him how great I was feeling that day or how he needed to think very hard about his technique.

I even wore my senior team singlet that day to be flashy. Our platforms were right next to one another so I would sit at the bottom of my Snatches and have conversations with Spencer. I tried everything I could think of to psych him out. Simply put, I was a real dick. We made some great lifts, talked a lot of trash and in the end Spencer took me down. I missed one of my Clean & Jerks and he did not.

That video with Spencer showed the fun, but we also had many videos that portrayed the real deal. Ones that gave an insight into the frustrations and failures that occur in hard training such as the one named "No Crying!. Inspiration from California Strength." Even professionals go through tough days. In that one you can hear Glenn yelling for me to stop crying on a set of Push Presses, Spencer missing Cleans and even Donny missing Jerks. It showed that we are human just like everyone else.

Today you can literally be lost on YouTube for hours watching videos on the California Strength channel. You have been warned.

♪ ♪ ♪

The videos of our training sessions were never really used for coaching purposes. Most of the guys did not think much of it; it was just funny. Eventually it just became part of the routine for them. I, on the other hand, thrived being on film. Every session I felt like Brad Pitt preparing for a big role. I used to receive a lot of shit from Coach and my teammates because I would not lift sometimes unless the camera was focused on me. I fed off of its energy and one thing I always found very interesting was the psychological aspect of being on camera.

Training with the same people every single day, boxed in by the same four walls can become depressing and miserable. However, when I was on camera, I came alive. That little red light came on and that was my cue. It created an atmosphere where training felt more like a meet. Coaching may not have been the intention, but in many ways that camera did more for me than almost any cue or technique advice had. It made me feel like I was always competing in front of hundreds of people.

Being filmed also gave me a physical high and made me confident. Donny and I would often talk about how ego in this sport is a positive thing. You have to have one if you are going to lift heavy and win. When I was exhausted, the camera gave me the energy to push harder. I knew people were going to be watching, so I stood a little straighter and smiled. There was no question about it, I was born to perform.

♪♪♪

Before the YouTube explosion, Donny and I had our blogs. They allowed us to be creative and relax between training sessions, almost like a digital cigarette. At our computers, the screens back to back and us drinking coffee, we would write about our lives. We shared our philosophies on Weightlifting with the world and each other. It was a continuation of our peaceful time from behind the gym and a break from the battles just a few feet away.

Donny and I always listened to music while we wrote. It is a tradition that I still honor today, and I have never written a blog without a song playing. The first thing I would say when I sat down was, "Donny give me a song." He would always respond with, "Oh, I've got one for you today, Jon." Once the melodies hit my headphones, and I started drinking coffee I was in another world. We played symphonies and other types of instrumental music. It helped to stimulate our minds and evoke deep emotions that we could cast upon the canvas of our empty screens.

Donny always had a way with words and would finish writing his post sometimes before I had even started mine. Our styles were so different, but that is a beautiful thing about art – each artist has their own way. After we finished our masterpieces for the day, we would read one another's work. We were training our minds and in between took breaks to train our bodies.

♪♪♪

Everything took off very quickly. We had large numbers of views on our blogs, videos, and website. It was clear – people wanted more California Strength. Emails asking for advice on training poured into all of our inboxes. We had become more than just a gym, we became a destination. Our product was well sought after and that led to the seminars.

Glenn started traveling all over the country and eventually the world. The very first international seminar was in Ireland and I had the honor of accompanying him. Sitting on the plane, looking out the window was very surreal to me. Not too long before all of this I was working at a McDonalds. I was living out of my car and trying to make a better life for Jessica and myself. Now I was sitting next to quite possibly the greatest coach in the world flying to another country.

The trip to Ireland with Glenn was a very maturing adventure. I had only been exposed to gyms in California, but I learned something important in Ireland. It does not matter where you train. Weightlifting is Weightlifting wherever you go. The barbell only speaks one language and has one culture. It makes no difference if you are training with guys from Ireland, Russia or China. You are all brothers and sisters engaged in the same fight for every kilo possible. Our shared world was hidden before, but now it is open and accessible to the world.

I admired and respected Coach Pendlay a lot. I was excited about the trip to Ireland the same way a kid would be to go to a Baseball game with their father. Having the opportunity to spend time with him on the plane and between seminars was something I cherished. The two of us spoke about so many things other than Weightlifting on this trip. I learned more about his past and told him about mine. I could tell that he cared about me and I returned to the United States with a new level of respect for him. I want it to be clear. I love Glenn Pendlay. He was and always will be like a father to me. It does not matter if we are at different gyms or teams, I will always respect that man.

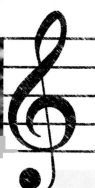

CHAPTER 5

WHAT IS A LIGHT DAY

What Is A Light Day?

N/A

I am going to tell you how to become a good Olympic weightlifter. I am going to tell you how to make The Pan American games in two years. I am going to tell you how to be number one in two years, and break records in two years. I am going to give you the secret free of charge. Grab a pen and paper and write this down, you won't need a lot of paper, mostly just guts, balls, and a lot of determination. The weightlifting program goes like this: snatch, clean and jerk, and squat. Maximum everyday. But you don't want to talk about that. You want to talk about double knee bend, breathing technique, grip width, percentages, and light days. What is a light day? Please someone help me with this! Why even come into the gym? Stay home and watch TV while my California Strength soldiers and I lift more than your max, daily. A light day to me is a sign of weakness. "If you have to run from a bear, you're not going to tell that bear that you need some time to stretch and only run 85%, you are going to run maximum every time" -Donny Shankle. Do you think that California Strength put three of our athletes on the Pan American team by going light? Do you think I win by training light? Haha. If you do, then you're not winning. I am numb to these weights, these kilo's I kill. This is what going heavy everyday makes you, numb. I don't care what's on the bar anymore, I just lift it. I love pulling on heavy bars. I hate pulling on light bars, what's the point it's light? Training like this

BEN
CARIDAD

turns me into a machine, I can go hard anytime, anywhere. I want
to point out something I get asked a lot, and that is how do you
train your body for such heavy loads all the time; how long does
the progression stage take? The answer is I don't have an answer,
just do it and stop talking. I use the giant chip on my shoulder,
and the hunger to be the best, what's yours? "You can bleat like
a sheep, or be the Shepard" -Donny Shankle.

- Jon North

Outside of the Olympics, The Arnold Sports Festival is the Mecca of the sports and fitness world. It is held in Columbus, Ohio and is named after the man who changed my life that fateful night back in a crack house – Arnold Schwarzenegger. The event includes a diverse variety of sporting activities such as Archery, Fencing, Gymnastics, Arm Wrestling, Boxing, Weightlifting and of course Bodybuilding. What truly makes The Arnold unique is that it brings athletes together from all over the world to participate. It provides fans the opportunity to see performances from those they would normally have to travel out of the country for.

After a few years in the sport, I qualified for the Arnold Weightlifting Championships in 2010. The competition was held at the Columbus Convention Center located in downtown Columbus, Ohio from March 5th to the 7th. Going into the meet I had two goals. First was to qualify for the 2010 Pan American Championships. The second (and possibly much more importantly) was to meet the man himself, my hero, Arnold.

The Fitness EXPO was intense. It contained well over eight hundred booths where companies were promoting the newest inventions in equipment, apparel and nutrition. A sea of people flooded the area for free samples and to talk with the Bodybuilders who would hang out at vendor booths to help sell products. I found it fascinating that so many people who loved fitness would come together and share ideas. I felt like this is how all competitions should be.

It was always part of our routine to arrive at the venue at least a day before a meet. It allowed us to relax, stretch out our legs and have a safety net if anything went wrong with our travel arrangements. I was particularly excited to be early for The Arnold because I wanted to explore everything the festival had to offer. After team meetings with Glenn concluded, I ventured out into the world of fitness. I spent a great deal of time meeting professionals like Jay Cutler who were behind supplement tables. I also walked away with a pretty hefty bag of free samples.

The highlight was when I finally saw Arnold. I had been watching the 77KG weight class with Jessica and a few of the other guys on the team. After a little while we decided to take a break from watching to hit the restrooms and grab some food. We politely waited for a weight change, and while the bar loaders were doing their thing – we walked between the space dividing the crowd from the competition stage. Our group was almost clear of the stage when I just so happened to look out into the crowd...and saw the main man himself.

Arnold was sitting there, no more than ten feet away from me enjoying the meet. My head began to swirl as a series of emotions over took me. I had a brief flash back to sitting in that crack house, holding the "Pumping Iron" DVD case while admiring Arnold's freedom. Had that movie not been played that night, I may not even have been standing there in Columbus, Ohio on that day. Instead, I could have been dead or in jail and the man who helped light the fire within me to follow a new path in life had no idea what he had done. He did not know the role he played in setting me free and I was compelled to tell him about it.

Weightlifters train to react because there is no time to think. In that moment, I had to be brave and just go for it. With my eyes misty from all of the thoughts cascading through my mind – I jumped into the crowd. To the horror of my teammates and those sitting in that general area – I quite literally crowd surfed my way to Arnold. Immediately, three massive bodyguards descended upon me. They tried to pull me away, but I struggled, one hand gripping the seat under me firmly and the other extended toward Arnold. It must have sounded like incoherent gibberish, but I quickly yelled "Arnold you changed my life!" He turned his gaze from the stage and looked at me with the calm reaction of someone who has experienced this exact situation many times over the years. He shook my hand, said "Thank You" and then turned again to watch the meet. Overjoyed I allowed the bodyguards to escort me away from the area. It had all happened in about the span of thirty seconds – the look, the jump and the handshake.

It felt very invigorating to tell Arnold that he changed my life. I now felt unstoppable. I was in Arnold's house and I would make him proud. My Snatch session went extremely well ending with a 141KG lift. If I wanted to make the Pan Am team, I needed to Clean & Jerk 184KG. Glenn planned everything out so that I would go for this lift on my second attempt. If I missed it, I would still have one more try to pull it off.

Chalking My Neck Before One f the Biggest Lifts in My Career.

I knew I would not need two attempts. Arnold had fucking touched my hand the day earlier. I now had his strength with me and I would use the emotions I felt to lift this weight or die. My name was called and it was my turn to lift. 184KG was loaded on the bar and I chalked my hands and neck with Glenn watching my every move. I stepped out onto the platform.

I was like a bull staring down the three red plates and some change in front of me. I nudged the bar closer to the front of the platform. My lower lip was pushed up toward my nose, and I had an angry face like De Niro puts on in the movies. Each time my foot hit the barbell I thought in my head, "not today you motherfucker…not today."

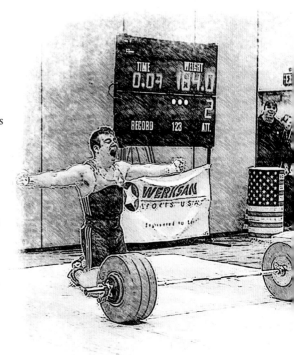

Celebrating My Qualification for the 2010 Pan American Championships

I let out a few small grunts. I walked forward with all the confidence of Arnold and all of the fearlessness of Donny. I put my hands on the bar and pulled. The Clean offered no struggle. Glenn yelled "Dip n' Drive Jon!" 184KG felt like warm up weight as it soared above my head. The judges gave me the down signal and I slammed my defeated opponent back to the hardwood beneath my feet.

I fell to my knees and yelled with my fist clenched, and arms outstretched from my body. It was a significant moment in my career, and I could not have wished for it to happen on any other stage. I placed my head on the plates and kissed the weight. The path Arnold set me on had finally led to my first Pan American team.

♪ ♪ ♪

The 2010 Pan American Weightlifting Championships were held in Guatemala City, Guatemala from May 26th to May 30th. Weightlifters from all sorts of different clubs and parts of the United States were now on one all-star team. We brought eight men: Kendrick Farris, Matt Bruce, Phil Sabatini, Donny

Shankle, Cody Gibbs, Patrick Judge Collin Ito and me. The seven ladies on our team were: Kelly Rexford, Rachel Churchward, Amanda Hubbard, Sarah Bertram, Erin Wallace, Sarah Robles and Holly Mangold.

International competitions are not like your typical local meet. I was not there to set a personal record or have fun – It was serious business. I might as well have been wearing a suit and tie instead of a singlet. I took representing my country very seriously and was going to give this event everything I had. This was not Weightlifting, it was war.

I was in awe at the different styles of technique I witnessed. I wanted to grab an interpreter and go around asking questions, but I needed to stay focused. The competition was fierce and I had to do my part so the team could succeed. I ended my Snatch session with a 141KG lift. For the Clean & Jerk I completed 177KG for my best lift resulting in a 318KG total.

Overall, Team USA had a fantastic showing. Everyone on the team finished at least top ten in their respective weight classes. Donny took home a Bronze medal in the 105KG weight class with a total of 358KG. My dear friend Kendrick Farris brought home three gold medals; one for each event and the total. He Snatched 159KG, lifted 203KG for the Clean & Jerk and totaled 362KG.

My numbers were a little more conservative from what I was accustomed to doing, but I trusted the international coaching team's decisions. I placed eighth in the competition beating twelve other lifters. I had done my duty, represented my country well and returned home with my head held high.

Him

Monday, May 14, 2012

It was sad to watch him leave. It truly broke my heart. I wanted to run up behind him and catch him before he disappeared through the front door. The way his head hung low with his droopy eyes and rolled over shoulders showed defeat; he knew it, and I knew it. He is now just another weightlifter who has been killed by rest. Another soldier who has been taken down by the brutal training that will either make you or brake you. Another soldier down. It was as if the sharp rays of the sun striking through the door were pulling him towards the bright outside.

Training was finally over and all the weightlifters seemed to gravitate toward the bench presses and free weights. Lots of grab-assing, laughing, and all around tom-foolery was taking place at this time. Coach joined in and gave a lecture about how we weren't

pushing ourselves hard enough in training if we still had all this
bull crap energy to fool around with this "curls for the girls" type
crap. Everyone laughed and so did coach, but me, I had my eyes and
emotions wrapped up in him, him being the soldier who desperately
needed a hug. You would of thought I was a part of the crazy loud
crowd by the bench, but I really wasn't. I wasn't laughing or
grab-assing. I wasn't talking about how big my chest "pump" was,
or showing everyone how much I can bench press. I was lost in the
lost world of "him." I watched his every move. It has only been
a week since he flew into train with us, yes, training has been
beyond hell, but already? Is he already breaking down? Is the
imagination and temptation of rest getting to him? These were the
thoughts that were racing through my head as I watched him slowly
walk around the gym picking up his stuff one by one as if he was
a prisoner on the chain gang. He grabbed his back with his right
hand as if someone just shot him with a paint ball gun. His eyes
closed as his pain flowed though the air and hit me right in the
face. I felt his pain, as I was once like him. He reminded me so
much of myself at that moment, he reminded me of the hell my mind
and body went through when I first joined the team and had to adapt
to the training. His pain seemed to leave his body as he bent over
supporting his weight by resting his hands on his knees. Sweat was
dripping down his face like a waterfall. In the first few days of
his arrival he was talkative, outgoing, and definitely would have
been down here by the bench press messing around. But no, not that
day, that day he only had one thing on his mind, and that was rest.

Then it happened, the most amazing thing I have ever seen happened
right in front of my chalky face. Rest walked in the front door
with her beauty blinding the room with light and love. In shock,
I started hitting Tom next to me keeping my eyes locked onto her
beauty. I told Tom to "Look, look Tom." But instead of the reaction
I though he would give, he simply told me to stop hitting him in
the arm and to leave him alone. To my surprise, no one in the gym
saw her. They were going on with their everyday business as if
nothing was happening. She wasn't walking, but floating across the
gym straight toward "him." I stood there like a deer in the head
lights, watching rest float across the gym with her smile, comfort,
and ease. He saw her and broke down into tears of joy. He put his
arms out like a kid wanting to be picked up by his mother. His smile
was long and desperate, desperate to be saved by her, desperately
wanting to leave this cold dark world that us weightlifters call

home. She put out her open hand, and he took it. His eyes were wide
open, completely focused on her every move. She smiled at him while
pointing at the door behind her. He nodded and returned the smile.
Rest started to lead him toward the front door and I knew I would
never see him again. He is with rest now. She will take good care
of him, or so he thinks. I wanted to say something, or even run up
behind him and tell him no, stay with us, don't fall for her beauty.
But no, I did nothing. I just stood there watching what others for
some reason could not see. I thought for sure he would see her long
red pointy tail. I guess her tail blended in well with the color
of her red dress, because he did not see it. Then he was gone. He
vanished outside into the bright sun never to be seen again. The
light vanished and a second later hundreds of rusty black prison bars
fell from the sky all around the gym. I was thinking about going
with him, but I guess there is no getting out of this hell.

Goodbye him, farewell my friend, it was nice training with you for
that short time. Tell rest hi for me and let her know that she
might have gotten you, but fuck it, she will never get me.

Train 2016

First and foremost, I have always been an athlete and a student of the sport of
Weightlifting. However, after finding success in the sport, an increasing desire to
share my knowledge had blossomed. I felt that there had to be more to all of this
than just being an athlete. I had experienced a great deal and trained under world
class coaches. It would be wrong for me to not give what I had learned to others,
so they too could better themselves.

I wanted people to know that there are more bad days (than good) in this sport.
The training is harsh and repetitive. You could spend the whole day doing the same
things: Snatch, Clean & Jerk, and Squat. There will be periods where you set personal
records every single day and then go through a drought lasting months or years with
none. Injuries are going to happen and you will be in pain and frustrated regularly.

I remember watching the Bulgarians training in the early days of California
Strength. In their sessions they would build to monstrous Snatch weights like
170KG or more. Some guys would fail to complete a repetition and be stuck with
it for the rest of the day. They would take a ten to fifteen minute smoke break and
then try the weight again. There was no stripping the plates and trying a lighter
attempt. Instead, 170KG stayed loaded on the bar and over the course of the day
it might take fifteen lifts to find a successful one finally. That way of training is
mentally taxing and it is not fun.

I saw a lot of people come and go, all with dreams of living the lifestyle of a Weightlifter. When they first start there is a lot of excitement. I would be happy to make a new friend. Then things would get hard for them. They were faced with the sobering reality that the fun times they see on YouTube is only a minuscule part of the lifestyle. I would make the mistake of becoming attached to my new friend which made it difficult for me when they would leave. It always left me feeling heartbroken, like after a breakup.

I wanted to share with them the knowledge that I had lost more than I had won. That there was such a thing as a good miss and that; in this sport, eighty percent of lifts are misses. They needed to know that **training would be extremely fucking hard**, but that is part of a Weightlifter's journey when en-route to the podium.

Before I could start to teach, I first had to find what worked best for me. If I could learn to coach myself; then I could eventually do the same for others. I think to be a good coach, an athlete first needs to master the craft they are trying to teach. That meant I needed more time under the barbell to fine tune my technique. I also had to develop a philosophy through trial and error that would be my foundation.

♪ ♪ ♪

I viewed coaching as life insurance. It was something I had an interest in that I could pursue when I retired as an athlete. Previously, I had dabbled in coaching at Hassle Free. After a brief hiatus, I found this craft again through the Cal Strength work-train program. I would tuck my coaching shirt into my pants, grab my clipboard and go to town training athletes. Dave gave me and others the authority to write programs for clients ranging from middle school up to the collegiate level. At any given time, there were thirty to forty kids training in the weight room.

I found my rhythm as a coach by teaching these kids. I was helping them, but they were helping me just as much. They were my guinea pigs. I could mold a kid, teaching him the technique I wanted to use and see firsthand if it were correct or not. In the beginning, there was a lot of trial and error. I tested cues, changed how I taught things and worked to discover how I could motivate my athletes.

I was bitten by the coaching bug when I coached my first athlete at Cal Strength. I found that seeing one of my athletes achieve a personal record was more gratifying than setting one myself. It was a new high that I had never experienced before. I loved helping others to develop. I enjoyed seeing the look on their faces when they accomplished more than they thought they could. When they would scream for joy, I would do the same.

California Strength is more than just a gym; it is a support system as well – it is a family. Dave created something special, where kids could come lift weights and be off the streets. They would do their thing in the weight room and then hang out in the back playing Xbox or doing homework. It was just as much a social place for them as it was a training facility.

The kids would often inspire me. I was not at the gym when I was their age. I was out partying and causing trouble. I would watch them and wish that I could go back and take sports and athletics more seriously. I know that everything I have done in life has made me the person I am today, but sometimes I had doubts. I would sit there shaking my head and say, "Damn it, Jon." Those kids had no idea, but they motivated me deep down as a human being to be the best person I was capable of being.

♪ ♪ ♪

The popularity of the YouTube videos and my blog continued to rise to new heights. I began to receive a lot of emails from people around the Bay area who wanted personal training. I viewed this as the next step in my development as a coach. Training clients one on one made me nervous. I had no idea how much to charge or how to structure my sessions. I sat down with Dave, Donny, and Glenn for guidance. With their advice, I developed a business model and put it into practice right away.

I remember my first client felt just like a first date with a girl. I had butterflies in my stomach, my heart was racing and my hands were sweating. It was real life shit. He was a man who had a job, a family, and was expecting me to produce results. It was very motivating. I felt like I was no longer just an athlete, but a professional.

Adam Hall was my client. He was a tall, lanky man who had never touched a weight in his life. It would be quite the challenge. Throughout the session, he did extremely well. I had him practice my technique drills that had him moving better with every repetition. Things were going great until the Cleans. Adam ended up chipping his tooth after catching the bar a little too high. Completely mortified, I thought he would never come back. I felt awful he was hurt, but to my surprise he returned the next day eager to learn.

My small personal training business took off after Adam. My inbox was filled with emails from people who wanted to learn Weightlifting. From 7:00am to 10:00pm, between training sessions, I was booked. Our gym was packed with athletes, coaches and clients all day. It came to the point where I started to book them together for group training sessions. My career in Weightlifting was progressing fast with new opportunities still on the horizon.

♪ ♪ ♪

The 2011 Arnold Weightlifting Championships held from March 4th through 6th was a very special meet in my career. I was an animal in training. No weight was a match for me and a graveyard of broken barbells could be found behind Cal Strength. I was going to be setting foot on Arnold's stage again. This time I planned my performance to be the greatest masterpiece I had ever created.

I opened with 152KG on the Snatch. That first lift was smooth. I slammed it to the platform and looked back at Jessica. She was filming me and cracked a smile as I posed for the crowd. Glenn made the call for 157KG to be put on the bar. I was thinking too much and I missed, the weight falling behind me. I had one more shot at 157KG. I set up on the bar trying to channel my emotions, but the speed just was not there. The bar crashed to the floor in front of me and sent my body flying back several feet.

I had to stay calm because even with those two failed lifts, the Snatch session concluded with me as the victor. Now it was time for the Clean & Jerk. I opened with 180KG to bolster my lead over my competitors and I put it away effortlessly. Someone should have taken that toy off the stage – I was feeling good – cocky even. The next two guys jumped to 184KG and then 187KG. It was not the time for games – fuck it – let's put 189KG on the bar.

My second attempt would be an all time personal record and seal the deal on my win. 189KG never stood a chance. I threw it on the platform, pointed at Glenn in celebration and danced around the stage, chalk dust filling the air as I clapped my hands together. Today was a big day, one that demanded a significant weight. For my final attempt, 192KG would be loaded on the bar. "**DONNY SHANKLE**!" I yelled as I stepped to my opponent. The Clean was grueling. It took just enough out of me and I missed the Jerk. That miss was okay – I had something more important on my mind now.

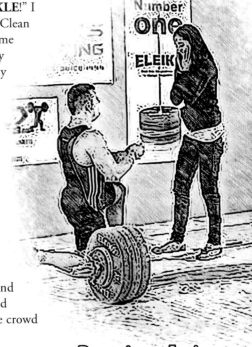

Having just won the Gold Medal with a 341KG total, I called Jessica out to the platform to help me celebrate. She joined me and I stood there staring at her. She had been everything to me. The one person who believed in my dreams and always said I was worth something. If the barbell was my life and I the plates, she would be the collars on either end holding everything together.

In front of her and everyone in attendance, I knelt down on one knee and presented her with a ring. Jessica covered her face in surprise and happiness as the crowd

Proposing to Jessica at the 2011 Arnold Classic.

howled and cheered. She walked closer to me and took my hand as I looked up at her teary eyed. "Will you marry me?" I asked. I had so much love in my heart – when she said yes I felt like I just won the Olympic Games. We were married later that year in a beautiful ceremony attended by family, friends and many Weightlifters.

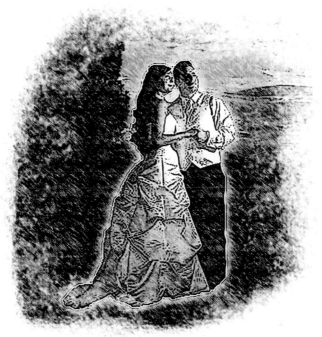

Jessica and I On Our Wedding Day.

♪ ♪ ♪

I am so honored to have been a part of the California Strength knowledge boom. I had the privilege to watch the journey they took from humble beginnings to a world class strength and conditioning facility. At first my passion was lifting heavy weights and climbing the rankings. However, as the gym matured, so did I. My focus shifted to a desire of growing the idea, the lifestyle and the sport of Weightlifting. These new ambitions led me to fine tune my coaching skills and of course create the Attitude Nation.

The birth of the Attitude Nation all started with the "What is a light day" blog. After I had written that post, Jessica and I thought it would be cool to put the phrase on a T-Shirt. We had the shirts printed at a local shop in San Ramon and needed a place to sell them. I did not want to use my blog. It is too personal of a space to me and I felt that plugging or selling things on it would tarnish its magic.

Jessica came up with the great idea of creating a new website. Back then it was called JonNorthAttitude.com. We launched it and the sale at one o'clock in the morning and we waited. There was no post on Facebook or anything. We just sat there staring at a computer screen waiting to see if anyone would by the shirt. I do not know what we were thinking, but we were excited and thought it would sell out in twenty minutes.

Eventually, when it came, I was very proud of our first sale. We were now business owners and people wanted to purchase our creations. Having another website gave me the freedom to expand my personal brand. On it I promoted my blog, new products and personal coaching services. It ignited an entrepreneurial spirit within me and provided yet another outlet to promote Weightlifting.

The YouTube sessions Dave and Glen filmed eventually evolved into live internet feeds. Anyone interested could tune in and watch us train in real time. I believe there was even a comment feature where viewers could chat with one another. Now we had two cameras rolling, one for YouTube and one for the live show.

I had two red lights on me while I was trying to get three white. Both cameras were always moving filming practices. I knew that the people watching the live feed were just like me. They were Weightlifters who could relate to what I felt in training. We shared in the emotional highs and lows of the sport and I wanted to speak to them directly. I thought about what I could call them – a name that would be easily recognizable. Eventually I concluded that since I was "Jon North Attitude" they would be the Attitude Nation.

I would call out to the Attitude Nation often. If I missed a lift, it was because I needed more of the Nation watching me. I wanted to feel their energy and support on every lift. Glenn would bust my balls about how it was not really a nation yet. "The Attitude Village" he would call it – population five. My following took off from there. We had a website, and I wanted to recruit more brothers and sisters of the barbell. I wanted to learn about their lives, educate them on technique and share in a mutual love of Weightlifting.

♪ ♪ ♪

Years of arduous training had gone. I had been kicked out of Hassle Free for that one punch. I had lived homeless in a Dodge Neon camped outside of local meets. Donny Shankle breaking me down just to build me back up. All my actions had all been culminating to accomplishing one goal. It was the one always lingering in the back of my mind...

The 2011 Senior National Championships was held in Council Bluffs, Iowa on July 15th to the 17th. Having just proposed to the woman of my dreams and winning the Arnold; I knew nothing could stand in my way. In the 94KG weight class, I would be going up against some big names in the sport such as Phil Sabatini, Coard Wilkes and Travis Cooper. They had no idea what was coming to that competition, a Weightlifting juggernaut that was set into motion by the Jeff Wittmer's poster.

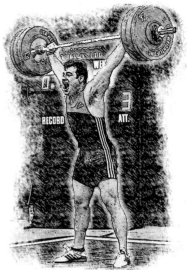

Coach Pendlay had me in prime condition. I was the last Weightlifter to make a first attempt in the Snatch event. I opened with 155KG, 7KG over many second attempts. We were there to take no prisoners and **WIN!** I missed my first try but crushed it on the second. Phil tried the same weight for his third attempt but missed. I was all alone and it was the last lift of the session. Glenn called for 160KG. It was time to send a message that the champ was right here. I smoked 160KG for a new competition personal record and victory in the Snatch.

Standing Triumphantly With 160KG Overhead.

The Clean & Jerk session turned into an all out fight. Coard opened with 180KG and Phil hit it on his second attempt. I began with 185KG and missed the Jerk on my first two attempts. This close to the ultimate goal and my mind was scattered. 185KG was in my head now and Glenn made a tactical move to 186KG. This weight was new, it was fresh and it was mine. I ripped it off the platform and threw it over my head without fault. Up until then, I may never have slammed a barbell harder.

Phil successfully completed 186KG as well, but his performance in the Snatch event was only enough for a second place finish with a 333KG Total. Coard missed both of his tries and finished the meet with a 327KG Total and third place finish. Out of fucking nowhere, Travis attempts and makes an 187KG Clean & Jerk to win that event. With his 137KG Snatch, he would ultimately not have enough points to earn a spot on the podium. With a 155KG Snatch and 186KG Clean & Jerk I

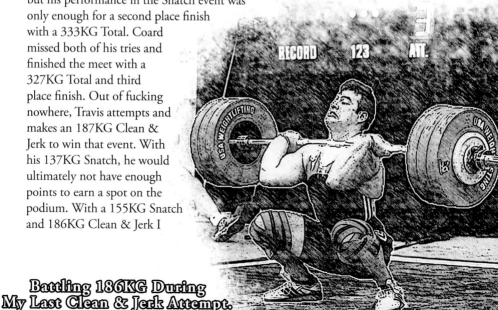

Battling 186KG During My Last Clean & Jerk Attempt.

finished the meet with a 346KG Total and earned the title of National Champion. I cried and hugged Glenn in the back room. My dream had finally come true, and I was the luckiest man in the world. Everything I had sacrificed to accomplish this feat had paid off.

I had to fight for my dreams and sacrifice a lot to obtain them – with the help of Jessica, Donny, Glenn, Dave and all the other coaches and teammates who came before them. I had to find the courage to open my mouth and boldly proclaim them out loud. Only then was I able to find the fortitude to keep believing it was possible when life presented obstacles. My first day of the sport; I said I wanted to beat Jeff Wittmer and win Nationals. Jeff may have been retired, but I never stopped training like I was going toe to toe with him. If I had I might not have achieved all that I did.

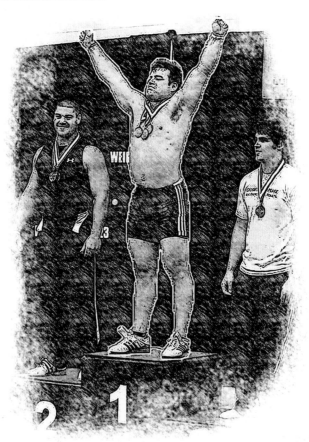

On The Podium After Winning The
2011 National Championship In The 94KG Class
With Phil Sabatini and Coard Wilkes.

Later that year, after winning the National Championship – I had the honor to once again represent my country on the world stage at the 2011 Pan American Games held in Guadalajara, Mexico from October 14th to the 30th. I was on a team of our country's finest lifters including: Chad Vaughn, Kendrick Farris, Jared Flemming, Donny Shankle and Patrick Mendes. It was quite literally a dream team and we all did very well.

I will never forget how electrifying the crowd was at this meet. Regardless of the country – they cheered loud supporting every lifter. I remember walking out on stage to chants of "USA!, USA!, USA!" which fired me up like nothing else ever had for my lifts. When the meet concluded I had Snatched 155KG, Clean & Jerked 183KG and finished in fourth place with a 338KG Total. I will forever be proud of my performance at this meet and grateful for the opportunity wear the team singlet and represent my country.

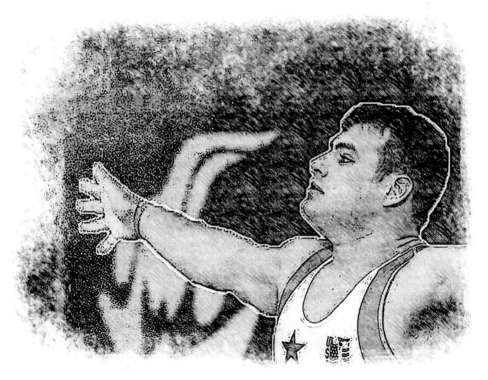

Doing My Best
LeBron James Chalk Toss
at the 2011 Pan American Games.

Hooters

Saturday, January 21, 2012

How many wings from hooters do you think you can eat? Do you
think you can beat Donny Shankle? If eating is a sport, then I
guess Donny is a pro at two things! When you train hard you need
to eat, and eating is what we all did, or some of us tried to do.
We all have never been the same after this battle took place. I
still have nightmares of fallen soldiers. I still will not eat
around Donny, and not a day goes by where that brown owl doesn't
haunt me.

It was a Tuesday afternoon here at California Strength, and all
the weightlifting soldiers and coaching captions battled hard all
day. On this heroic day Coach Glenn Pendlay coached well and
hard, Donny Shankle hit big weight, Caleb Ward moved fast, and I
yelled out some bad ass phrases before I lifted my bar full of red
Kilo plates.

After practice was over, everybody agreed how hungry they were and
how we should all go out and eat. We all had a big meet that we
were getting ready for, so eating was very important. There was
silence in the big gym, as we all looked at each other back and
forth waiting for someone to speak up about where we should go
eat. Finally, Coach Pendlay made a suggestion, only if we knew
how much this suggestion would change our lives for the best, or
worse, I haven't figured that one out yet. "Hooters has all you
can eat wings today," Coach Pendlay said with a little smile on
his face, like a kid getting ready to enter a candy shop. Without
any hesitation, we all said "ok" and started off to the land of
boobs, wings, and more wings, and even more boobs, but mostly
wings! We all rode in coach Pendlay's big Texas truck, with
the Captain Pendlay driving, the team leader Donny in the front
seat and the two soldiers Caleb and I in the back. I remember
the whole Texas truck ride over like it was yesterday. It was
dead silent as if we were heading into war, and the truck was our
tank. This was not lunch, this was a mission. Donny and coach
Pendlay take their food very seriously, like it's a job, like it's
a sport, like its game time baby. I on the other hand, view and
approach food with much less intensity, and I eat just because I

have to; but these guys are on a whole different level. I tried to spark up a few conversations in the car but was quickly shut down by coach and Donny, "Jon no time for talking, just preparation," Donny said in his deep southern voice, as if he was saying his most famous line, "Kids these days" hahaha I love it. I soon came to the realization that this was not just a fun team lunch, instead this was a battle, and I was caught right in the middle! I found myself scared and nervous like maybe I should have just went and got lunch by myself! I took a deep breath and thought to myself, "come on Jon, its only hooters"!   And boy was I wrong.

When we walked into Hooters two very big-boobed girls greeted us at the front door ready to seat us, but Coach Pendlay and Donny pushed them to the side, knocking them both down while keeping their focus completely on the task at hand. Coach Pendlay started looking around in circles, with his arms out to the side like he was being surrounded by a group of ninjas. In a panicky manner, Coach finally found the table he was destined to find. Coach and Donny sat down like knights at the Round Table, while Caleb and I just sat down like normal people wanting to eat lunch. Caleb and I had a great little conversation while Donny and coach stared at each other from across the table. Their four heads were already sweating, their napkins tucked in their shirt, their hot sauce just inches from their hands as if they were cowboys ready to draw at any moment. The innocent happy little waitress came skipping over, as if it was her first day. Let me skip forward by telling you that after we left the war zone of Hooters, that little innocent happy skipping waitress on her first day, was no longer innocent, happy, or skipping and that first day was probably her last.

The hot wings started coming out in trays one after another. Waitresses where running around the restaurant like the building was just hit by those North Korean commies. Donny and coach never took a breath. Their hot sauce never left their hands, while each wings soul rode the grooved tracks to their final destination into the abyss. Both of these crazed men never took there eyes off each other. Both of these men were in another world, and each of these magnificent creatures refused to be beaten by the other. Wings kept piling up as if they were building a fort of bones to live in. Kids were crying and women were running for safety as Caleb and I could only sit back and watch this massacre. Donny was approaching 80 wings when Coach finally had to throw in the towel at a very impressive 87 wings, not because he was full and couldn't eat anymore, but he was late for a meeting he could not miss. While coach stood up to leave, Donny's eyes followed. There were no words spoken, coach just left.

Donny was at 93 wings, and at this point the whole restaurant was watching in amazement as Donny kept fighting those chickens one after another. His goal was to eat one hundred, and he could already taste victory. At 96 wings the most amazing thing I have ever seen happened, he stopped eating and spoke. The whole place went quiet and Donny said, "I am full" as he looked over at me like he needed help or even a hug. He quit at 96 wings, but I refused to see my team mate lose; a soldier was down and I needed to pick him back up, that's what team mates are for. So I leaned across the wing grave yard, and
looked at him right in the eyes and said, "don't you quit on me Donny, don't you even think about stopping when you are this close, you pick up those last few wings and you eat them with everything you have boy"!! This California Strength soldier finished those last 4 wings, stood up with pride and we walked out of that restaurant like he owned the place. That day changed my life, and I will never forget it. We never did see Coach Pendlay again, some say that after his defeat on that sunny Tuesday afternoon at Hooters, he packed up his stuff, bought a pair of board shorts and joined a Crossfit gym near a retirement community in Miami Beach.   100 wings 2012

The end

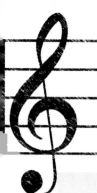

CHAPTER 6

I GO WHERE COACH GOES

Midnight Train

Thursday, May 9, 2013

His thoughts rambled in his head with the swaying of the train.
Side to side as the train slid his duffel bag across the floor with
every turn, as his forehead stayed stuck to the window looking out.
The window was now warm against his head from the small ten minute
naps he would take before being woken from his new found reality.
A reality that went against everything he has been working for
over the years. A stable and successful career, wife and kids,
a dog and a hobby, all that would make him come alive again like
his first year in college. None of what his teachers told him when
he graduated from college ever came true, just empty dreams and
a piece of paper that says "your ready for the world young man".
He was, he truly was ready, but the world didn't seem ready for
him. His parents pushed old fashioned, as his friends pushed a
more outgoing night life than he had wished for. A girl wearing
a bright red coat across the isle, seemed to be writing
with the night light on above her head. What was
she writing about, he thought to himself, as
he turned back to the midnight adventure that
could end anywhere, or start somewhere.
A midnight train ride after an
11 hour flight across the world
made his eyes heavy, and his
thoughts blurry. How he ended up
flipping burgers for Wendy's he
didn't know, or couldn't get
to in his head. His hand
washed over his face
as if he was getting
out of the shower in
the early morning while truly
realizing that a big day awaited
him. He felt empty and broke,

BEN
CARIDAD

lonely and lost, confused and weak. Hunched over in his hard but
fuzzy seat that had now turned into his own apartment from boredom
and lack of people traveling to a place called I don't know. 50
bucks, a pack of cigarettes, and a duffel bag of clothes to his
name as the train whistled down the tracks guiding him to what he
had been looking for for so many years now......him.

He guessed she was 23 years old, getting a better look at the side
of her face from him leaning forward while staring out from the
corner of his eye. He thought he was safe from sight as his long
hair waterfalled over his eyes. Her face was bright and glowing,
maybe from the reading light above her head, but most likely
from her bright red lip stick that matched her coat. She reminded
him of the girl he always had a crush on, but never gained the
courage to introduce himself to, as he sat on a train in Europe
introducing himself to the world.....odd how life works. Odd how
courage only shows itself when your never expect it. Her eyes
flickered to the side catching his, as he threw his back against
his seat while ducking his chin downward for shelter and comfort,
all while still keeping an eye on hers. Her eyes moved back to
her book that laid over her crossed legs. He was caught red
handed, and felt so much like a moron that he felt like moving
seats away from hers. She was the most beautiful girl in the
world, and he was the jobless stalker that had no plans nor goals.
Right before he grabbed his army style bag with more pockets than
he would ever need, she broke a small smile and soon after started
biting her right index fingers nail that of course was painted
bright red. She never glanced over this time, but a body language
that made his heart race for the first time in a while. His eyes
stared forward as if a weight just lifted from his back. His
breathing relaxed, and his hands began to stop twitching from bad
thoughts. He soon closed his eyes, and fell asleep.

Small chatter swept the train car, as a smell of coffee and
buttered bread made its way to his little apartment bench he
called home. His forehead hurt from resting it against the window
of the train. He missed the sunset which was fine with him, he
knew a few good hours of sleep was much needed. The sun blasted
through the window making all the lint and dust in front of his
face appear clearly. His squinted eyes moved around with his
hands feeling his pockets, bag, and passport, yep, everything was

intact and still with him. There was one thing he wish he could
look for and then touch, the girl. He almost forgot. Before
looking over he wiped his eyes and pulled down his wrinkled
sweatshirt before the rude realization that she was gone. His
hand turned white from him leaning against the seat looking up and
down the isles. In an odd way he felt good. He felt they knew
each other perfectly, and understood each other better than any.
He thought how amazing it was just to have that moment that rang
friction between them both. She would from that point on never
leave his thoughts.

"Hello.....Sir, are you awake?" The train conductor asked as
she leaned over like she was a volleyball player preparing
herself for a serve. She had to be at least 6' 2", red hair, and
with teeth as long as his travels so far. "Yes, I'm awake,"
he said snapping out of a day dream of relaxation. Something
he was not used to feeling. "We are at our final stop Sir,
you must exit the train now". She said with a smile, that
ended with more of a hurry up kind of head nod. His head fell
back against the seat with such a careless motion. "OK," he
said quietly. A street made of rocks met his feet, as the sun
hugged his entire body. No where to go, no job to get to,
no burgers to flip, no judgmental friend and parents looking
down upon him. Just a cobbled street with people who had no
idea where he came from, or who he is. His degree no longer
mattered, and his athletic ability meant nothing in this big
world of compass chasing and soul searching. He must have
been in a small farming town. The air was cold, but the sky
was bright blue. Green grass filled the hills that supported
houses and farm animals. Children were playing tag with a bouncy
ball, throwing it at each other to tag one another, he thought
this was an odd game, as he hiked his bag up higher around his
shoulder beginning to walk forward with nothing but possibility
and land that layed in front of him. He walked, thinking of the
girl in the red coat, how tall the train conductor was, and how
beautiful the landscape was he was walking in. He didn't take
the time to ask where he was, because frankly he didn't care.
This was the whole point of his journey, to get away from maps,
roads, and time. No more nine to five, no more opinions from
others. No more gambling on a life that was blocking happiness.
A full day of freedom stood in front of him.

The night closed in as he found himself settling down on a bench outside of an old shut down steel mill that looked as if the only life around the area was mold, plants and the occasional deer that would wind itself inside and out of the fallen posts and cracked open walls that once lived and gave a living to so many. His bag as a pillow, and his clear mind as a nighttime song, cool air from the river below, as ringing bells from the fishing boats helped him close his eyes. Some would call this being homeless, but he called it freedom. This is something that he wanted to do. A necessary path in finding himself. What would the next day bring, he asked himself out loud. Who will I meet and what opportunity will I find? How much better will I know myself tomorrow, he asked the bug crawling near his arm that rested under his bag he layed his head on. He knees to his stomach, and his heart as open for the world to see. He fell asleep with freedom by his side.

Freedom 2016

The Weightlifting world is a small one and word travels throughout it quickly. After winning the National Championship, the spotlight was on me and the Attitude Nation was clamoring for more. Jessica and I had posters made that featured me and the tagline **"I Slam Bars!"** up for sale on my website. I continued running my personal training business and the increase in clients eventually led to the next step in my development as a coach.

One day I received a phone call from a guy named Jeremy "JJ" Jones. He is one of the owners of Diablo CrossFit™ located in Pleasant Hill, California. Apparently I had been training some of his members and he was interested in starting a class at his gym – an "OLY" class as you board short wearing sons of guns would call it. I was thrilled at the opportunity and with Dave's blessing, Jessica and I began structuring the course.

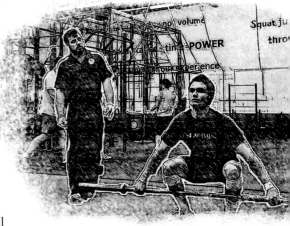

My stomach was filled with butterflies every day leading up to that first class. When I assisted Glenn at his seminars he always did the talking and I was the back up. I would demo movements and help people one on one. Now everyone was going to be looking at me for all

Coaching the Snatch at Diablo CrossFit™.

of the information. It is funny how sometimes the more nervous you are about something, the better you perform. The day of the class arrived and as soon as I started those butterflies went away. I was confident as I spoke about my passion for Weightlifting.

Our class was a tremendous success! Jessica and I were invited to continue teaching to once a week. Eventually it became so popular that we had to add more days to accommodate all the athletes. Jessica would post updates and links to the schedule on our website. These classes were the precursor of the Attitude Nation seminars.

♪ ♪ ♪

Even with the success, it became increasingly difficult for me to coach at seminars. I was only allowed to teach how Dave and Glenn wanted movements to be taught at the Cal Strength and Pendlay seminars. I could not completely show the passion I had for the technique they coached because it was their baby not mine.

Having to suppress all of my ideas made my mind spin a million miles a minute. I craved for the ability to share my knowledge with the world and that desire led me to film a video for my Hit and Catch drill. I just said, "Screw it; this is what I want to teach." Donny filmed me in the Cal Strength parking lot and I put it on my YouTube channel.

I had been coaching the Hit and Catch to my personal training clients, but this was the first time it would be introduced to the public. The video spread like wildfire and I was receiving so many emails every day that I did not know what to do with myself. Some were negative, *people who had closed minds,* but the vast majority of the responses were positive. I released a few more videos and began to make a name for myself as a coach not only in the local community, but the international one as well via the internet.

♪ ♪ ♪

My frustration with other seminars continued to grow until I eventually posed the question to Jessica. "Why don't we do our own?" She agreed and together we set out to develop our own curriculum. We had no intention of copying Cal Strength or Glenn. Our seminar would be original and unique to us in accordance with our Weightlifting philosophies. All of what I know is based on what I felt, saw and heard as a Weightlifter. I want to make it clear that I did not just win a few medals and then decided to do seminars. Building up to that was a slow process.

We held the very first Attitude Nation seminar at Cal Strength on a Sunday. There were twelve attendees and I gave them every trick in the book. The word spread quickly and Jessica and I had emails pouring in asking, "Can we please host an Attitude Nation seminar?" Originally, we had thought we would host a few seminars at Cal Strength a year. We never planned on going to other gyms.

The idea of hopping on a plane and traveling to other cities was a wild one. Hell, I never thought people would want to host one, but I was very wrong.

CrossFit™ Redding, owned by Bryan Schenone, hosted the first Attitude Nation seminar outside of Cal Strength. It was very different from our initial seminar and other classes we had instructed. Our goal was to make every seminar better than the one before it. The more we did, the more things evolved.

We never claim to have all the answers. One of the best coaching tips I can give someone is to say, "I don't know." Then it is my homework assignment to research the answer. At a seminar I was once asked if I release the hook grip when I Snatch. I honestly had no idea. I never thought about it before and did not want to give that athlete some cookie cutter, textbook answer. I wanted my response to be honest, so I reviewed videos of myself and found half the time I did not release the hook grip. Two days after the seminar I emailed the guy back with my answer. I think it is crucial to be a good coach that you have to admit at times you do not know instead of feeding people bullshit.

I approach coaching like a Weightlifting meet. That is why I am very intense when I lead athletes through technique drills. Coaching is not something I take lightly. It does not matter to me if you are Snatching ten pounds or three hundred pounds. Each session is as if my athletes are on the Olympic stage. I coach to help people lift more weights; in this sport that is the only way you can win. During this time I wore many hats – I was a husband, a coach and a high-level athlete training to break records and win championships.

♪ ♪ ♪

In this sport repetition is king. You want to become a robot. A machine that is numb to the pain and performs when the switch is turned on. I trained my body, beating it down into the ground until all it knew was how to react and not think. The second you start thinking too much, the lift has already been lost. In our gym the expectations were always very high. Pushing myself to the limit and setting personal records was my job. It was this philosophy that guided me to unofficially break the American Snatch record.

The 1997 National Championships was held in Blaine, Minnesota from April 25th to the 27th. At this event the legendary Tom Gough, representing Team Southern California, set the American Snatch record at 165KG. At that time, the 94KG weight class did not exist. In fact, all of the current weight classes were much different and Tom competed in the 99KG category. A few years later, the International Weightlifting Federation changed the classes and the 94KG class was born.

The record stood at 165KG for the Snatch. Tom also held the Clean & Jerk record of 210KG which he set on the same day. That record would later be broken by Kendrick Farris when he hit 211KG well over a decade later at the 2013

Summer Universiade in Kazan, Russia. The Snatch record; however, had not been touched in the 94KG category since it was initially set.

It was just another day on the job at Cal Strength. The day before the team had maxed out both lifts. I was supposed to be doing percentage work – lifting weights calculated off of my current personal best for the Snatch and the Clean & Jerk. I felt good and proclaimed that I "Ain't got time for percentages." I was just going to go heavy again and coach allowed it.

I started by working up to a heavy weight in the Snatch by working off of the "high board." Standing on a board increases the distance you have to pull the bar during the lifts. That is because elevating your body a few inches causes the barbell to start lower on your shins. I quickly hit 150KG followed by 155KG. These weights were falling before me like dominos and I felt like I could do no wrong.

After that, I took the board away to go for an all time personal best of a 162KG, my previous being 160KG. I lined it up in my crosshairs and pulled the trigger. Dave should have called the police and had me arrested after that lift because I straight up murdered 162KG. I needed to ride this momentum for one more lift. Glenn suggested we go for the big one – 166KG the American record.

The house music was blaring. The red light of the camera was on and I felt I had to give the Attitude Nation something special. I setup on the barbell pulled and fully committed to this lift. I rocked down to the bottom and caught it over my head. I stood up and held it for all to see. I had unofficially **(I would need to do this at a sanctioned meet for it to be official)** set a new American record, beating the previous one by 1KG and improving my personal best by 5KG.

I honestly believe there is not another gym in the country where I could have done that. The magic in that building at Cal Strength is one that could never be replicated.

My Black Hat

Sunday, May 27, 2012

A week in a small and far away Country called Siskiyou County. A local bar is where I sit, writing to you while I occasionally ask the bar tender for more coffee......please of course. Everyone is bent over the bar drinking their bud light, as I take out my ear piece from time to time to catch small parts of their "when I was a kid" stories. They all know each other, and they all are

probably wondering who the city guy in the corner is drinking
coffee on his liberal Mac computer. I smile and nod when we
catch eyes, some nod back, and some just turn away. A parking
lot full of trucks outside surrounding my little black on black
Audi, as if the trucks are about to kick my car's ass. It's
almost embarrassing. I love my car, but a truck is much needed
right now. I stick out like a sore thumb. I envy them, I envy
their lifestyle. I wish I was a Country man, a farm owner, a
bucking hay and riding horses guy, a hard working man, a Cattle
hand man who meets his buds up after work and grabs a beer or
two man, a go home to the wife after a long day man, a do it
yourself man, a kids these days man, a move boy I don't have all
day man. Wranglers, like it wasn't even a choice. Camo hats and
cowboy hats line up straight down the bar like music notes.......
Awesome. Chew spitting, unshaved face rocking country music
dancing mother fucken bad asses. Attitude Nation soldiers, and
they don't even know it. I think I might order a beer so I don't
look like such a pussy. Some of the cowboys are quite, and some
are loud. Even though they are all mysteries to me, I would love
to hear some story's from the quiet cowboys. I bet I could learn
a few things from them. I guess in a way me and all these Cowboys
are the same. We both work hard in our own profession. We both
love the down time with friends after a hard day's work. They
wear jeans, I wear adidas sweats. They lift bales of hay, I lift
bars. Their hands are rough and callused, mine are as well. They
wear boots; Donny wore boots in the war. Salute Donny, thank you
for serving this great Country, in weightlifting and with a gun.
They dosey doe, I do the cat daddy. They rope cattle, and I like
to rope up Coach when he gets grumpy. I love this place, I love
these people. But this is their world, not mine, and visiting
their world makes me miss mine. The air is crisp and clean. The
stars at night are bright and loud. The sea of rolling hills
and flat land goes further than the eye can see. No freeways, no
buildings, no Starbucks, no Priuses, shit........no weightlifting
for miles.... Heaven.

Five hour drive to a whole new land. Every hour that went by, my
body seemed to become more and more weightless, my eyes lids drew
like shads, my heart slowed down, and my worries and stresses seemed
to catch the wind from the half rolled down window, taken away by the
air never to be felt or seen again. I have never been more relaxed.

I have been in a weird place lately, and you will soon figure out
why. That's all I can say at this point. It's good to get away
and visit my wife's family for a while. A place where we met, a
place I played football at and graduated college from, (aka) my
associates degree. A great achievement for me. How I got my AA,
I still don't know. Seeing my old football coaches and teachers
is something that I needed to do for some time now. A place that
brought me friends for life, and memories that will stick with me
until the day I die. Pause my life for a second and go back to
what made me the man I am today. Take a breath of fresh air, and
try to figure out what has happened to me the last few years. I
look in the mirror not recognizing the face looking back at me.
It seemed like yesterday I was just a punk college kid flipping
burgers part time at McDonalds to pay off a high school DUI. A
kid who watched weightlifting videos and dreamed of becoming a
National Champion. Day dreams in class of representing my Country
in this sport. Dreams of meeting Coach Pendlay, and hopefully
getting an autograph and picture with Donny Shankle. Wow, now
this has all happened and I have no idea how. It still has not
set in yet, and I have trouble comprehending it. Now I write
blogs with Donny and get hugs from coach if I do well in a meet or
in training. What? This is crazy. I need more coffee, one sec.

Yes I will still train. Don't worry coach calls, texts and even
seems to pop up in my dreams at night asking me how the workout
went and what numbers I hit in training. I swear I can still feel
his presence all the way up the windy road of I-5. I can still
feel the famous Pendlay look staring through my soul wondering why
I just missed the lift. "Hey coach what happened?" "You missed
it". "What do I need to do to make it"? "Make it" "Yes Coach"

I will be training with the man who got me into this sport, the
man who saved my life from going down hill, and down hill fast. A
man who was really my first coach before Jackie Mah. A man who
I look up to and admire. He is Eagle football, he is the best
football coach, strength coach, and linemen coach in the world.
His name is Coach Tim Frisbie. I will be here training away
with him in the football weight room. Coach Frisbie is the mad
scientist who invented the crazy, man in black, champ, most hated
man in USA weightlifting, slamming bars, jumping Jonathan North,
Attitude Nation soldier, me......Jon North. Thank you Coach Friz

for everything. Thank you Siskiyou County for the peace you have
brought me on this trip.
I bought a black Cowboy hat at the local thrift shop in Mt Shasta.
You ask why? Why, I have no idea, I have no care in the world
right now. I just walk around wearing
my funny hat with a smile over my face.
No cameras, no live feed, no one on one
coaching, or weightlifting classes. Just me
and my black hat.

Here is a video of yours truly performing
a clean back in College at College of the
Siskiyou's under Coach Friz. Go to 1:20 to
see my clip. I was even more crazy back
then! Arnold!

Coach Friz 2016

Our little Weightlifting family had made so many great memories that
will no doubt stay with me until the day I die. But, if there is one sobering
lesson that I have learned it is that good things seldom last forever. One day at
a team meeting, Glenn sat us all down and announced that he would be leaving
California Strength.

My heart dropped to the pit of my stomach. Glenn was my mentor, my
coach and was like a father to me. Nothing would be the same without him.
Glenn told us that he would be moving across the country to South Carolina to
work at Muscle Driver USA.

Muscle Driver USA is a corporation that manufactures strength and
conditioning equipment. In 2008 they merged with Glenn's successful company
Pendlay Barbell. Glenn still had ties to the company and the Pendlay brand
was alive and well. In 2012, they sought to build their Weightlifting team and
founded Team MDUSA. Muscle Driver requested that Glenn come coach their
team and he accepted the opportunity.

I sat in that meeting with my face cupped in my hands. I could not believe
what I was hearing. The greatest coach in the world was leaving our team. The
man who helped me fulfill my dreams to win a National Championship. He was
always there to say what needed to be said. I tried to imagine training without
him sitting in his chair yelling, "C'mon Jon!", but could not. Glenn did not ask
any of us to go with him. He knew we all had lives there in California that we had
worked hard to build.

During the meeting he simply stated that he would understand if we decided to stay. But, if any of us eventually wanted to go to South Carolina, we would be welcomed. I listened to these words and nodded. It was one of the hardest things I have ever had to do in my Weightlifting career. I had to think about what it was that I wanted. Donny said it the best: "You have to be selfish if you want to be a great athlete." That is why I left California Strength – I would be selfish because I wanted my coach. I go where Coach goes.

♪ ♪ ♪

Yes, I was sad to be leaving California, the gym, my family and friends, but at the same time I was thrilled about the new adventures the move would bring. I wondered how it would affect my career, where we would live and who would be on the team.

Jessica and I had so much fun driving across country. All of our stuff was packed tightly into two vehicles. We were staying in a different place every night, meeting new people and enjoying this beautiful country. I lost my cell phone during the trip so we had to develop hand signals to communicate. Different fingers meant things like stop for gas, pass me, slow down or I love you.

Glenn had already made the trip out to South Carolina and we were meeting him there. It took us a full week to make the trip and during that time we hardly had any money. Along the way we stopped at CrossFit™ Magna owned by Brian and Katie Kunitzer. The gym is located in Phoenix, Arizona and was the host of our fourth Attitude Nation seminar. It would be our very first one outside of California. We had a great day and they loved learning from us.

Leaving our secure lives back in California was a huge risk and we knew it was not going to be easy. After the seminar the banks had already closed for the day so we had to spend the night in our cars (something we were not strangers to). Without that seminar we would have struggled greatly to make our way across the country. It funded our trip and I cannot thank them enough for their support.

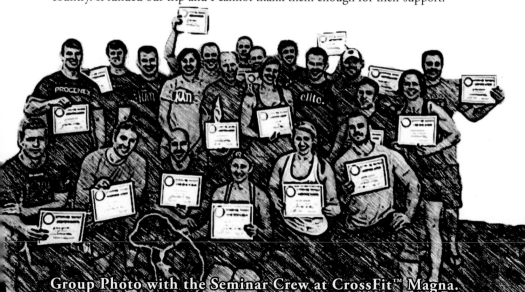

Group Photo with the Seminar Crew at CrossFit™ Magna.

We were driving across country to a whole new life. It was an exhilarating experience. We had no place to stay when we arrived in the new state. We ended up crashing at Glenn's house for the first two weeks.

♪ ♪ ♪

When we arrived at MDUSA, the gym was still under construction. The team was a mix of Cal Strength veterans and several new faces. From the Cal Strength group there was only Donny, Kevin Cornell, Tom Sorka, Jessica and I. The new guys were: Travis Cooper, Kaleb Whitby, Mike Szela, Christopher Gute and James Tatum.

In those early days, everyone went crazy running around the facility looking at all the new equipment. They wanted to see the office and other exciting parts of the building where they manufacture products. Donny and I had a different agenda. We needed to find a new place where we could decompress after tough training sessions, and smoke cigarettes. We were still very much in Cal Strength mode.

We had stepped outside of our comfort zones. No longer were we in our supportive, light-hearted, but competitive gym in sunny San Ramon. Now, we resided in a severely intense environment where money was on the line. California Strength had been like Arnold's gym in Pumping Iron; it had a bright and happy atmosphere. Muscle Driver on the other hand, was sort of like Lou Ferrigno's gym. It was dark, serious and harsh.

There was no work / train program at MDUSA. Instead, all athletes were paid a stipend to be on the team. I received a paycheck just like any other job. We were all professionals, but I felt like I should have been wearing a tie and carrying a suitcase when I walked into the building. Tensions were always high and it was by far the most competitive team I had been on.

Guys were training hard to make "A" team, "B" team or any team just to make more money. It was taken way more seriously and personal. You break someone's balls a little bit and they wanted to fight you over it. With the exception of Travis, who is one fucking cool dude, these newer lifters wanted that exposure we had at Cal Strength on the YouTube videos.

We were like little celebrities and the new guys wanted that status. They were trying to put on a damn show to make money and a name for themselves. I ended up in multiple fist fights off camera, and had been in scuffles with Chris. Donny and I even reached a point where we threw chairs at one another. I can only speak on what I was personally involved in, but we had fights every week. That was the stuff that went on when the red light turned off.

You cannot put nine guys in a room full of testosterone and lifting heavy weights (with money on the line) and then be surprised when there are confrontations. We all went a little stir crazy being enclosed in the same four walls with the same people all day every day. I think we should have filmed it all. That drama would have probably received a million views on YouTube. At the end of the day when practice was over and the battle done, we all shook hands. We would go out to dinner and laugh about it – that was the only way the team could survive.

♪ ♪ ♪

I truly love the Attitude Nation and could always rely on its members to cheer me up if I was feeling down from the tension at the gym. Like me everyone is on the same mission of rising to the occasion and accomplishing goals. Each member has a different incredible story to tell. I wanted to get to know each person, to be able to talk to them and share ideas. The idea to start a platform where I could do this came to me while I was listening to the Joe Rogan podcast. I thought to myself: it would be cool to host a live podcast where the Nation could call and ask questions or just chat.

My relationship with Donny reminds me of the one shared by Dmitry Klokov and Evgeny Chigishev. They are both Olympic level Weightlifters who represent Russia. Klokov is very vocal, loud and energetic. Chigishev is quiet, blunt and keeps to himself. They complement each other very well and I have a very similar chemistry with Donny. He is Chigishev and I am Klokov. He **HAD** to be my co-host.

Sitting in the MDUSA facility, I was going crazy brainstorming all sorts of ideas of what to call the show.

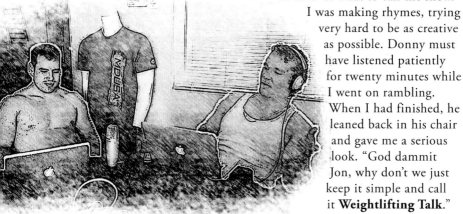

I was making rhymes, trying very hard to be as creative as possible. Donny must have listened patiently for twenty minutes while I went on rambling. When I had finished, he leaned back in his chair and gave me a serious look. "God dammit Jon, why don't we just keep it simple and call it **Weightlifting Talk**." "Donny you're a genius!" I replied.

Donny and I live on Weightlifting Talk.

Donny is a very private person who keeps to himself. But, when he is in coaching mode, he is a social butterfly – a fierce, confident machine. The beautiful thing about the podcast was that although there were hundreds of people listening all he saw was the phone and me. It allowed him to open up about topics and the listeners could hear a side of Donny not many had the privilege to.

It was natural. A real conversation just like the ones we had during our smoke breaks. The show started on a website called blogtalkradio.com. We used my cell phone as a microphone and the sound was terrible. The show can currently be found at a new web site: Spreaker.com.

"The old show "

Wednesday, August 17, 2011

I need a coffee like I need to win the Olympics. I need a coffee like I need to break the American records. I need a coffee like I need coach to call in sick one day so I can finally rest. Damn I need a coffee. Training has been hell, shit....training is always hell. I remember in College there would be days that I would just lay around all day and play video games...heaven. Now its barbell in front of my face, barbell in my hands, barbell on my back and even in my head. This fucken barbell follows me around everywhere, now that I found my bar I am almost wishing it would float away from me again. Maybe I shouldn't have wrote the "red Balloon".

Train train, that's all I know these days. It's almost like I have forgotten who I am. I sometimes sit in the gym watching other people come and go thinking I am missing out on life. Am I? Then I am woken up from coach telling me to lift the barbell, that fucken barbell. I don't know if that barbell is my friend or my enemy, Sometimes I don't want to lift, sometimes I want to go play outside. I slammed the bar down at nationals winning me the national tittle, and making the Pan Am games all in one lift, but for some reason I didn't feel the same joy and accomplishment that I did last year at the Arnold. If you youtube my name you will find me winning the 2010 Arnold and putting me on the USA team for the Pan Am Championships. That moment was the best moment in my whole career, possibly life. But why not this year, you would think that this years nationals would have brought me much more happiness. I kept looking for the rush of joy, I

thought it would come any minute. It never did. Maybe my first
coach Jackie Mah was right, she always said that "its the climb up
that will be your best moments in this sport, the top will never
feel the same." I now understand what she means.

I have a long ways to go in this journey, but the higher I climb
the more dark it gets, the less excitement I have, the less I
yell, slam bars and call weightlifters names out before lifting.
Maybe I have let people's negative comments get to me without me
even knowing. Maybe The bar is just set higher, or maybe reality
has kicked in, that I could make an Olympic team. Its weird how
you want something so bad, and you fight for it for so long,
but once it is in reach you hesitate to grab it. I am like an
act that is getting old. The show is dying and the people are
leaving. You are once a breath of fresh air, you are the crowd
favorite, you are the talk of the group. Intel time goes by and
you succeed, the hype goes way down, the bets start to turn else
where and you are just another top weightlifter sat next to by the
other top weightlifters. Now I am categorized, jumping Jonathan
North is dead, UN original, just another. Maybe this is why I
was not more excited lately. I will watch others laugh and fool
around in the gym all day, while I am leashed to the platform. I
am fine with that, they can do what they want. I have coach to
talk to and my team mates who seem to come and go over the years.
I will still be here, training away, in my corner. If you want to
find the old race horse, the old act, the old show, I will be in
the back of the gym with coach Pendlay.   see you there someday.

Champ 2012

CHAPTER 7:

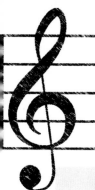

A MILLION MILES

A Million Miles

Monday, March 4, 2013

Feet dangled from the tree branch, as he sat and stared. A
million miles with a million thoughts were lit up from the sun
that slowly drew the night closer and closer up the tree's
trunk, reaching for his bare feet. Cold, but inviting. Quiet
as a mouse, with nothing but the sound of the boy whispering his
thoughts out loud. All it took was a snap of a branch for the
boy to become startled. But soon back to a non-blinking stare
into a million miles that sat upon another tree facing back some
where a million miles away. The sound of constant chatter with
himself, the boy felt at ease on this empty tree. A buddy named
Max appeared beside him as they admired the view of challenges and
triumph, rolling hills and windy trees, while never once talking
nor looking at each other. Max, sitting beside him, stopped the
boy's chattering amongst himself. A full conversation with no
words, just the smell of cooking from the town people
below that caused their eyes to close while their
heads tilted back catching all the scent had
to offer. The breeze from the trees ahead had
finally met their arrival as friendly mother
nature whistled through their
toes like a subway train in New
York. Max soon disappeared, and
the boy was then alone. His head
sunk and his stomach turned.
The whole time Max was a
branch. The shadows from
the sunset can play
tricks on your mind.
Jared appeared to the
right side of the boy and
pointed out a giant deer that
was sprinting across the field.

BEN
CLARIDAD

The boy never once asked himself where Jared came from, or how
Jared got up the tree so fast. Frankly the boy didn't care, he
was just excited to point at a deer with him. Simple. They both
laughed at the exact same time, in the exact same way, sitting
on the exact same branch. A tree that makes you see things in a
whole new perspective. The boy didn't want to climb that high,
and sit on the branch that far out, something just told him to.
Situations that led to an outcome that no one will ever know, led
him to this branch looking over a million miles of thoughts and
ideas. Jared swung his feet and told stories of the old times. A
tear dropped from the boy's face splashing down upon the dark that
was rising further up the tree and closer to his cold feet. The
cold hard truth is hard to make warm at times, and this was one
of those times. Jared's stories reminded the boy of just how long
true happiness had been detached from his life. Jared didn't seem
to see the boy's sadness as Jared soon vanished and the night sky
started to close over the boy's head, making branches and leaves
look like past friends and funny stories. Jared was never there,
and the boy knew this all too well. The boy could only sit on the
branch and remember when Jared once was there, as a journey of
memories played over in his head.

A man named Shankle came across the boy's path pulling a wooden
cart full of rocks and stones behind him. The horns from his
viking helmet were bent sideways as if he had been in a few
battles himself. His voice was deep and his body was covered in
tattoos. "What are you doing up there young man!" Shankle asked
as if he was giving a speech in front of a handful of town's
people. The boy's feet stopped swinging, the boy looked back out
into the million miles of land, and this time noticed a group of
swordsmen practicing battle in the open hay field below. Roughly
1,000 feet away. The boy's head didn't move, but his eyes shifted
down. Reality can be hard to face. The boy noticed his sword
upon his waste was becoming rusty laying in its case, and the
possibility of it sticking in battle could be costly. The boy
spit on his light brown leather vest that had signs of wear and
tear all over it, and wiped his sword clean. Reality can sting,
but the breeze that passed through his toes snapped him out of
his trance, and back into the question the man with the viking
hat asked him. The boy confidently and proudly replied, "I don't
know". The viking below leaned up against the tree with one arm,

and began to eat an apple with the other. "What do you want to
do?", replied the viking. The boy wanted to take another gaze
into the millions of miles, but knew that the answer to this
question could only be found in his mind and not through his
eyes. Big Ben appeared beside the boy as the boy was in a battle
of thought. Big Ben slapped the boy on the back and chuckled,
"this viking's really got you thinking doesn't he?". The boy
thanked Ben out loud, for Ben was his first coach, the start of
it all. The viking asked the boy who he was talking to. "Big
Ben" Shankle looked at his apple in a funny and confused way, and
then violently took a heaping bite out of the shiny red apple,
while rocking his head back and forth. Ben leaned over and laid
a Sac State towel in the boy's hands. Then before he disappeared,
turning into another tree branch, he said fast and upbeat,
"Start from the beginning". The boy cracked a smile that even a
scientist with a microscope couldn't find. The boy kicked his
head back and grabbed one of the branches above his head with his
left arm, while letting the right arm clinch onto the branch as if
he was going to leap at any minute. The boy replied to the viking
eating the apple, "I want to be a weightlifter". Shankle smiled
while nodding his head. The boy smiled. The viking patted the
tree a few times as if he was praising a horse, and then continued
pulling his rocks and stones to where ever his destination may
have been. The boy looked back out into the now dark fields of
the million miles. There were no more swordsmen practicing battle
in the distance. The deer was no where to be found, and this time
there were no branches that came to life in the form of an old
friend, just the boy and a small light from the ideas and plans
coming from his head.

The boy shed a tear as the black faced man he once fought for
walked away, his pigeoned toed feet swaying him side to side.
The black faced man disappeared over the hill from afar. No
more tree branches came to life. Just a real man and a real
scar. Real sadness with a lot of respect. The boy took a deep
breath.....black.

Train 2016

107

I was a seasoned athlete, who had known loss and gain in competition, but nothing could have prepared me for Donny leaving Muscle Driver. Getting kicked out of Sac State – I can handle that. Getting banned from Hassle Free – I can bounce back. Living homeless out of my Dodge Neon – no problem! Now you tell me Donny Shankle, my best friend in the entire world is leaving? Get the fuck out of here.

He left five months after the move to South Carolina. A lot of people speculate that there was bad blood, but that was not the case. Donny is a free spirit. He is a traveler and at that point he felt like he had to spread his wings and explore the world. The man wanted to experience what was out there and enhance it by sharing his knowledge. I understand he had to go do his own thing, but coping with it was another story.

Donny had been my friend and teammate for close to four years. He taught me how to be mentally strong and find the focus of a champion. He had become so much more to me than just a coach, but a dear friend, a brother. I looked up to him and I wanted to be just like him and now he was gone. No more co-host on Weightlifting Talk. No more training partner to push me. No best friend to smoke with behind the gym. I would write my blogs alone and the Orchestra grew darker.

♪ ♪ ♪

Donny's departure came just a few days prior to the 2012 American Open. A gold medal in this event had eluded me for years. In backward fashion, I had won the National Championships first. I would have to be mentally strong going into the competition. That is why Donny broke me down all those years ago – so he could build me back up again, stronger, and able to deal with situations like this one.

The event was held in Palm Springs, California from November 30th to December 2nd. It was bittersweet going back to the Golden State after everything that happened. I still had Glenn and Jessica and together they helped me focus on why I was there – to win. As the number one 94KG Weightlifter in the country, my confidence was extremely high. I would be lifting with a lot of aggression and I was pissed that Donny was not there. When I eventually returned to Muscle Driver, his platform would be empty.

My quest for gold was almost halted at the weigh-in. As I got older, it was harder for me to drop weight for competitions. The 94KG category ranges from 85.01KG (187.002 pounds) to 94KG (206.8 pounds). On meet day, I weighed 97KG (213.4 pounds). It is best practice the day of the meet to be 1KG over and cut weight before registering. I was a whopping 3KG above the cut.

Drastic measures were taken to drop the pounds. The first thing was putting on multiple sweaters and running laps in the parking lot. I was trying to sweat out the extra water weight in the hot California sun. Next, I went into the bathrooms and gagged myself. I was throwing up everything I could purge. People must have thought I was bulimic. Finally, coach threw me into a hot shower.

The water was scalding hot and Glenn was still wearing his khaki shorts and black Muscle Driver polo. He forced me to stay under the water even when I complained. The room was full of steam – all I could see was Glenn's big black beard floating in the mist. This went on right up until the last second before weigh-ins were going to close. I toweled off and hopped on the scale completely naked. Glenn was still in the shower room soaking wet. Thanks to his persistence and quick thinking I made the cut.

♪ ♪ ♪

I opened with 156KG in the Snatch. I walked on-stage and motioned for the barbell to get away like it was an annoying fly bothering me. I made gestures to the crowd insinuating that this weight was a joke. It certainly was and that first lift was for Muscle Driver. Glenn called for the jump to 160KG and that lift was for America. I paced around the stage and shouted **"USA!"** It felt lighter than 156KG and I slammed it hard enough to break the stage had it not been so well reinforced.

That lift was 20KG over the next lifter ranked below me. As long as I did not bomb out on the Clean & Jerk, I had already won the American Open. Now I wanted to take the challenge Tom Gough had laid out over a decade earlier and attempt to beat the American Snatch record. Glenn instructed the meet officials that we wanted 166KG to be loaded on the bar and I took a seat in the back room. I knew I could do this – I wanted to break this record for everyone who had helped me throughout my journey.

I had a towel draped over my head and was in deep thought staring at the floor in the back room. I heard my name called, snapped out of my daze and made my way to the competition floor. It was dark in the venue and when I walked on the stage I could not see the crowd – only the platform and the barbell. The spotlight was on the both of us and I was determined to not be outperformed. I raised my hands in the air to prompt the crowd to cheer. I needed their energy to help me with this feat. I set up on the barbell, pulled and went under. For a brief second I had the weight securely over my head, but the bar wavered and fell behind me.

I jumped forward to avoid the crashing barbell. I had set a record for a brief moment, and then just like Donny it was taken away from me. I heard the barbell crash to the floor behind me on the platform. I sat down in a squat, cupping my face in my hands. So many feelings and emotions suddenly surged within me and I would have to regroup before the Clean & Jerk event.

I won the Gold medal after completing a 188KG Clean & Jerk resulting in a 348KG Total. My attempts were the last three for my weight class. I was in full control over my destiny, just as Steiner was in Beijing. It was a major win in my career, but I was still frustrated with myself for not breaking the American Snatch record. Being that close to completing a goal only to have it not come to fruition was torture – that is the cruel nature of the sport.

♪ ♪ ♪

I felt like I went away at summer camp and my best friend did not come this year. I did not know anyone and the other guys did not understand my antics. I found it difficult to stay motivated. The only thing that made it bearable was that I still had Glenn. He came on to host Weightlifting Talk with me, but it was a different dynamic. I felt it was a good thing for listeners who did not know him like I did.

Donny had left and then soon after, Kevin left as well. Had Glenn not been the coach I would have left right when Donny did. He tried hard to help me settle in, but my frustrations grew daily. It was well documented in the YouTube video "Attitude Nation - Get Off Me Bro." I was working on the Snatch and had built up to around 145KG. It is a weight I should be able to hit cold turkey as it was well below my minimums.

I missed the weight behind me multiple times. I grew angrier with every failed repetition. I had reached my boiling point by the time the camera had made its way to my platform. I ripped the plates off of one end, picked up one of them and hurled it at a squat rack. Glenn was furious. I had never seen him so angry and he scolded me for not acting like a professional. I stormed out of the room to cool off.

A little while later I came back inside to apologize to everyone for my behavior. I wanted my teammates, Muscle Driver and especially Glenn to know that I had meant no disrespect. Glenn was very much a father figure to me and I felt awful that I let him down. It was important that he knew that my anger was not directed toward him. Everything was just starting to affect me negatively and I felt confused about how to deal with it. Later that day, on the car ride home, I began to contemplate my future at Muscle Driver.

Jessica and I decided to leave Muscle Driver a few months later. We needed to push the pause button on life and reevaluate. Looking back on it now, I think I was just searching for a home. The MDUSA adventure was exciting at the start, but I missed my family and I missed California. Donny was my anchor during those times. He kept me grounded and focused on what I needed to do to be a great Weightlifter. With him gone, the new atmosphere and a few new injuries I had sustained, my focus was more on finding what made me a happy person than Weightlifting.

We parted ways with Muscle Driver on good terms. They are good people and I have a lot of respect for the hard work that goes on there with their team and company. It just was not the right fit for Jessica and I. I had dreaded telling Glenn. I ended up in tears several times in my apartment thinking about what I would say. In the end, I found the courage and we sat down to discuss how I felt.

I was very emotional. I told him how I felt about the new gym, my training and Donny leaving. I talked about how I wanted to try something new and that I felt like I had something to share with the world. He never pressured me to stay and only offered me understanding. Glenn knew I was in a bad way and needed to change things in my life. Yes he was disappointed, but one last time he coached me and wished me good luck, not goodbye. I hugged him and thanked him for everything he had done for me. Thanked him for caring so much and that we would see each other again soon.

♪ ♪ ♪

Crossroads in life can be difficult. The first couple of times you find yourself at one you might feel pretty vulnerable. Maybe even a little lost. I have found the best road maps to guide myself through the process are things I already have – my gut and the people who love me. I never ignore either one.

I admit that while I am always confident everything will work out for the best, it does not mean I am not scared during the process. I find that being scared is almost necessary for success in a way. The fear keeps you on your toes and makes you stronger because there is something to lose. It has happened to me with each big move in my career. When I left Cal Strength and then MDUSA, I feared losing the Attitude Nation.

I thought I would wake up the next morning and find that you were all gone. I feared that people would stop reading my blog or listening to my podcast – that no one would care anymore. In the end I am always proven wrong. At the times when Jessica and I felt like we had nothing, I was always reminded that the Attitude Nation was still right behind us. It showed us that we had everything we needed. The support you give me always helped to quell my fears of an eviction sticker over the Attitude Nation doorways, something I often have nightmares about.

The loading Dock

Grey paint drips from my paint brush as I stand on the ledge of
the warehouse's loading dock. Heels on the rusty metal edge,
while my toes hang over the 4 foot drop that leads to a black
concrete ocean which separates me from the world that I once knew.
My hands hurt, not from training, but from normal people work.
Painting, moving, building, and cleaning. My back aches with
pain as I stand over the dock watching boats and cars flash by.
My back hurts while I watch my old life disappear, and a new one
bloom under my feet. Creaks, drips and cracks echo throughout the
gym, as if the gym is welcoming me. I stand in a clean gym after
many days of work building an idea, but my body is covered in webs
and dust. My white eyes brighter than ever from the dirt that
covers my face. My shirt stained from the coffee that has dripped
from my mouth. My jeans wrap around my legs with much insecurity
from not being worn much. Weightlifters don't wear jeans, they
wear sweat pants. This is a fact. Hot or cold, rain or sun. The
Adidas stripes make us proud, make us feel as if we are a part of
something bigger than us. A weightlifter only trains in shorts
if he or she doesn't have sweats available in the closet. People
ask me why weightlifters only train in sweats. I answer, "The
same reason why weightlifters don't use clips on the bar when
lifting.......there is no method to the madness, no one really
knows the answer, we just do".

Holes in my black Adidas sweats cover my shoes as if oil was
dripping down my leg. Oil from my rotting back leaking down my
spine, dwindling all hopes of ever getting back to where I used to
be. Every pinch of pain my back gives off, a kilo drops from my
eye, falling into the black ocean of pavement below the loading
dock I hover over. There is no where for me to go. If I step
forward I fall off into the ocean of forgotten and normalcy. If
I step backwards, I am met by a familiar friend and enemy....the
bar. Maybe this is why I have been standing on this ledge looking
out for so long. I wonder.....are we really in control of our
own destinies, or does a greater power already have a path laid
out for us? If I step forward, was I supposed to step forward?
Or would I have made the wrong choice and should of stepped

backwards? Is moving to the side even an option? If so, what the hell is to each side? My paint brush feels heavy from all the paint it has collected, and I just noticed that I have been hook gripping the handle this whole time.

Am I a coach, or am I a weightlifter? Will my back ever let me be the athlete I have grown to love over the years? I miss Jon North, I miss the freak athlete that gave myself more confidence and energy than anything ever has. My gym is coming alive as I am dying. The gym is becoming clean as I build rust. Yes, I have built a fresh new life around me. The gym is filled with rolling hills covered in green grass, and trees the stretch across the gym roof as if they were creating a bridge of branches that hold a crossing for those who walk by without noticing the underground world of weightlifting that lies beneath the shadows. My knuckles bloody from frustration, my forehead wrinkled from thought, my legs heavy from standing, my back hurt from 7 years of training. The sound of the paint dripping off the paint brush wakes me out from my trance. I chug a muscle milk with little finesse, noticing my forearms have a lot of blond hair on them. The sun has drawn down creating an orange glow that has pierced through the gym and into the lobby in front. This orange world reminds me of a blog I wrote some time ago called "The Orange Room". One of Shankle's favorites, I might add. Yes, I miss training with Shankle, but I mostly miss writing with him. Computers back to back, no words spoken besides the occasional, "How's it going? Good, how about you? Good".

I am in my third day of training full time. AM sessions and PM sessions. Wow, I am out of shape. I didn't realize that my absence from the bar the last two months would have affected me this bad. I had a few "day one" come back sessions, but they ended with a hurt back every time. I soon felt like Michael Jordan constantly making the come back but falling short of the big bang. The gun went off, but my feet stuck to the blocks while the others took off like race horses out the gate. The cheers from my corner lowering in volume, and my dreams of making an Olympic team seemed to taste like salt water by the ocean tide. Yes, I am feeling better these days, and yes, I am making my come back. My back seems to be doing alright. The oil leaks down my rusty back at times, but I have just enough juice to keep fighting. One more round, one more round, keep punching, keep your hands up to protect your face. I am lifting more weight everyday, this is the program I am on. Lift more than the day before, written by the skeletons that watch me train. I can hear all the coaches throughout my career giving me advice, coaching me, motivating me. This makes me smile to myself at times, as I push my elbows to my knees while sitting and anchor my head toward the ground; I miss them all.

Finally moved into the gym. Finally have all my ducks in a row. My back seems to finally be better. I am tired of talking about the future. I am tired of talking about the what ifs, whens, can't waits, and so forth. I am ready to do. I am ready to walk the walk again. I am ready to start lifting big fucking weight.

Paint Brush 2016

♪ ♪ ♪

Jessica and I found ourselves in a very familiar place again, sitting in our apartment and asking "What are we going to do?" We spent a few days in limbo trying to come up with ideas. Eventually, we decided to open a gym of our own. The idea of opening a gym had always been in the back of our minds. We thought it would be a project to embark upon when I retired from the sport. I am sure it is something every athlete thinks about. The idea comes up in those "what if" conversations you have after an excellent training session. In our minds, it was never a question of if we wanted to, but could we and when.

We were in a unique situation of being financially stable to the point we could go any route we wished. It was new because previously we had to resort to borrowing money from my mother; God bless her. However, the seminars had changed all of this. After the one we did in Arizona, we were booked well into the next year. Word hit the streets and took off like a match hitting gasoline.

Now we sought to put our stamp on the world. No more would we work for a company that was not our own. Places where we could not preach our methods and philosophies. I started to have a new outlook on life, that if you are happy you can be a good Weightlifter. I decided I would rather be a happy person and not a Weightlifter than an unhappy Weightlifter. It was that philosophy that brought us to opening the Attitude Nation gym.

We wanted to build a place that was very intense, high energy and where anyone could come and train. In our gym, it would not matter who you were or what ability you had. You could just show up, get your shoes on and train right next to Jessica and me. The house music would be turned up, we would workout, have fun and get better together. I did not want a training hall that was closed off to the public. Instead, I wanted a destination of freedom that was open from 9:00am to 9:00pm.

♪ ♪ ♪

I do not need someone to lift big weights to motivate me. I need a gym full of happy people working hard to achieve their goals. That is how I can become a better Weightlifter. That is something that I really admire and love about the sport of CrossFit™. At seminars, I enjoy seeing the brotherhood, sisterhood and family aspect they have in their communities.

Everyone at those gyms has each other's backs. Instead of organized crime, it is organized motivation. That was the kind of community I wanted to create. If I look across the gym and see someone going all out, pushing themselves to the limit doing pushups, then I am going to be fired up and Snatch 160KG. I knew nothing about this style of training, so I needed to find a coach who did.

That path led us to Ryan Grady. Ryan is, in my opinion, the top CrossFit™ coach in the country – probably the world. In his younger years, Ryan was an All-Star Soccer and Baseball player. He found the sport of CrossFit™ in 2008 and has since guided countless athletes toward personal glory. Before we found him, he was the Head Coach at CrossFit™ Koa located in Cranford, New Jersey.

Ryan is the nicest guy I have ever met. I do not know what it was, but I felt such a powerful connection every time we spoke. His energy was through the roof and I found we had the same thought process on what a gym should be to its athletes. We had the same outlook on life and sparks grew into flames. The cherry on top was that he is a Skeleton (what I call those who read my blog) of The Dark Orchestra. He read every blog I had written and loved the Attitude Nation.

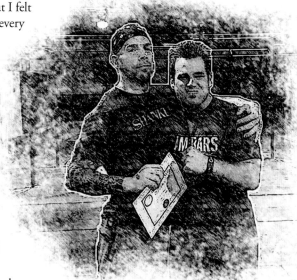

THE Ryan Grady.

Jessica and I interviewed close to thirty different CrossFit™ coaches for the job. They were all qualified individuals, but we kept hearing Ryan's name pop up when we had conversations with other gym owners. He had great street credit, was certified in the Attitude Nation ways of Weightlifting and knew his stuff when it came to CrossFit™.

Finally, we took him out to dinner in Charlotte, North Carolina. We were there for four hours just talking about training and life until the manager had to kick us out. If he had not, we probably would have stayed there all night. After that dinner there was no question, we needed to hire him as our Head Coach.

♪ ♪ ♪

Ryan is a perfect example of how to do it right. Throughout all of our talks, he never once mentioned money or taking high-level athletes to the games. Instead, he spoke at great lengths about how he wanted to change lives. He wanted to make people better through building a supportive community – if you do it that way, the money will follow.

I want to make it very clear; I know nothing about what those board-short-wearing sons of guns do. The experience Ryan was bringing to the table was going to be pivotal to our success. Usually, when you are the owner of the gym you are in charge. You do the programming, make the rules and set the prices. That is not how we were going to run things.

We put a lot of faith in him and that was something huge for us. Ryan was going to have full reign over the CrossFit™ side of the gym. It was very scary to put the Attitude Nation into someone else's hands, but in the end we believed we were making the right decision. He took a risk himself moving from New Jersey to North Carolina, where we just had an empty warehouse space. He is a phenomenal person and someone that I have a lot of respect for. He is a handsome devil and a great friend – *even if he is a Giants fan.*

There we were, standing in the doorway looking out at our new home. Jessica stood to my right holding my hand tightly. Ryan was to my left, arms crossed with a grin on his face. It was dirty and empty and cold, but we would clean it, fill it and give it love. It was our blank canvas to which we would paint our new dreams.

It was a long journey leading us here, but the journey was not over yet. There were still countless hours of training ahead with bars to slam and personal records to kill. I was excited for what the future would bring and the friends I would meet.

♪ ♪ ♪

Life is one tough son of a bitch who does not play by the rules. When you are not looking, it will knock your teeth out and stand on your throat leaving you gasping for air. There was a time when I did not think lifting that boot from my neck was possible. All I wanted to do was breathe and be free from the prison of drug addiction, but life's thick rubber heel kept sinking deeper. I only heard muffled voices, and as my vision started to fade, I saw a flicker of hope. A gleam of light dancing on metal drew my attention.

I reached out my hand and found the barbell instead of drugs. Iced steel in my clenched hand, I swung back at life and broke its fucking leg. Staggering back to my feet, spitting blood from my mouth, I took a deep breath, and I was free. I found Weightlifting and this great sport has saved my life by giving me a new road to follow. I will forever be grateful for everything Weightlifting has given me.

My years in the trenches of training have led me to realize that Weightlifting is a lot like life. There will be dark times; you will struggle and have to make sacrifices if you want to succeed and be a champion. I want **YOU** to know that no matter where you came from or your current circumstances; you can achieve anything if you put your head down and keep pushing forward. Never stop pushing until you can stand tall and breathe again because the only other option is death. I have been blessed to have met and gained the support of many amazing people throughout my career who have helped me redirect my path in life. They laid the bricks guiding me towards National titles while I supplied the mortar made up of my blood, sweat, tears and a fiery desire to reach the top of the greatest sport in the world.

I want to say thank you to all of my past teammates. Thank you to all of my coaches. Thank you, Attitude Nation. You all helped Jessica and I make it through the tough times. Thank you for believing in us and for loving us as much as we love you. Skeletons, grab your violins and let us embrace our path together in the dark.

THANK YOU

Jessica North - Lincoln North - Lezlie McConnell - David North - Jim McConnell
Kim North - Lexy McLellan - Leah North - Tim Frisbie - Les Courtemanche
Ben Claridad - Kathy Bowling - Paul Bowling - Jackie Mah - Paul Doherty
Kari Doherty - Donovan Ford - David Garcia - Kyle Hasapes
Matt (owner of Nutrishop) - Rob Earwicker - Jasha Faye
Dave Corbin - Freddie Myles - Kevin Doherty
Jim Schmitz - Dave Spitz - Kathryn Spitz
Donny Shankle - Max Aita - Jo Ann Aita
Glenn Pendlay - Caleb Ward - Jared Enderton
Spencer Moorman - Rob Blackwell - Kevin Cornell
Adam Hall - Danny Lehr - Charlie Zamora
Alex Krychev - Martin Pashov - Pete Bauman
Tom Sroka - Kyle Pierce - Pete Roselli
Kayleigh Gratton - Travis Mash
Kendrick Farris - Jeff Wittmer
Jared Fleming - Phil Sabatini
Christopher Smith - Matt Bruce
Travis Cooper - James Tatum
Ryan Grady - Kevin Houston
Dean Saddoris - Aaron Landes -
Sam Holmes - Janet Thomas
Steve Thomas - Jerry West
Jordan Aguilar - Pat Mendes
James McDermott - David Katz
Charles Shipman - John Stevens
Nathan Apsel - John Brown
Mykala Butts-Hord - John Broz
Greg Huston - Jimmy Duba - Bryan Schenone
Rob Chicano - Janet Gass - Bill Gass - Emile Garcia
Bobby Smith - Mark Hazarabedian - Martha McDermott - Joanna Toman
Jason Murphy - Jason Ackerman - Patrick Regan - John Thrush
Juanita Smart - Rick Buro - Dean Leber - Kiera Taylor - Ian Wilson - Darcie West

JON NORTH AND JAMES MCDERMOTT

PRESENT

THE DARK ORCHESTRA

PART II.

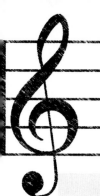

CHAPTER 8:
A PHILOSOPHICAL RECKONING

Camp Catapult

Tuesday, April 30, 2013

Little rocks looked like giant mountains, untouched, and laying peacefully at rest. Flying fish circling though the green sea weed as if birds to a tree. The water was cold as ice, but as clear as his beliefs. His long hair was dancing in front of his face as his eyes stayed open and wide taking in the whole experience. Quiet like the early morning, with small mumbles of deep echoes coming from the outside world like a morning fire place cracking from the night before. His eyes finally blinked as bubbles started to escape his tightly locked lips. His face was turning pale from the lack of oxygen. He wanted to stay longer, but he knew the calm would eventually lead to the heavy storm that awaited him above water.

His long hair was heavy as he pulled his head out from the shallow stream water that snaked past his camp. His eyes closed and his feet planted in the rocks below for support against the water's weak current and strong winds that swept down from the mountains above. His head thrown back as if life was pulling him down violently from the back of his hair. His brown matted hair swooshed back like a whip to a horse. This was happening in real time of course, but to him, the last few minutes felt like slow motion, including the mist from his heavy breathing meeting the cold air outside as it swirled around his face only to disappear seconds

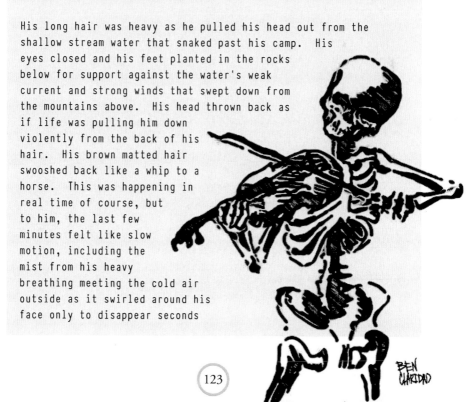

123

later. His hair now fell straight down behind him, besides the few hair locks he had tied with tree bark gathered over the years. The end of the locks held teeth from the people he had once killed. There were handfuls of teeth woven in his hair that fell from his forehead chattering amongst each other every time this quiet warrior moved. Black eyes and chapped lips. Skin burnt from the once hot sun, now replaced by a cold foggy day that felt cold upon his wet face. The small gusts of wind made him cover his face with both hands, but not from the cold, but from the actions that he knew would haunt him for the rest of his life. He knew what was awaiting him in the mountains above, and what the outcome would most likely be for both prideful camps. The sound of children playing tag around the tents that were held up by rope and tree branches made him lower his hands and squint his eyes in concentration. A true warrior must have control over his emotions, or else his emotions will be the death of him.

The Catapult camp was located on the sandy beach at the bottom of the tall green hill that twisted and turned beyond the lingering fog and past the chanting warriors hanging from the large broccoli trees. Ooowwaa! Ooowwwaaa! The echoes rang loud as if King Kong was climbing the hills. Birds scattered fast all throughout the tall grass, while mothers scurried their children into the tents. Bear coats dragged upon the ground as the warriors grabbed their daggers from the muddy ground below them. Chatter rang, not from the men talking, but from the medal blades that were being past around from one man's hands to the next as if they were passing bread before supper. The man's teeth were chanting loudly from the wind picking up. His body was facing toward the tent where his family laid safely, while his head was still facing the broccoli trees high in the hills that awaited his arrival. The handle of his dagger smashed against the ground, as he sharpened the other side where his arrow head was tied tightly, all without ever breaking concentration on the high pull dagger camp that has been on top for too long. "Fight for what you believe in, or die trying," his good friend said right before drinking a cup of dirty water. The man's beard was long and red, braided and half burnt off from battle. His body was shaking from the cold, but his long beard and reluctant eyes stayed motionless, a friend he has been in battle with for decades now. How they are still living has amazed even their deepest enemies. Little words were ever spoken between the men that stood a hundred plus lined up in a single line one behind the other. Only actions could determine the outcome of this ongoing battle between the triple extension and the catapult. Both sturdy in their beliefs, both have seen success in battle, both will die with pride as they both stab one another with daggers until the blood runs dry and their hearts stop beating. Big pull towards greatness.

His hair was still wet as water ran down his dry back and into his tightly laced up boots that ran almost up to his knees. The morning fog started to break as he had a better view of the high hill before him. He could of swore he made eye contact with one of the triple extensions looking down in almost the same stance he was in. Both with blood stains around their thumbs, both with dreams to achieve. Both with pride in their heavy hearts. The black eyed viking thought to himself what the other camps at this exact time must have been thinking. Were their families hidden away in tents as well. Were they at peace before battle as well. Were they ready to die as well. So different, but so much alike, he thought to himself. A different path of the sword, but the same deadly result. The same deadly goal. If either camp laid down their sword, then all in the world wouldn't be right, and days of sun and family wouldn't feel as sweet. Each camp was an enemy much needed to push the other camp to become better at their craft. Enemies that fuel motivation and constant progress. Worlds apart on their methods, but as close as brothers on their goals. Passion and love is what he and the others on the hill fight for, love that ends in death. Love that starts with cold water and sounds of children being echoed for all of eternity.

Small strings of rain fell from the now dark sky as the warriors from camp Catapult gathered their weapons and kissed their loved ones goodbye. The man with teeth in his hair started to hike up the long windy hill.

The Battle Continues 2016

Grow Your Melting Pot

I have acquired a world-class education in Weightlifting throughout my career. I am also the man I am today because of the influences countless coaches have had on me – they each played a part in transforming me from a rookie to a professional. Donny Shankle, Dave Spitz, Jackie Mah, and Glenn Pendlay, to name a few, have all contributed to what I refer to as my Melting Pot of Knowledge. The Melting Pot is a harmonious mixture of experiences and influences I have personally had while Weightlifting. When I teach a seminar these coaches and one hundred others might as well be standing in the front of the room alongside me – you just cannot see them. I want to give them credit because credit is most certainly due. For me to develop my methods, I first had to become a student of some of the greatest minds in the sport. I listened to every coach I had completely and when they gave instructions I did the work. **"YES COACH!"** I would say – objections or questions never crossed my mind.

I want you to understand that much of what I know has been filtered through the grueling trenches of competition and training. I have learned more from being beat than by winning. I witnessed the beauty of human movement and gained a desire to teach it by training with Caleb Ward whom in my opinion has the best technique in the world. Each time Phil Sabatini denied me a gold medal he fueled a fire that made me train harder and be hungrier for the next meet. The opportunity to be on a Pan American team with Kendrick Farris and Matt Bruce taught me the importance of representing my country on an international stage. Experiences like these were invaluable and helped teach me the ins and outs of being a Weightlifter – the things that every rookie must learn on their way up through the ranks. That is why every athlete I have competed against or trained with also stands with me at the front of the room as I coach.

We are all artists. When we read a book or take a seminar we are just purchasing more paint and brushes to use on our canvas. You should never stop growing as athlete or coach. Take a Mike Burgener or Greg Everett seminar. Read other books, articles, and watch videos. I am a true believer in trial & error and I encourage you to experiment with the methods other coaches are preaching. See if you are a thigh or hip Cleaner, pull with straight or bent arms, triple extend or catapult. If it is something that can add more weight to your bar then keep it, if not, at least now you know.

Keep experimenting even if what you are doing is not considered "common practice." The vast majority of athletes perform the Snatch with a wide grip, but if you wanted, you could walk out on the Olympic stage and perform the movement with your hands one foot apart and win a gold medal. Now, not a single person in the world is lifting record breaking weights in this fashion. Yet if there was such an athlete, who are we to say what they are doing is wrong if it is safe, successful and within the rules of the sport. I have attended too many seminars where the first discussion point is about how something is "wrong." I even used to be that asshole, who believed it was my way or the highway. Over the years, I became more open minded and realized I had been wrong. The truth is that every athlete is original and unique in their way of expressing their hard work when on the platform.

I one hundred percent believe there is no wrong way to lift weights if the methods you practice are safe. All that I will teach you is based on my experiences in the sport and is just one of many methods that are available. As a coach, meld my methods with your own to become more diverse. As an athlete, take this as an opportunity to learn from someone who has been where you want to go. If you are a beginner, use this text as a resource to help bring greater understanding to the sport you are embarking on. I know in my heart that my techique can help you. That is why I coach it. Why I use it. I am thrilled to share it and help you grow your melting pot.

The Technique of Oscillation
(The Attitude Nation Catapult Method)

Weightlifting technique is something that is widely debated throughout our community. Seldom, are there topics that we can all agree on. Much of what you read will go against what is considered the norm because I want to tell you the truth. I want you to know what athletes really do, behind the curtains, in the warm up national events. My sole purpose is to teach you how to be a Weightlifter and lift big weights the way others did for me. If these are your goals then I present your first and most important lesson: <u>You must learn the art of how to move your body around the bar and not the bar around your body.</u> That line needs to be the mantra you live by in the weight room. Say it over and over in your head. Write it on your bathroom mirror as a reminder every morning. To have success, you first need to understand that fundamental aspect of this style of lifting and teaching method. Within this chapter, we will discuss at great length the following topics:

- O Weightlifting Terminology
- O Weightlifting Pedagogy
- O Barbell Oscillation
- O Peaking the Barbell
- O The Philosophy of Opposites
- O The Weightlifting Catapult

As we continue through the text, we will gradually build upon these themes. Forming a clear understanding of what it means to move around the barbell and be a catapult lifter.

Weightlifting Terminology

Our definitions may differ from others out there in the Weightlifting community. There are many terms in this section and throughout the text that are unique to our methods. At this point, we are going to focus our attention on the ones that are most relevant to the topics discussed in this chapter. The Snatch and Clean & Jerk are defined as they appear in the International Weightlifting Federation's official handbook. That document is one that new and veteran Weightlifters should regularly read. You need to be familiar with the rules of the game if you plan on playing.

The Snatch

According to the IWF, the Snatch is defined as:

"The barbell is centered horizontally on the competition platform. The athlete takes the start position behind the barbell. The athlete grips the barbell and bends at the knees. The barbell is gripped; palms downward and pulled in a single movement from the platform to the full extent of both arms above the head while either splitting or bending the legs. During this continuous movement upward the barbell should remain close to the body and may slide along the thighs. No part of the body other than the feet may touch the platform during the execution of the Snatch. The athlete may recover in his/her own time, either from a split or a squat position. The lifted weight must be maintained in the final motionless position, with both arms and legs fully extended and feet on the same line and parallel to the plane of the trunk and the barbell. The athlete waits for the Referees' signal to replace the barbell on the competition platform. The Referees give the signal to lower the barbell as soon as the athlete becomes motionless in all parts of the body." (1)

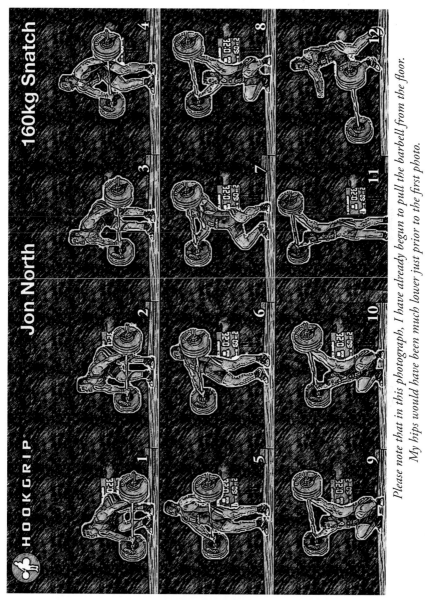

Please note that in this photograph, I have already begun to pull the barbell from the floor. My hips would have been much lower just prior to the first photo.

(Figure 8.1)

The Clean & Jerk

According to the IWF, the Clean & Jerk is defined as:

"The first part, the Clean:

The barbell is centered horizontally on the center of the competition platform. The athlete takes the start position behind the barbell. The athlete grips the barbell and bends at the knees. The barbell is gripped, palms downward and pulled in a single movement from the platform to the shoulders, while either splitting or bending the legs. During this continuous movement upward the barbell should remain close to the body and the barbell may slide along the thighs. The barbell must not touch the chest before it stops at the final position either on the clavicles, chest or on fully bent arms. The athlete's feet must return to the same line and the legs must be fully extended before starting the Jerk. No part of the body other than the feet may touch the platform during the execution of the Clean. The athlete may recover in his/her own time and must finish with the feet on the same line and parallel to the plane of the trunk and the barbell." (2)

"The second part, the Jerk:

The athlete must become motionless after the Clean and before starting the Jerk. The athlete bends and dynamically extends the legs and arms simultaneously to move the barbell upward in one motion to the full extent of the arms, while either splitting or bending the legs. The athlete returns his/her feet to the same line parallel to the plane of the trunk and the barbell with his/her arms and legs fully extended. The athlete waits for the Referees' signal to replace the barbell on the competition platform. The Referees give the signal to lower the barbell as soon as the athlete becomes motionless in all parts of the body." (3)

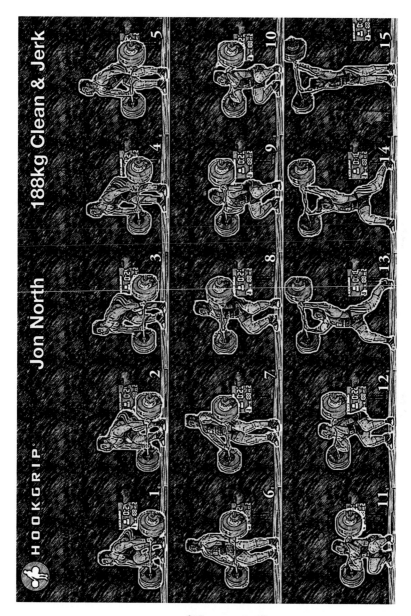

(Figure 8.2)

Other Important Definitions

○ **Bar Body Contact:** The violent striking of the barbell with the hips or upper thighs when completing the Snatch and Clean. This can be seen in **Figure. 8.1 - Frame #5 and Figure 8.2 - Frame #6.**

○ **Barbell Oscillation:** A product of bar body contact where the pliable nature of a barbell assist in the completion of the Snatch, Clean & Jerk.

○ **Barbell Peak:** A period during the lifts where the barbell is momentarily rendered weightless via barbell oscillation and the forces applied to it by an athlete. A fully peaked barbell can be viewed in **Figure 8.1 - Frame #7 and Figure 8.2 - Frame #8.**

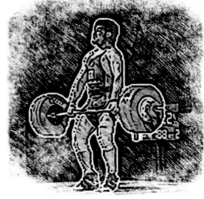

(Figure 8.3)

○ **The Double Knee Bend:** The action of the knees that helps to aid in transitioning from the first phase of the lifts to the second. This point of transition can be viewed in **Figure 8.1 - Frames #3-4 and Figure 8.2 - Frames #5-6.**

○ **Early Arm Bend:** The gradual act of rowing the barbell into your hips or upper thighs to produce a greater amount of barbell oscillation. It occurs throughout the entirety of the Superman Pull.

○ **The Finish:** An umbrella term for the three phases of the lifts that aid in the extension of joints and firing of muscles to create the force necessary to peak the barbell.

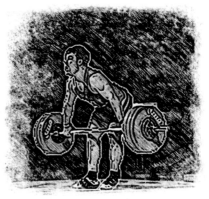

(Figure 8.4)

○ **The Power Position:** The middle of the Finish. The point of contact between the hips or upper thighs and the barbell. **As seen in Figure 8.3**

- ○ **The Superman Pull:** The act of breaking the barbell from the floor and guiding it to the hips with the late initiation of the double knee bend. This phase of the lifts has completed when the barbell ascends to around the mid-thigh. **As seen in Figure 8.4.**

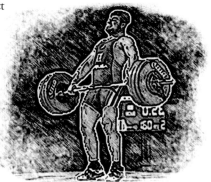

- ○ **The Superman Pause:** The first phase of the Finish. An athletic position in which an athlete has achieved optimal leverage over the weight in hand and can begin to exert maximal force. It occurs at the exact moment the Superman Pull ends.

(Figure 8.5)

- ○ **The Arched Angel:** The last phase of the Finish. It is the extension of joints and follow through of the hips after successful bar body contact. **As seen in Figure 8.5.**

- ○ **The Catch:** The receiving position for the Snatch, Clean & Jerk.

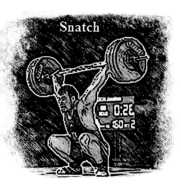
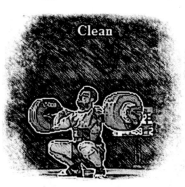
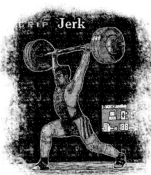

(Figure 8.6)

Weightlifting Pedagogy

When teaching the Snatch or Clean it is common practice to use a Top-Down method. This method utilizes movement progressions starting with an empty barbell in a standing position. Individual aspects of movement mechanics are focused upon until athletes attain competency. Teaching lifters in this manner allows coaches to instruct small or large groups efficiently while ensuring safety. Barring the presence of limitations such as coordination, flexibility, mobility or strength, an athlete may move to the next step of the progression. Through this process, we can teach athletes how to find positions during the lifts as they begin to develop their technique.

The relationship between positions and technique is an important one. Positions are the visible structures of a lift. They are the part of a Weightlifter's anatomy specific to the sport. Each athlete has to go through the same positions, but there are differences in how they look. This notion is similar to how most people have eyes, ears, and noses, but with variances in size and color. Technique, on the other hand, is what occurs before, during and after an athlete achieves positions. It is the individual physiology of a Weightlifter. The inner workings, the style, and mentality of an athlete, which allows them to thrive. Technique is performed to lift the weight. Through strength and with the help of technique, positions can be held leading to the successful execution of the lift.

The movement techniques section of this book is designed much like my seminars. You will learn about drills, the precise breakdown of essential positions and explanations of the inner workings of our method. Most importantly, you will learn **why** each aspect of our technique is the way it is and how our view further differs from classical thinking. The centerpiece of the text will be the Snatch. In our seminars, we spend a great deal of time refining the movements of the Snatch. We have found that once athletes become more familiar with the Snatch, the Clean is developed much easier. The repetitive nature of practice and the similarities between the two movements help newer athletes learn how to move their bodies. There is much to learn; however, before we start to talk about drills or tricks to fine tune skills. First, the philosophies which provide the foundation of our methods and how they aid us in moving around the barbell must be understood.

Barbell Oscillation

Quite possibly one of the most remarkable things to happen in our sport is the creation of Hookgrip.com by Nat Arem. In 2010, he launched his now famous website which features photos depicting lifting sequences and slow-motion videos of top lifters in the world. These videos have opened my eyes to the small nuances of technique each person possesses. This resource allows us to see movements which typically happen in seconds much more clearly. Significantly slowing them down exposes things we would normally never be able to see such as barbell oscillation.

Barbell oscillation is the product of bar body contact where the pliable nature of a barbell assist in the completion of a lift. It occurs when the forces placed upon the bar, by either the athlete or attached weights, cause it to bend. Many coaches out there would like to pretend it does not exist and do not teach it because they are stuck in the old ways. I, on the other hand, feel it is a topic that is not talked about enough!

This phenomenon is possible because of a pivotal point in the history of Weightlifting. In the 1960s, the two events that dramatically changed this sport forever were:

1. The International Weightlifting Federation's decision to change the bar body contact rule.

2. The development of a barbell capable of withstanding the demands of Weightlifting by the Eleiko Sport Company.

Years ago, when the sport was young, the rules stated that the barbell could not touch your body when performing either of the contested lifts. For the Snatch, the barbell had to be lifted from the ground in one continuous motion overhead. The Clean was the same except the bar had to be taken to the shoulders first, then the weight could be brought overhead via the Jerk. The barbell was not even allowed to touch the shins when you initially addressed the bar. In the early 1960s, the rule was changed to allow the barbell to "brush" the thighs, but not "bang" or "bounce." The type of violent bar body contact we are used to today was eventually allowed later. Weightlifters figured out that keeping the barbell close and using bar body contact was stronger and more efficient. These changes to the rule book led to heavier weights being lifted than ever before and posed a new problem.

Barbells would frequently break during competitions. A combination of heavy loads and the impact forces of lifters striking the barbell with their hips / thighs caused this problem. The Eleiko Sport Company worked to rectify this complication. They developed a barbell, comprised of unique pliable steel and it made its debut at the 1963 World Championships in Stockholm, Sweden. This new barbell was able to withstand the demands of high-level competition without bending permanently or cracking. The new bars sent shockwaves through the Weightlifting community and catapulted Eleiko into the limelight as the premier barbell supplier for the sport. A few years later the company revolutionized Weightlifting again when they introduced the first rubber discs, replacing the metal plates that were common at the time.

Today, barbells are designed to bend. In conjunction with body contact, we can use this to our advantage when performing the lifts. The amount of weight you load on the bar does not matter; even an empty barbell will oscillate. To demonstrate this point at my seminars, I perform the following demonstration: A barbell in hand, I squat down until my thighs are parallel to the floor. I raise the bar in the air about a foot, aiming for the middle of my thighs. I drop it (applying a little downward force). The barbell bounces off my thighs and back into my hands.

Look at that as barbell oscillation on a miniscule scale. To put this concept into perspective on the Weightlifting platform, we can turn back to Hookgrip. com. Go to your computer, visit the Hook Grip channel on YouTube and pull up a video of your favorite Weightlifter performing the Clean. Watch the plates loaded on the bar carefully as they rack the weight on their shoulders at the bottom of the squat. See how they move up and down? That is barbell oscillation. In the catapult method, we can use it to peak the barbell, standing out of the catch and on the Dip & Drive portion of the Jerk.

Peaking the Barbell

A barbell has peaked when it reaches its highest point of ascension from the ground. There it is momentarily weightless, floating in the air as if it were a fixed object attached to the walls. As the bar is achieving its peak an athlete is allotted time to pull themselves underneath and receive the weight. Everything we do revolves around bar oscillation – without it we could not achieve a weightless bar in the way that we desire as catapult lifters. The barbell is going to peak regardless of the style of technique used, but there are different ways to achieve it. This brings us to the topic of Triple Extension vs. Catapult methods of Weightlifting. There are a lot of differences between the two styles, but for now our focus is how and where the barbell is peaked.

- O **Triple Extension Method:** In this form of technique, athletes use a combination of forces from the legs and pulling up with the arms to peak the bar. After the drive with the legs has finished, athletes using this method pull the bar up, with the goal of having it peak high, around the solar plexus. In my opinion using the arms to peak the barbell is the devil in a red dress. Sure, it will peak higher than in a catapult method, but for not nearly as long. Pulling up on the bar causes the bar to lose its peak and make gravity a factor again. When that happens, you will be hard-pressed to beat the bar as it descends, and catch it. When you pull up on the barbell, you risk it losing its peak and falling like a meteor back to the platform.

- O **Catapult Method:** As a devout soldier of camp catapult, I firmly believe in driving my hips through the barbell instead of pulling it high with my arms. When peaked with the hips or upper thighs, the barbell will be low, no higher than the belly button in the Snatch and the groin in the Clean. It will also "float" for a much longer period in contrast to the other method. That is due to the force generated by the hips or upper thighs which helps to produce oscillation. Here the time the barbell spends in the air is only possible because of the oscillation we create by bringing it to the hips. The barbell will bow as your hips or upper thighs continue to drive through it (Arched Angel). When the bar snaps back and straightens, it is no longer touching you. That moment that the barbell snaps off your body is when it begins to peak and is your opportunity to pull yourself underneath the bar. I could care less how high the bar peaks. I want it to peak longer. I want to be able to leave, take a sip of my C4 pre-workout drink, come back and find the bar still floating there.

Catapult Weightlifters are some of the fastest athletes in the world and if it is speed under the bar that we need the lower peaking bar is always going to better. A low bar equates to more torque being produced to pull underneath it. More torque translates to violent speed. That is why lifters like myself are so fast. That is how Donny Shankle rips the head off a motherfucking lion every lift. You need to pull under fast and waste no time doing it. Lifters like myself and Ian Wilson produce so much bar oscillation that we are a quarter of the way under the barbell before it has reached its full peak. This can be seen in Hookgrip videos as the bar appears to still be traveling up while our feet are off the platform and we are going down. In reality, by the time the barbell has reached optimal peak, we are already a quarter of the way underneath it. In the Snatch the bar ascends to a higher peak because the weight is so light, but in the Clean, the extremely heavy weights will go no higher than the groin. The more time you spend pulling the bar up higher equates to less time you will have to pull yourself under to catch it.

My performance at the 2012 American Open Championships is an excellent example of peaking the barbell. In the 94KG class, I would be going up against Romanian National Team member Istvan Dioszegi. Dioszegi was the favorite to win, but not without a fight from me. The competition at any meet starts in the back room. So much goes on back there such as mind games and politics, all to win. My strategy was to get into Dioszegi's head well before either one of us stepped on stage. Most lifters will sit a lot in between warm up sets. I never sat throughout mine. Instead, I paced back and forth like a fucking caged lion on my platform staring directly at my opponent. His warm up platform was across from mine, and I wanted him to see I had no fear. My teammates, coach, and everyone else in the back room thought I was crazy. I never went underneath one bar in my warm ups leading up to my opener for the Snatch. Instead, I would set up on the bar, pull it from the floor, strike it with my hips…and then take my hands off of it. With the bar still raising to its peak in front of me I made fists, raised them over my head and smashed it back down to the ground. Then I paced around my platform looking Dioszegi right in the eyes.

I ended up defeating Dioszegi and winning the American Open. I finished the meet with a 160KG Snatch,188KG Clean & Jerk and a 348KG Total. I honestly believe that my display of power in peaking the barbell in the warm up room not only gave me the confidence to win this meet, but also got into the minds of my opponents.

The Philosophy of Opposites

The Philosophy of Opposites is the belief that each position of movement is the exact mirror opposite of another. A perfect example to illustrate this philosophy would be the relationship between the Superman Pause and the Arched Angel. These two phases of the Finish are the Yin to the others Yang. To put this philosophy into perspective, we will examine the differences between these two positions in greater detail. As seen in **Figure 8.7.**

Joints	Superman Pull	Arched Angel
Shoulders	In front of the barbell	Behind the barbell
Elbows	Slightly bent	Bent Slightly and in-line with the Shoulders
Hips	Flexed, Behind the barbell, High	Extended, Driving through the barbell, High
Knees	Pushed back (extended)	Pushed forward slightly flexed
Foot	Flat, weight 100% on heels	On balls of feet, pushing through the floor

The hips play a significant role in helping Weightlifters abide by the Philosophy of Opposites. As the hips move, transitioning through each phase of the lifts, the changing in location of the hips influences the movements of the other joints and the bar. For example, as the hips rise, the knees move back and as they move back the shoulders move in front of the bar. The lower the hips start at the beginning of the movement results in a more dramatic expression of each position of the lifts. That is why we teach our athletes to setup on the barbell with their hips very low.

If we look at the Snatch as a whole, we can see how the rest of the body is affected by the movement of the hips. **Figure 8.8** on the next page shows the start position of the hips. From there, during the lifts, the hips will move through the following sequence: low to high, to low, to high, to low. This concept can be seen more clearly and be broken down on the next page and in **Figure 8.9.**

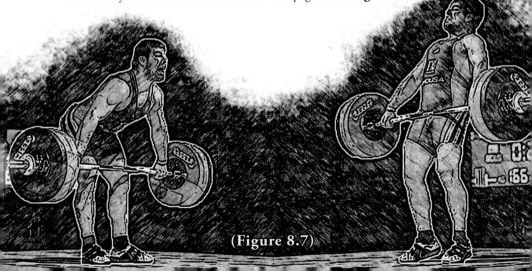

(Figure 8.7)

- **Low – Frame #1:** The lower the hips start, the higher they can go throughout the pull. That is because the hips must now travel a longer distance before they reach the point of transition to the next phase in the lift (the Finish). Higher hips in the pull also equate to more loading of the hamstrings. Since the hips are low, the shoulders will start on top of or behind the barbell, and the knees are bent. **Figure 8.8** more accurately demonstrates the proper start position. In **Frame #1** the hips have already began to move high.

- **High – Frames #1-4:** As the hips raise the knees go back (extend), and the shoulders travel out in front of the barbell. As with the hips, the shoulders must also go a long distance to move out in front of the barbell. That allows us to stay over the bar, covering it with the torso, for a much longer period. The result is a longer lever to pivot from when executing the Finish. It would not be possible to do this if you set up on the barbell with the hips high and shoulders already out in front. You would initiate the Finish much earlier than what we are looking to do in our method. Athletes who start with the hips high and shoulders already in front of the bar typically initiate the finish when the barbell reaches the knees instead of the mid-thigh.

- **Low – Frame #5:** The double knee bend has initiated. That aides the hips in dropping low again in the transition to the Power Position. As this happens the shoulders move back directly over the barbell. At this point in the lift bar body contact is successfully achieved.

- **High – Frame #6:** Transitioning from the Power Position to the Arched Angel, the hips drive up and through the barbell. The bar oscillates from the forces created by bar body contact.

- **Low – Frames #7-10:** The barbell has lost its oscillation and peaks. I pull myself underneath the bar to receive the weight. I end relatively in the same position I started, with the hips low, shoulders behind (if the bar were on the floor), a vertical torso and bent knees.

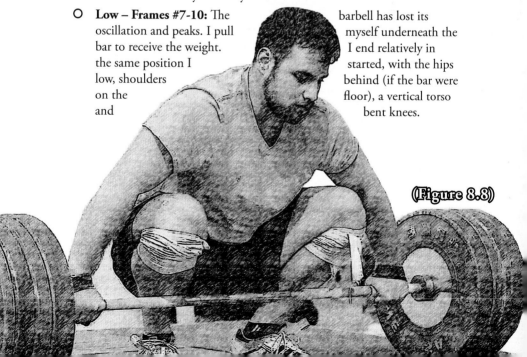

(Figure 8.8)

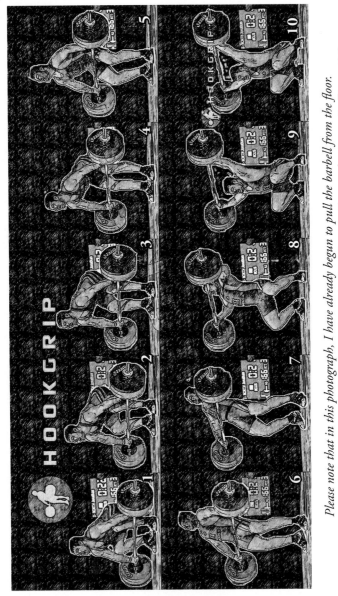

Please note that in this photograph, I have already begun to pull the barbell from the floor. My hips would have been much lower just prior to the first photo similar to what is seen in Figure. 8.8.

(Figure 8.9)

The Weightlifting Catapult

A catapult is an apparatus that can be used to hurl objects a great distance. Our model, as seen in **Figure 8.10**, is a representation of a Mangonel catapult. Its purpose is to illustrate how a catapult operates. Once we understand the mechanics involved in this machinery we can then broaden our view of the catapult philosophy in relation to ourselves. The Mangonel uses a bucket (1) to hold its payload that is attached to an arm (2) connected to the rest of the machine. The arm is loaded by using stored energy via the torsion bundle (ropes) centrally located at its base (3). As the arm is cranked (loaded) down the ropes of the torsion bundle twist together tightly creating stored energy. When released, they unwind, in turn rotating the arm at a high velocity. The payload launches into the air, but the arm will stop further movement by contacting the crossbar.

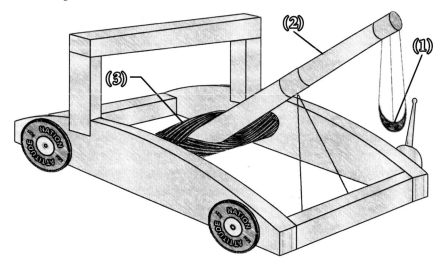

(Figure 8.10)

The Mangonel catapult abides by the philosophy of opposites. The bucket starts high because it must go low. After it goes low, and the time is right, **WHAM!** It goes high again. Yes, there is a slight variation in the sequence of movements when we apply this to Weightlifting. There are also fewer steps involved in the movement, but human beings are more complex than a medieval siege weapon. On the platform, you are the catapult; the barbell is the payload. If we keep an open mind, inferences can be drawn on how you can act as a Weightlifting catapult to move big weights. First, let us look at the parts of our body that perform the actions similar to that of a Mangonel.

Comparisons to the Human Catapult

- **Barbell:** The Payload.
- **Hips:** The bucket that holds the payload.
- **Torso:** The arm attached to the bucket.
- **Arms:** Cables attached to the Arm (Torso).
- **Hamstrings:** The torsion bundle that stores energy when loaded.

We have discussed quite a bit in this chapter thus far. You now have the knowledge of terminology; barbell oscillation, peaking the barbell, the philosophy of opposites and how a catapult works. Let us put all of this information together and see how it relates to the human catapult. The photograph on the next page depicts the Attitude Nation Catapult Method, in sequence, perfectly. What typically happens in seconds can now be examined frame by frame.

- **Hands:** I hold the barbell (payload) within my hands.
- **Arms:** The cables that will help bring the barbell from the floor to its next destination.
- **Frames #1-4:** I perform the Superman Pull. My hips start low, but then go high. My shoulders were back, but now move out in front of the barbell. The knees also go back (extend). These actions cause my hamstrings (torsion bundle) to create stored energy.
- **Frame #4:** My hips are as high as possible. The barbell has reached the mid-thigh and I have completed the Superman Pull. In the Superman Pause, there might as well be a handle sticking out from between my shoulder blades. All you would need to do is slam it down and **WHAM!** I will activate the double knee bend to begin to complete the Finish.
- **Frames #4-6:** My hips drop low again as I transition into the Power Position. I have achieved optimal leverage over the weight in my hands. I begin to exert maximal force by driving my hips into the barbell while simultaneously pulling it back into me. Right here the payload is in the bucket (hips), and the arm (torso) is moving at a high velocity.
- **Frames #4-6:** I continue to drive my hips through the barbell. As that happens, my hips will go high again, and I will transition into the Arched Angel. As the two forces (me and the barbell) collide, the barbell will oscillate. If it were even more pliable than it is, the barbell would wrap around my hips like the finish line tape at the end of a marathon.
- **Frame #7:** By now the Mangonel Catapult would have released its payload, but I do the opposite. I hold onto it instead. The barbell has snapped back and straightened. A straight barbell that has come up and away from a lifters body is a sign that it has lost oscillation and is now

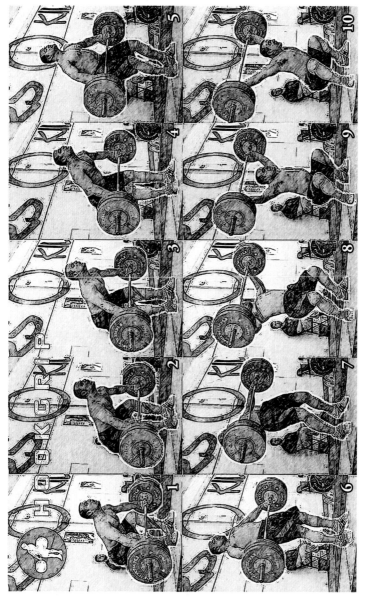

Please note that in this photograph, I have already begun to pull the barbell from the floor. My hips would have been much lower just prior to the first photo.

(Figure 8.11)

peaking. Wasting no time, my hips go low one last time and I begin to pull myself underneath the barbell.

- O **Frames #8-9:** I continue to pull myself underneath the barbell. Take a look at the circle on the wall behind me and where the bar is in relation to it. You can see that once my feet have planted, and I continue moving beneath the barbell, it rises no higher than the very bottom of the circle.

- O **Frame #10:** The bar was weightless for a moment. I did not pull it up. I pulled myself down. My body moved around the barbell; the barbell did not move around me. The lift is over. Triumphantly, I stand and lay waste to my enemy. I slam that bar back to the dusty wooden platform from whence it came!

The Technique of Oscillation (The Attitude Nation Catapult Method) is extreme. It requires a strong posterior chain, patience, and violence. There are several points throughout the movements where errors can cause you to miss the lift. Did you initiate the Finish a little too early? You might miss the lift. You did not completely drive your hips through the bar aka pass through the Arched Angel? You might miss the lift. Be patient…Wait a little longer. Be patient…drive all the way through the barbell. Everything you do from the start is just a setup for the next step so complete all the steps entirely. As a Weightlifter, you are a unique machine that must master the Philosophy of Opposites. If you do that combined with bar body contact, barbell oscillation, speed and violence then you will be unstoppable. You will make lifts and lift big weights.

WELCOME TO CAMP CATAPULT!

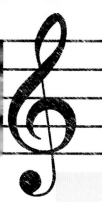

CHAPTER 9:
THE POWER OF POSITION

Trap King

Friday, June 22, 2012

Yes, the traps activate. Yes, they try so hard, and yes they are as worthless as tits on a bore. It's a sad story of how this came to be. A story that drew a tear to my eye, a story that will make any man grab his heart with pain. But don't feel too bad, for once he was happy, once he stood proud, once he was King.

Chapter One

Once upon a time, in a far away land where the bar wasn't allowed to touch your body, the trap was king. The trap ruled the weightlifting world with his big stick and his large high crown. He never got tired of the attention, as a matter of fact, he took in every bit of it like it was Christmas morning. They talked about him as a legend from coast to coast, as myths and stories began to pile up about his power and strength. He was conquering world records. He was winning Gold medals in the Olympics. He was kicking ass on a daily basis. Scholars wrote hundreds of books about his efficiency and power. It was once recorded that he stood 15 feet tall, and could chop down the tallest tree with one swish of his sword. Athletes and coaches spent years trying to mimic his greatness. Some felt and understood his beauty, and some fell short only to stare hopelessly at the podium. Others tried to defeat him with different tactics and methods. He was constantly challenged from others

BEN CARIDAD

who envied his power. But they fell short, and nothing seemed to
please the King more than victory on the Platform and off. His
way was the best way, the only way. He knew it, and everyone else
knew of his glory. The traps could shrug any bar higher than
the eyes could see. He made weight disappear into the blue sky,
only for the birds to enjoy. The scarecrow some called the king,
which fit him well, and explained the position he was always in.
Upright, straight, and elbows high as if the scarecrow was showing
a young kid where the sun was. The crowd went crazy, and the King
grew an inch with every lift that was made. The King was happy,
and I am happy for him.

Years went by, decades passed almost with a blink of an eye. He
sat on his silk green thrown growing older and older while the
sport grew old with him. They were two peas in a pod, they shared
war stories together until the orange afternoon fell dark. The
King had no idea what was about to happen next. The King was
about to be turned upside down.

"Siar we have a problem, come quick!" "The Weightlifters are
starting to make bar body contact!" "They are breaking the rules,
they are going against you Siar!" The king woke from his gold
thrown in a panic, as his crown stumbled into his lap with frantic
hands. He tried everything in his power to stop this craziness,
this reluctant rebellion. But the lifters kept at it. The coaches
scratched their heads and talked amongst each other with smiles
and approval. Once the lifters found this new way of throwing the
barbell over their head, there was no stopping the ease and joy
they got out if this new found relationship with the bar. The
sport was chattering with new ideas. The trees were swaying from
the swift change in the air. A monster was being created, and the
King was feeling its bite. The chatter from the towns people kept
the king up at night, only to fall asleep with his pillow over his
head. Only to find his presence slowly dwindling. The committee
spoke, and the rule of no bar body contact was changed to bar
body contact. A shift in the sport that changed everything,
including the King's masterful power over this great sport. A
rule that drew a single tear from the king's face that with ease
and patience fell from his right eye and splattered onto his high
golden crown.

Chapter Two

The scarecrow was taken down from its high perch in the middle
of the town, and replaced with an arched angel that struck such
beauty and rhythm. An image that turned people's head to the side
as the sun glazed over her bent body. A sling shot type movement,
a catapult machine the weightlifters turned into. That same year
a record of world records were shattered. The weight went up, and
fast. The bar had much more color on each side. The competition
grew fierce, as weak lifters were now able to battle with strong
lifters. Mad scientists is what they were, the coaches that
is. Blue prints of how their athlete can move their body to lift
more and more weight, even if they had weak legs. Yes, strength
building is always a must, but a new found creature was going to
help build the athlete to new heights. Their arms grew skinny as
they hung like cables. The traps grew smaller as they held less
of a purpose. The back grew bigger and stronger from staying
over longer and longer. The weightlifters moved faster, as their
hips drew blood against the bar with a large amount of force and
determination. The weightlifter is now a machine of some sort,
and there is no stopping what its capable of performing next.
Who knows, the Arched Angel may someday be replaced with another
statue for the towns people to talk over.

The King is still with us today, he is still a part of this great
sport. The King will never leave. Every part of the body plays a
part in this great fight. All parts of the body belong and serve
a purpose. The athlete must not think, just do. Letting the body
perform such elegance and strength. "What foot do you step forward
with in the jerk?" A question that cannot be answered, a question
that only the athlete must do without thinking, for then he or she
will find out themselves. In my opinion, this is how the bar body
contact was born. An athlete just moved, just lifted, and then
found a comfort that worked in unusual ways compared to the norm
back then. The sport is always growing, and the King will live
on forever. He might now smile as big and bright as before. The
King may not stand 15 feet tall anymore, but he is still proud of
what he created, and proud to see lifters achieve greatness to
this day. Long live the King, and welcome to the new and possible
ideas of a weightlifter.

The King 2016

149

The Power Position

As the middle of the Finish, the Power Position is the point of contact between the hips or upper thighs and the barbell. It is a universal position that every Weightlifter, regardless of the style of technique used, must pass through to continue exerting maximal force into the barbell. Paul Doherty said it best "everything in Weightlifting is back, up is back." You could stop reading right now and add twenty kilos to your lifts with that knowledge. There is no such thing as "up" in Weightlifting. Yes, the bar will rise off the ground during the pull. That obviously needs to happen to complete a lift. However, too many people focus on pulling the bar straight up instead of pulling the bar back into their hips or upper thighs. Focus on "back" not "up."

Everything done when pulling the bar from the floor is just to set the stage for our arrival at the Power Position; to pull the barbell back into the hips or upper thighs. Creating good habits by reinforcing this position is crucial for new and veteran athletes alike. That is why we start here when teaching the lifts, working from the Top-Down. Drilling the Power Position will help develop essential skills that will be necessary for bar body contact. It will transfer over to and be a prerequisite to almost every drill cataloged within this text. Take your time and perfect this aspect of your technique. Too many lifters out there falter here, and the result is kilos left on the table, makeable lifts missed and a lot of frustration.

The Power Position is going to teach you:

- How to move your body (develop kinesthetic awareness), as needed when Weightlifting.
- How to actively pull the barbell back into your hips or upper thighs.
- Body weight distribution and using it for leverage when completing the Finish.

The Snatch

Let us begin. Grab your bar, get your shoes on and follow along as you read. Go through the checklist below as we break down the Power Position. Make sure your body meets these standards for the position or better yet, read along with a friend and coach each other. Start building your melting pots!

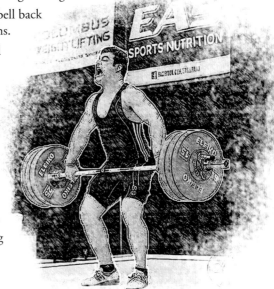

(Figure 9.1)

150

Position Standards:

- **Stance:** Your feet should be directly under your hips roughly six to eight inches apart. It may take some trial and error to find what is comfortable for you. The toes may be pointed straight ahead or turned out slightly.

- **Weight Distribution:** Your body weight should be shifted back 100% on your heels.

- **Grip & Bar:** You will want to have a wide grip on the barbell. The Barbell should be deep in the crease of the hips.Below the pelvis or "ouch" bone and above the genitals.

- **Arms:** In this method we want all athletes to utilize a slight arm bend. This will help to keep the upper back tight and teach you how to drive the bar back into your hips on the Snatch or upper thighs on the Clean. A tiny (slight) arm bend is all you need, but increase it as needed.

- **Hips:** Your hips are going to drop straight down towards your feet.

- **Knees:** The knees will bend allowing the hips to drop low four to five inches depending on your flexibility. They will also track over the toes.

- **Torso:** Your torso should be as vertical as possible with the back arched.

- **Shoulders:** Actively pull your shoulders back and down. Spread your chest and squeeze the shoulder blades together.

- **Head:** Look straight ahead. Never look down because it can lead to sacrificing your posture.

The Clean

The Power Position for the Clean is exactly the same as in the Snatch except for one small variance. Instead of the barbell making contact with the crease of the hips it will instead hit the upper thighs for most athletes. That is due to the much narrower grip that many Weightlifters typically use when performing the Clean.

Position Standards:

- **Stance:** Identical to the Snatch.

- **Weight Distribution:** Identical to the Snatch.

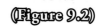

(Figure 9.2)

- **Grip & Bar:** You will have a much narrower grip than in the Snatch; approximately a thumbs distance from the smooth part of the barbell. Experiment to find out what is comfortable for you.

- ○ **Arms:** Identical to the Snatch
- ○ **Hips:** Identical to the Snatch.
- ○ **Knees:** Identical to the Snatch.
- ○ **Torso:** Identical to the Snatch.
- ○ **Shoulders:** Identical to the Snatch.
- ○ **Head:** Identical to the Snatch.

The Early Arm Bend:

The Early Arm Bend is the act of gradually rowing the barbell into your hips or upper thighs to produce a greater amount of barbell oscillation. It occurs during the lift throughout the entirety of the Superman Pull. I recommend those using the Technique of Oscillation (The Attitude Nation Catapult Method) to do this on both the Snatch and Clean. Classical methods of technique do not promote the utilization of an early arm bend. That makes sense for that style of lifting. If they are going to use the arms to help peak the barbell higher, then of course they would want to save the arm bend for the very last second after utilizing the legs and hips. However, in our method we want as much bar oscillation as possible. We use the arm bend purely to hit the barbell.

Rowing the barbell into the hips has many benefits. First, it aids us in pulling the bar **BACK** into the hips or upper thighs instead of straight up thus ensuring that we make bar body contact. Second, this rowing action helps to contract the muscles of the mid and upper back. Tightness in these areas contributes to adding stability to the Catch Position or regain posture if lost, during the Superman Pull. Third, if you are someone who has very long arms, this technique will help you bring the barbell to its correct destination. I have worked with many athletes whose bodies were built for Basketball and not Weightlifting. Grabbing the bar collar to collar when performing the Snatch was still not enough for it to make contact with the crease of their hips. We cannot make the barbell longer, so to find success, we made their arms *shorter* with the arm bend.

Coaching Cue: "Row your boat" when practicing the early arm bend.

The Hip Clean:

While the Thigh Clean is what many athletes do, there is another style out there called the Hip Clean. Many of my Weightlifting heroes such as Donny Shankle, Spencer Moorman, and Andrea Aramnau have mastered it. Hip Cleaners make contact with the barbell higher in the hips relatively in the same spot they do for the Snatch. I have unsuccessfully tried countless times to convert to this method. If the Hip Clean is something that comes naturally, and you feel comfortable with it, then consider yourself blessed.

The advantages of the Hip Clean are enormous. First, you will be able to produce more powerful bar body contact hit by bringing the barbell into the hips and closer to your center of mass as opposed to the high thigh. Second, if the point of contact is higher, then so is the location the barbell when peaking. To catch the Clean we only need to bring the barbell to our shoulders. A shorter distance between the Clean Catch position as opposed to the Snatch, coupled with more powerful bar body contact equate to increased time to get under the bar. I remember when Spencer Moorman first started to develop the Hip Clean. He had so much time to catch the bar that he would pull under, sit in the bottom of his squat, and the barbell would still be peaking a few inches off of his shoulders. The barbell would often crash down on top of him. It took a lot of patience and practice for him to relearn the timing needed for a successful catch on the Hip Clean. I recommend at some point you try to Hip Clean. A great deal of arm bend will be necessary for those attempting to learn this unless you have baby T-Rex arms. If it feels great and you love it, perfect. If not then go back to what you were previously doing.

Common Errors in Performing the Power Position.

Make sure that you are not committing any of these common errors for both the Snatch and Clean that could put you in an inefficient position.

○ **Error #1 – Allowing the barbell to slide down the thighs:** Make sure to pull your shoulders back and that your grip is wide enough on the barbell for the Snatch. With a narrower grip on the Clean this is usually a more apparent problem. Since we do not have the landmark of the hip crease, it can be easy to let the barbell slide down the thighs too much.

Coaching Cue: "Avoid the slope."

○ **Error #2 – Letting the barbell hang loosely:** I never want to see any daylight between the barbell and my athlete's body. Engage the muscles in your back and your Lats to actively pull the barbell into your hips or upper thighs.

Coaching Cue: "Pull Back."

○ **Error #3 – Not paying attention to your posture:** Remember we want a vertical torso in this position. Leaning forward can also cause the barbell to travel down the thighs. If you are doing this, then your hips may be too far back than what is necessary for this position.

Coaching Cue: "Get Shoulders On Top of the Bar - or - Get Shoulders In Line with the Bar."

- ○ **Error #4 – Shifting your body weight onto the balls of your feet:** If your body weight shifts forward then so does the weight of the barbell. That can pull you out of position. Lift your toes up towards the ceiling and lean back slightly moving your body weight back to the heels.

  Coaching Cue: "Toes up, lean back."

- ○ **Error #5 – Shallow hips:** You need to be comfortable moving your hips low. A two inch descent of the hips is not enough. Push your hips down deeper toward your feet four to five inches and increase the bend at the knees.

  Coaching Cue: "Sit deeper."

- ○ **Error #6 – Allowing the arms to be straight:** In this method of technique we one hundred percent want to use the early arm bend. A slight bend at the arms is sufficient to assist in keeping the back tight and increasing the power produced by bar body contact.

  Coaching Cue: "Bend the Arms."

- ○ **Error #7 – Not tucking up or down:** This is mainly a warning to the men out there reading this. You want to make sure you do not hit your penis when making bar body contact. I made this rookie mistake back in 2009 at a local meet. For the Snatch, you tuck down and for the Clean you tuck up (unless you are a Hip Cleaner). After the Snatch session, I completely forgot to tuck up for the Cleans. I ended up smashing my penis with the barbell and had to be taken to the emergency room.

Technique Drills:

Learning to Pull Back: Part One

You will need a partner for this drill, but no barbell or dowel yet. The goal is for you to feel what it is like to engage the muscles of your back and Lats while pulling the barbell into your body.

- ○ **Step One:** Assume the Power Position. Perform a double check of the position standards and make sure you are not committing any common errors. Move your hands out to the left and right of your hips mimicking the width of a Snatch grip. Your palms should be facing behind you.
- ○ **Step Two:** Next, your partner, will stand on your right side and put their hand up against the palm of your right hand.

- ○ **Step Three:** They will apply pressure and try to push your hand forward.
- ○ **Step Four:** Your job is to not only resist them, but to maintain the Power Position as you apply pressure back into their hand. Take note of the tension you feel in your back as you do this. That is how it should feel when you have a barbell in your hands.
- ○ **Step Five:** Switch sides and repeat.

Learning to Pull Back: Part Two

The second part of the Learning to Pull Back Drill builds on the one previously performed. Its goal is to help you maintain proper mechanics in the Power Position while being challenged by weight and the forces of gravity. A heavy barbell is always trying to pull you down while you are lifting it. That is why it is crucial that we practice pulling back so much. It is also going to help you work on staying back on your heels when in this position. Expect to do a few variations of this drill as we progress to other aspects of our method. With a partner perform the following:

- ○ **Step One:** With a Snatch Grip on the Barbell; assume the Power Position.
- ○ **Step Two:** Hold this position while a partner stands in front of you and places their hands on the barbell just outside of your hips.
- ○ **Step Three:** From here after they communicate with you that they are going to start; your partner will **gently** pull the barbell away from you in their direction. They should not be fighting hard to overpower you.
- ○ **Step Four:** Your job is to resist the force applied by your partner and pull back hard on the barbell. The bar should not leave your hip crease, and you should remain solid in the Power Position. Squeeze the muscles of your back and dig into the floor pushing through the heels at an angle as if a rug were being pulled from under you. That will aid in stopping your partner from pulling the barbell away from you. If you lose your balance and are pulled forward on your toes stop, restart the drill and try harder.
- ○ **Step Five:** Repeat.

George

Monday, March 26, 2012

Mr. High Hang is a tall man with dark hair and a curvy long black mustache. Mr. Hang has actually named the creature above his upper lip, and he takes much pride in the grooming, smell, shape, and overall relationship he has with it. His name is George, and George is constantly smiling at you even if Hang isn't. Now that we have gotten the mustache out of the way, let's chat about the gunslinger himself. His hands move dramatically when he talks, his eyes never blink much, but his forehead moves up and down like a pogo stick pretty much at all times. His big white eyes open as wide as an alligator's mouth when he is talking about a matter that has importance to him, or better yet when he is lifting weights, a sport he has been doing for many years now. His nick name is the finisher, because he has the strongest finish around. His finish is faster than most, and some say his explosion is more powerful than the A bomb. There are actually many storys of Mr. Hang breaking logs in half to build his cabin out in the hills of Oregon. He is an impatient human that curses anything that takes longer than his liking. For example, long bus rides, waiting for the bus, and then waiting for people to exit and enter the bus from the horrible stops it makes throughout his long impatient ride in the bus. The worst of them all is the dreaded pull in weightlifting that now some underground army is calling the superman pull. He can't stand it! I watched him snatch once and right in the middle of the pull he became bored so he dropped the bar and started playing his 1997 Nintendo game boy that I think was Mortal Combat by the slamming of buttons and mouth expressions that were happening in his chair behind the platform. This struck me in an odd way considering this happened just a few days ago, and I haven't seen one of those bad boys since.....well, 1997.

The old hip slinger, the smoking hips, the bar breaker, the lady's man, and the last but not least, the tree cutting pickle jar opening nail gun shooting slug hammer house plowing hips attacker. Yes people, these were only a few of his nick names, and the last one is my favorite. Mr. Hang and his fuzzy snake friend George only snatched from the high hang. They would compete in meets but never put up a total because they would stand tall and then go from the high hang right above the knee. Some people said "give it to them, that lift right there is even harder than the full snatch"! But most people, including myself, said "no way Jose, that right there is illegal". But they didn't care, training or meet they went from above the knee where there is hardly any momentum, and a very small pull, which some called the room 2 pull or the special pull, a pull that never really completed its full potential.

Here is a video of Mr. Hang and George completing their high hang snatch with 140kg!! Oh, and by the way, after chatting with them both, I soon found out they are a part of the ATTITUDE NATION! Salute and see you guys tomorrow.

Hang snatches are hard 2012

CHAPTER 10

GO UNDER

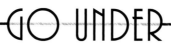

Go Under

Saturday, January 26, 2013

Pull my head out of the sand and go under. Sometimes your
thoughts don't look good on paper, and right now my paper has
been stamped defeat. What am I so scared of anyway? The boogie
monster? What's under that bar that has me doubting myself? What
lies underneath the bed that makes me hang upside down before
falling for cover underneath the blankets? I pull the shades up
for light, only to slam the door in front of my own face. I play
peek a boo with going underneath. Every time I peek, the crowd
boos throughout my head, leaving me feeling gutless, shameful.
I have always said that weightlifting is like going to Vegas, your
odds of making the lift go up significantly when committing. In
a sport where I truly believe is based on 95 percent skill, and
5 percent luck, we must at least go under even if the weight feels
like a dead body. Go under and cross your fingers for the
5 percent that could land in the palm of your hands,
sending a shock wave of surprised emotion to our
face. Go under for nothing more than respect, to
show others and yourself that you are a warrior
amongst droids.

I realize this is easier said
than done. It's very easy for
me to sit in front of a computer
screen while sipping tea....but
I'm aware that its one of my
biggest problems at times,
the balls to go under,
or better yet, the wits
that stopped me from
going under. This can
leave you turning in your bed
while sheltering your thoughts

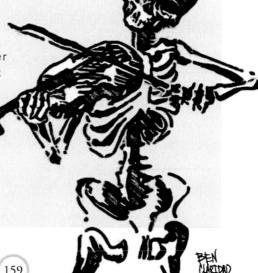

BEN
CLARIDAD

with a pillow. I don't "clark" as much as I used to, I have
mentally trained my body to go under no matter what. I have come
to the conclusion that I would rather break my arm than bathe in
my own shame. And yes, I have missed thousands of lifts, but I
have made hundreds as well. It only takes two lifts to win, just
like it only takes two white lights for a make. Give me two made
lifts with two white lights and a million misses, over a million
makes and two misses. I would rather lose knowing I went under...
than win knowing I left something on the platform.

I came to this realization about a year back when the bar landed
on my head, splitting a small part of my skull open. As the blood
dripped down my arm I realized something fascinating....I was
ok. Like a kid who has fallen and scrapped his knee, the kid is
not hurt, but will cry if others around him panic. I wiped the
blood with my shirt, and began to finish practice. "A bloody bar
makes for a strong heart," Shankle replied to my confused face
expression. Confused in a way that has helped me to this day.
Confusion led to understanding, and understanding led to realizing
that the bar is all talk and no chalk. The bar doesn't hurt. The
bar looks mean, but hits like a girl. I smiled and kept lifting
like a kid getting released back to recess. Shankle winked at me,
coach nodded at me, and the bar wouldn't look at me. I slam you
bar, you don't slam me. I am in control, not you. Now don't get
me wrong, the bar put up a fight, and it still is. Landing on my
back, my head, spitting me out from the bottom like a baseball
player and his chew. The bar ain't got time for me, and I ain't
got time for the bar. Now I don't give the bar respect, I stopped
giving it lunch money years ago. No more bar, fuck you. Now miss
or make I go under, and the bar hates it. Going under means make,
means success, means good. There is such thing as a good miss,
and no matter how bad the miss might look, going under will get
you one step closer to your goals in the bitch of a sport.

Under, under, under, make it, miss it, squat it, press it, get
red lighted, get white lighted, who really cares? The only thing
that really matters is going to bed knowing you left everything
on the platform. Bleed from your head and piss blood from
striking the bar so hard. Stab your legs with squats and beat
your shoulders up with a hammer. This means you are getting
strong, and not just physically, but mentally. Thick skin means
strong legs, bloody skulls and bruised backs means big balls,

standing tall and ripping the heads off lions. This blog is what
I have learned throughout my career, what I have learned from the
streets of weightlifting. A melting pot, dark and light, misses
and makes. Anybody that says this is not a technique blog....
well then they are dead wrong. Dead like the dead weight of the
bar at it crashes on our backs. Dead wrong like how our bodies
will feel the minute we retire and have to become normal sheep.
Technique comes in all shapes and sizes. Learning how to become
a weightlifter is technique of its own. Training your mind to go
under weights you are scared of takes hundreds of mental hours of
training. Never ever listen to your body. Listen to your mind.
Train your thoughts to paint a picture...then fucken paint. Paint
what works. Paint a miss and put it up above your bed. Stare at
it, get to know it. Understand that misses will occur more than
makes, and this sport holds more bad days than good. It's the
athlete than can understand and cope with this that will succeed.
Miss a weight or make, at the end of the day we are training, and
training is what will rise us above the rest. Train hard, and
always go under.....no matter what.

Ain't got time For The Bar 2016

The Catch is the receiving position for the Snatch, Clean, and Jerk. It occurs
after the barbell has peaked and involves the athlete pulling their body underneath
(or pushing in the case of the Jerk) the weight without error. Development of the
catch position will be essential for success in Weightlifting. There is a lot of debate;
mainly for the Snatch, on the technique used when under the bar. We believe our
style offers the most efficient way, but you need to know other methods so you
can decide as an athlete what works best for you.

A proper Catch Position will help to:

O   Receive the weight safely and avoid injury.
O   Keep the weight being held stable and controlled.
O   Provide a bit of insurance for saving lifts.

The Snatch

I want you to participate in a little experiment right now. Like a true soldier
of the Attitude Nation, I know that you have this book in one hand and a big
cup of Miss Brown Eyes in the other. I am going to need you to put down that
delicious cup of coffee so you can follow along with this exercise. I know this is
hard, but consider it an important lesson. You have to learn to make sacrifices if
you want to be a good Weightlifter. Now if you think of yourself as a tough son of

a gun, feel free to do this with your cup in hand, but don't you dare spill a drop. Assume the Power Position. Now raise your free hand overhead with your arms in line with your ears as if you were asking a question. **Keep your arm in this position and do not put it down until I tell you to.**

Right now your arms should be in line with your ears; elbows locked (extended) and wrist straight. That is where new, immobile, or lifters who have been taught a more conventional way catch the barbell. It is a hard position to hold even without any weight. The weight of your arm and hand overhead is supported by the shoulders instead of the stronger muscles of the upper back. That is why so many athletes out there have shoulder injuries. You will also have a greater chance of missing lifts in front of you or press outs during competition. Back in my "Jumping Jonathan North" days, when I was still a young rookie, I lifted with this style of technique. Frequently, I would be called for press outs in competitions. This problem was not corrected until I changed to the form used in the Attitude Nation Catapult Method. I have not had a lift taken away due to press outs ever since making that change.

Hopefully, you are still staying strong with that arm overhead. If I were to come over to you, grab your hand and push down the elbow joint would bend. Let me offer you some relief. Rotate your arm as if you were screwing in a light bulb. That will help to create external rotation at the shoulder joint. Next, pull your arm back a few inches so that it is behind your ears and push your head forward as well. Not only is this a more stable position to catch the bar, but the arms cannot physically bend when holding onto the barbell. They will quite literally break before bending; press outs are now an afterthought. That is why I want you to catch the barbell here. **Okay…you can put your hand down now.**

Position Standards:

- **Stance:** When you catch the barbell your feet will move out wide. That is different from one individual to the next.
- **Torso:** As vertical as possible.
- **Arms:** Behind the ears.
- **Shoulders:** Externally rotated.
- **Elbows:** Fully extended with the biceps pointing up toward the ceiling.
- **Wrist/Bar:** Completely cocked back. The barbell will rest in the palm of the hands.

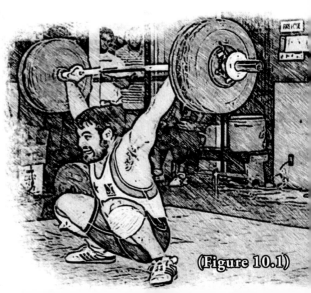

(Figure 10.1)

- ○ **Head:** Pushed forward with the chin anchored and eyes looking up. I call this the Turtle Head because it mimics a turtle poking out of its shell.
- ○ **Feet:** Take note of my left foot. I am doing whatever it takes to get as low as possible. Professional athletes take risks and while this foot position may not be anatomically correct, it was necessary for me to successfully complete this Snatch. I was trying to win at all cost.

Weightlifting Insurance:

Weightlifting insurance is the utilization of your head to create a counter balance that helps with the weight distribution of the barbell overhead. That provides athletes with the ability to save lifts. Shit is going to happen when you go under the bar, but it does not have to be as black and white as miss or make. If you want to be a good Weightlifter, then you need to know when to call the Allstate guy for some insurance to get you out of a bind. A unique and powerful tool you can use for this purpose would be your head. That is why it is important that you turtle head on the Catch. When you catch the barbell, with the weight supported by the shoulders, you have little room to save it if it drifts forward. However, when the bar is behind your head, you gain the ability to keep pulling back on the bar or reposition yourself as you stand.

Another way you can save a lift, utilizes the chin more directly. With the head pushed forward we do create better weight distribution, but sometimes it needs to be adjusted by moving the chin around. I do this by anchoring my chin to my upper chest. I can then move my chin, head and body to change my position under the barbell and find improved balance. In many videos, you can even see me with my chin almost touching my knee in an attempt to save a lift. Chin positioning is **THAT** influential during the Snatch. While I am moving my chin around I always keep my eyes looking up.

Your eyes help to control what the rest of the body is doing and looking down while in the catch would start a chain reaction of the head, and then chest and finally barbell dropping. **Figure 10.2** to the right is an example of how I repositioned my body to save a Snatch. The full lift can be viewed in my video titled "Tyson" at the 5:06 mark.

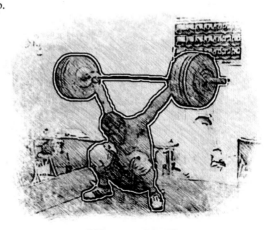

(Figure 10.2)

The Castle

How am I going to stand up? This is the only question you need to
ask yourself before squatting. Seeing the bottom of the world is
like inception, it is a lost world of unknown and forgetfulness.
Your rep set scheme becomes lost, and all recollection of time
itself vanishes as you free fall into a grave yard of missed
attempts, all screaming for you to take them with you. The dead
attempts stretch their arms like tight ropes, and their fingers
flail like sea weed in an ocean storm as they pull you down,
only for hope they can be pulled up. A castle of broken bricks,
hunched backs, and pale bodies lay at rest under a gray sky, all
surrounded by bloody rivers that carry dreams and hopes away
right under our feet. Grab your flash light of goals, and your
gym bag of tools my friend, you will need all the help you can
get when trying to save one of these failed attempts. The only
way to save these once strong soldiers of chalk and weight, is to
fall millions of feet down - lowering the bar just low enough for
one to grab on to your butt, back, bar, or whatever else the weak
hands can somehow hold onto. Yes you will see the castle, and yes
you might become one of them, but as weightlifters we never leave
a soldier down. We always keep pulling, pushing, and standing.

A deep breath, for deep is where we are going. Feet so close
your heels are almost touching, lining up your butt and calves
perfectly to bounce off of each other in the very bottom of the
deepest darkest depth of the squat. Without the bounce, you will
live in the castle, you will drink from the bloody rivers that
fill up from your own tears. Toes pointed out, directing your
knees away from the crumbling hotel on the journey down and up
called "missed lift inn". A place you never want to go. Your
knees will go in slightly no matter what, so by taking them out
wider than usual, the inn will not be the missed inn, but more of
the "made inn". The squat is a full commitment, the lower you go,
the better chance you will save an attempt. The lower you drop,
the faster you will rise. The faster you drop, the more your belly
(aka) "power belly" will kiss your thighs to help you stand up.
Yes I said it my friend, this is another trick from the tool box
that will improve your squat, and just another reason why I squat

with such a narrow stance. I call it the double bounce. 1.) butt
to calves. 2.) belly to thighs. The more narrower your feet, the
more bounce you will be able to create.

Your toes wiggle as if waving the weight away to your heels that
now crack the platform floor from its burden of importance. Your
back so arched that a waterfall has found a new home like moss
on a rock....nature has run its course perfectly. My heart hurts
many times throughout the day. You will not see this by watching
my videos, or by seeing me lift. The masked man that hides inside
of me pierces his thorn into my heart to remind me of the pain I
have left behind. By keeping my chest high during the squat, it
drains the pain downward toward the gray skied castle. Not only
do I save a dead attempt, but I leave behind bloody eyed demons
that bring me so much heartache. Goodbye masked man, hello stand.
Every time I stand, I feel more alive. Every time I save a lost
attempt, it brings me pride. I stand from a squat to someday get
the chance to fix the bricks that lay at rest, turn the river
into water, and the sky into blue. I hope to change my life and
others, one squat at a time.

Tools 2016

A Word on Depth:

In Weightlifting, whether it is at a local meet or on the Olympic stage, the
lowest man wins. You leave precious kilos on the platform every inch higher you
catch the barbell. That is why no one Power Snatches in the Olympics. Those
athletes are lifting weights so heavy that they need the ability to receive the weight
as low as humanly possible. Gold medals and record-breaking lifts would not be
possible without catching low with your ass two inches off the platform.

For the Snatch and Clean you will have two stances; a pulling and receiving
stance. Finding both are easy, and we are going to do it together right now so
stand up if you are not already. The receiving stance will be the same stance
you take when you Front or Overhead Squat. Move your feet out to that stance
and squat down as low as possible. Chances are unless you are an experienced
Weightlifter, what you **THINK** is low is not that low. Sink and let your hips
continue to drop down, feel out this position and if it does not feel quite right
make an adjustment. That is your receiving stance. Stand up, move both feet in
one inch each, that is your pulling stance.

Squat back down as low as possible again. What is holding you up? The
Earth, **stay down here with me and let us take a look at why.** At the bottom of

165

the Catch, your stomach should rest on your thighs, and your thighs rest on your calves. I call this the **Double Rest.** Here you are strong, stable and connected to the Earth, which in turn connects the weight to the Earth through you. That is why lifters such as Donny Shankle, Kendrick Ferris or myself can receive a 160kg Snatch and stay down there all day while we talk shit, take a nap or watch a movie. You need to be just as comfortable down in the bottom of the catch as we are.

Rock bottom in the Snatch is your friend, a haven, home. When you arrive there after pulling yourself under the bar, with the weight securely overhead, the lift is done. Conversely, catching the weight high at ninety degrees is the **DEVIL.** It is unstable and wobbly because of how far back the hips are pushed. **You should still be down here with me in the bottom, if not get your ass back down here!** Right now we are comfy, and all is good in the hood, but let's do an experiment. Rise up one inch and hold that position for a little while…**That is hard!** That is because now **YOU** are supporting the weight and not the Earth. Catching low, low, low is the only way to go, and you should be doing it often if you plan to be successful in this sport. Squatting does not exist in Weightlifting when you are performing the lifts. When you perform a Snatch or Clean, you are just catching low. Like squatting, there is no such thing as a Power Snatch; you are just simply catching higher. You can do that in the Olympics, but that would not be ideal because of how heavy the weight needed to win is in that environment. Catching heavy weight high is not impressive. Touching your ass to the platform is.

The Clean

The Front Rack is the catch location for the Clean. The weight being lifted here is so much heavier than in the Snatch. We need to bring it to the shoulders first before bringing the barbell overhead with the Jerk. If there is one thing, everyone in the Weightlifting world can agree upon it is the necessity of a safe front rack position. Unsafe front racks are a huge pet peeve of mine. I have seen too many teammates, and other lifters hurt themselves because they do not take the time to develop a solid front rack. If you do not possess the required mobility to catch weights safely on your shoulders then, you are putting yourself in a potentially dangerous situation.

If the elbows are low, you risk them coming into contact with the knees. Not only will this earn you three red lights in competition, but potentially a broken wrist as well. **This shit has to stop!** With all the resources available these days; there is no excuse to be in this sport and have mobility issues. Go take a Kelly Starrett seminar, buy his book and subscribe to his website. Even if you have a great front rack the potential for injury is still there. Other ways, to help keep yourself safe, are to wear a t-shirt instead of catching the barbell on bare skin. Also, chalk the bar, your neck, and shoulders. That is to prevent the barbell from slipping when you are sweating.

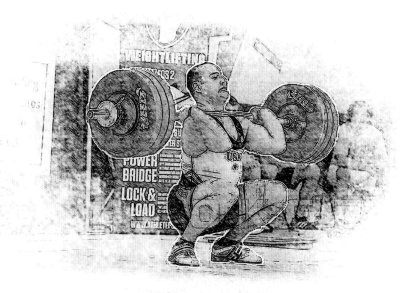

(Figure 10.3)

Position Standards:

- **Elbows:** They are high pointing to the horizon. Your upper arm is parallel to the floor.
- **Barbell:** Should be right up against your throat. It should practically be choking you. Every inch the barbell is caught forward down on the chest dramatically increases the likelihood of a missed lift.
- **Shoulders & Clavicles:** The more points of contact the better. With the barbell resting on the shoulders & clavicles, you will have an easier time driving into the barbell as you stand.
- **Hands:** Some lifters like me can keep a full closed grip on the barbell in the front rack. Others, who are not as flexible, allow the bar to roll back on the fingers a little with an opened hand.

Front Squats:

Once you have a safe front rack under your belt; you can start developing the bottom position of the Clean. Front Squats are an excellent tool that will strengthen your legs for heavy Cleans and make you more comfortable holding weight in the front rack. Now I will be honest with you. Front Squats are not something I typically use in my training. Almost every time I have tried to incorporate them, I end up hurting my lower back. The most noteworthy event occurred at the 2013 Arnold Classic. I was Front Squatting in the back room and severely tweaked my back. It was a major disappointment both to me and those who came out to watch me perform. If you are like me then, I suggest sticking to Back Squats. If you are lucky enough that Front Squats are no problem then use them. I recommend that for those of you who are flexible enough; to try holding the barbell with a full closed grip during the Front Squat. It will give you more points of contact when standing with the barbell, and that is what we want on the Clean. However, I do realize that not everyone can do this so try it, if it works keep it, if it does not then go back to what you did before.

Hotel California:

The bottom of the Clean is not your friend, it is a death trap. Just like in the famous Eagles song, once you check in, you may never leave! You need to catch the barbell and stand up immediately. That is so important that I even make it a point at my seminars that anyone, who pauses at the bottom of the Clean, will have to do Burpees. The weight is just too heavy to stay down there like we would in the Snatch. Instead, we need to use the oscillation of the bar to help us drive out of the bottom of the Clean. As the weight makes contact with your body in the front rack, it will oscillate.

Both ends of the barbell will bend creating what we call the **Frowny Face**. As the bar snaps up, it smiles, helping you to stand. It will help you all the way to ninety degrees…Then it will stab you in the back. That fucking bar will betray you and take your girlfriend (or boyfriend) too if you let it. If you find yourself in a situation where you are stuck at ninety degrees, stay calm. Go right back down to the bottom and try to bounce out of it again. That is entirely legal in competition. You need to get low. Lower will equate to more bounce and more bounce is everything in the Clean. If you are relying on just pure strength then, you risk not having anything left for the Jerk. The easier you make your Clean will in turn make the Jerk far less painful.

Common Errors in the Snatch:

- **Error #1 – Not pulling the barbell back behind the head:** A lot of lifts are missed by simply not placing the barbell in the correct spot. Typically this happens because lifters are either inexperienced or timid doing so.

  Coaching Cue: "Turtle Head!" or "Pull Back."

- **Error #2 - Tilting the chin up when receiving the weight overhead:** Tilting the chin up pushes the head back which will cause the arms and barbell to drift forward. That can potentially cause a missed lift in front of you. Every inch that the head moves back is an inch the bar will move to an undesired position.

  Coaching Cue: "Tuck the Chin."

○ **Error #3 – Missing the barbell in front:** A number of issues could cause this. If you are missing lifts in front of you frequently then you may:
  ○ Not be keeping the bar close enough to your body.
  ○ Not be bringing it back into the hips as much as you should.
  ○ Not committing to pulling under the bar.

○ **Error #4 – Missing the barbell behind:** This is the most desirable way to miss a lift. It shows that you tried to catch the weight, but a minor error in balance or timing needs to be adjusted.

Advice: Missing lifts can be frustrating. If you require help you can **A)** find a local Weightlifting Coach, **B)** take any Weightlifting seminar out there, **C)** film yourself online or email the video to Info@TheAttitudeNation.com. I would be more than happy to help you.

○ **Error #5 – Not catching the barbell low enough:** Start spending serious time down at the bottom of the catch until it is home.

Common Errors in the Clean:

○ **Error #1 – Low elbows in the catch:** When the elbows drop they take everything else with it. Posture crumbles, and now you are looking at the floor instead of at the crowd before the Jerk. Not to be a broken record, but it is also very dangerous.

Coaching Cue: "Elbows Up."

○ **Error #2 – Not racking the barbell fast enough:** The faster the elbows whip under the bar the faster you will complete the lift. Slow elbows can lead to a sloppy or unsuccessful catch.

Coaching Cue: "Violent Elbows."

○ **Error #3 – Spending too much time at the bottom of the Clean:** Make your stay in Hotel California very brief!

Coaching Cue: "Stand Fast."

Technique Drills:

Development of the bottom position is crucial to your success. I am not going to go into a great amount of detail on all the stretches, band exercises and the lacrosse ball mobility you can do. Kelly Starrett already has that covered. If

Weightlifting is important to you seek out his knowledge. However, what we will cover are just a few exercises that will help give you some flexibility for safety and more confidence at rock bottom.

Overhead Squat Stretch

The goal of this stretch is to loosen up tight areas in hips, knees, ankles and shoulders. Depending on where you have the most dysfunction you may feel it in a different spot than others do. To perform this stretch, you will need a partner and an empty barbell or dowel.

(Figure 10.4)

- O **Step One:** Move your hands out to the grip you would perform a Snatch with, your feet to your squat stance and bring the barbell overhead.
- O **Step Two:** Squat down as low as you can go and hold that position. Your partner will stand behind you to perform the stretch.
- O **Step Three:** Once you are at the bottom your partner is going to put one of their shins up against your butt so that you will not fall over during the stretch. They will also put one or both of their hands on the barbell to control its location.
- O **Step Four:** Holding the barbell and supporting you, your partner will then put their free hand on the small of your back and push down. You are keeping your arms locked out and trying to sink lower as they push your hips down. As someone's partner be sure to not push them forward on their toes. You want the hips to drop lower and lower progressively between the feet. If your partner focuses on pulling the bar back with their hands the stretch will be felt more in the shoulders.
- O **Step Five:** Repeat. You can hold this stretch for thirty seconds to a minute and then go back down and do it again.

Achilles Tendon Stretch

The Achilles Tendon Stretch is one of the most significant stretches a Weightlifter could do. I use it every time I warm up. It will help to develop comfort and balance in the bottom of the Catch. It will also assist in loosening up the ankles as well as the hips and knees to some degree. The ankles are often an enormous contributor of an inefficient bottom position. Flexibility down here allowing the knees to come forward while maintaining an upright torso is the hallmark of a Weightlifter. You can find a video of it on the Cal Strength YouTube channel called "Lower Body Flexibility for Weightlifting."

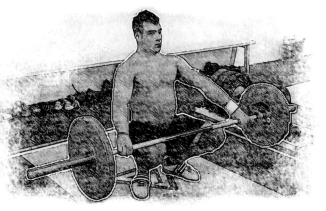 

(Figure 10.5)

- ○ **Step One:** Grab a barbell and squat down as low as possible.
- ○ **Step Two:** As you squat the barbell will slide down your thighs. Stop and allow it to rest on top of the knees.
- ○ **Step Three:** Hold this position, ideally with good posture. There is no sense in stretching while allowing poor mechanics elsewhere in the body. Teach your body now the place you want it to be in when in the bottom, from head to toe.
- ○ **Step Four:** As this becomes easier you can start to enhance the stretch. I like to roll the barbell slowly up and down my thighs a little to loosen up some of the tissue above the knees. I also like to push my knees forward and rock side to side searching for tight spots.
- ○ **Step Five:** Repeat.

Tigger Squats

The Tigger Squat is a fun way of easing your way down into the bottom of the Catch. It helps you develop trust in yourself that all will be okay when you land at the bottom with speed and a bar over your head. You will gain a small degree of strength when using even just the barbell. Trust, strength and finally learning how to move athletically in the Snatch will all help make you a well-rounded Weightlifter.

- **Step One:** Bring the barbell overhead into your Catch Position, move your feet to your receiving stance and squat as low as possible. Down here keep your body tight, arms locked out and your head up.

- **Step Two:** Start bouncing by raising your body up and down while keeping your feet planted on the ground. These are small, but violent bounces. Try not to come up too high yet because right now you are just learning to control the weight. As you bounce, the barbell should remain steady and not sway forward or back. Your body is bobbing up and down, and the barbell follows suit. Almost as if you are a puppet whose strings are being tugged on.

- **Step Three:** Once you start to become comfortable you can progress and add another piece. Begin with a few small bounces and then bounce higher and higher until you reach ninety degrees. From ninety degrees, drop down fast like an elevator and immediately bounce back out of the bottom.

- **Step Four:** You can add weight to this drill if you are ready for it, but ultimately it does not matter how much you can do here. I would never max out a Tigger Squat. Eventually, you can start to play around with shifting side to side, ducks walk or just simply holding the bottom. The easier this becomes, the more prepared you will be to pull under without hesitation.

- **Step Five:** Repeat.

Front Rack Stretch

One of my favorite exercises for improving the front rack is one that Coach Pendlay used to do with me all the time. There is even a video of it on the Cal Strength YouTube channel called "Upper Body Flexibility for Olympic Weightlifting." Grab a training buddy or coach to help you out.

- **Step One:** Setup a barbell in a squat rack.

- **Step Two:** Address the barbell as if you were going to Front Squat, but do not take it off the rack.

- **Step Three:** Your partner will stand facing you, lower their body a little bit and put their shoulders under your elbows. They will place their hands outside of yours on the barbell.

- **Step Four:** From here they will stand and drive their shoulders into your elbows pushing them higher. It is important that they keep their hips back

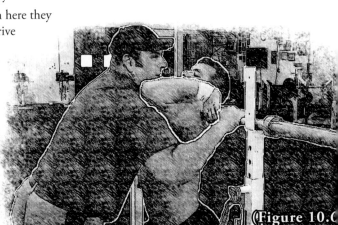

(Figure 10.0

to give themselves proper leverage in the stretch. This stretch can be intense so communicate if the stretching is too much.

○ **Step Five:** Repeat.

Jack Hammer Drill

The Jack Hammer drill is something fun I created messing around at the gym one day. Move slowly through this exercise and master one piece before moving on to the next because each piece builds upon the next. The drill can be viewed in my YouTube video "Vlog #6 Jack Hammer" at the 3:07 mark.

It will help you to do the following:

1. Feel the oscillation of the barbell.
2. Practice pulling yourself under the barbell.
3. Show you how the barbell springs back once it makes contact with the body. At the top of that spring, it peaks then you pull under.
4. Moving your feet as you pull under.

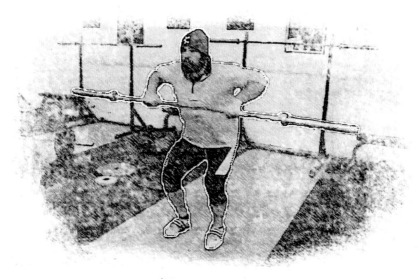

(Figure 10.7)

○ **Step One:** Hold a barbell with your Clean grip and squat down to about 90 degrees.

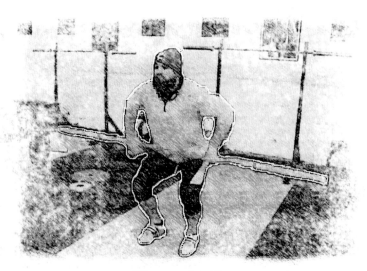

(Figure 10.8)

○ **Step Two:** Bend at the elbows and raise them up towards the ceiling as if you were operating a Jack Hammer. Push the barbell down and hit the upper thighs. As soon as you make contact allow the arms to bend again and raise the elbows for the next repetition. Continue to practice hitting and bouncing before moving to the next step.

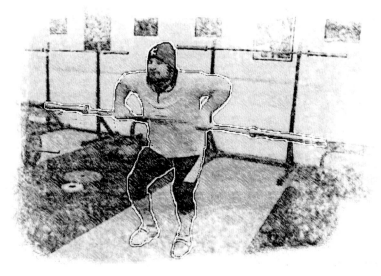

(Figure 10.9)

○ **Step Three:** Bounce the barbell off the thighs. When you feel the barbell is at its max height, pick your feet up and punch the elbows through to rack the bar. At the same moment, you should be picking up your feet and stomping them on the ground. That all happens in a very short amount of time. Your feet should slap the platform at the exact second the bar is being received on the shoulders. Continue practicing and working on your rhythm.

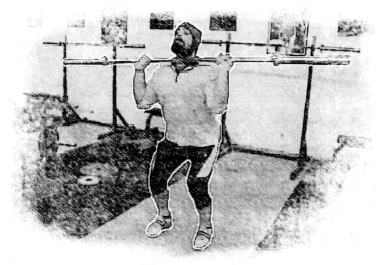

(Figure 10.10)

○ **Step Four:** If you are comfortable you can try bouncing the barbell off the thighs and letting go slightly. If you have done it correctly, you will be able to see the barbell floating in the air for a millisecond. Quickly, grab the barbell again and drive it back into the thighs for the next repetition.

○ **Step Five:** Repeat this drill as you begin to improve upon mastering barbell oscillation and pulling under.

CHAPTER 11:

ARCHED ANGEL

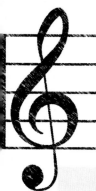

The Arched Angel

Tuesday, February 14, 2012

The way she bends makes you want to get under her...and fast. Her black wings open wide and her body stretches out as if she was being raised by God himself. A sudden pause in the gym occurs, a half second pause of beauty. A gust of wind hits the wide eyed watchers as they gaze upon her remarkable bent shaped arch. She rises higher and higher onto her toes as her hips come through like a 3D movie. Her shoulders are so far back that a cup could balance on her chest without spilling. Somehow, her eyes are still staring straight ahead, even though her body would tell you different. What a remarkable position. What a great athlete. A site that is kind on the eye, and would make a grown man cry from the beauty she holds. She is the Michael Jordan of weightlifting. Her finish is greater than Lance Armstrong finishing his race. Her arch is more famous than the golden arch we know so well from our childhood.

Her wings are now black from the hell she has been through, before weightlifting they were diamond white. Before weightlifting she could fly, now her back hurts so she only leaves the platform for a split second. Some call this (Ali Feet), and others say imprisonment. Every time the angel tries to fly home, the weight pulls her back down, like the Godfather trying to get out, but they keep pulling him back in.

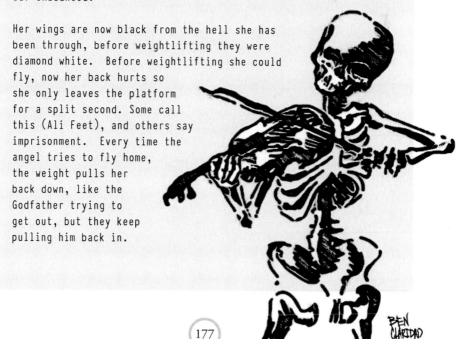

BEN
CLARIDAD

Yes Caleb Ward's video below shows he is
Married to her, but me.........I am married
WITH KIDS! ha! Get off me Caleb. Pause
around 26 seconds. Oh, and I almost got
kicked out of this meet for "exiting from
the front of the platform". I replied,
"Johnny Cash".

A kiss and leave relationship. How long do
you kiss before unlocking lips? This is
impossible for me to answer, only you and
her can figure this out. We need her; the
Attitude Nation must have her to succeed. We need her in this
sport to achieve greatness. Without love she would die, I would
die. She plays the part of my step mother, beautiful eyes and a
Julia Roberts smile. Hugs that smell like new car and a laugh
that dulls pain. She misses her old life with other angles, but
now she finds herself in a love web. One day she can fly home,
but not yet. First the Nation needs to make the Olympics; we need
her grace and her beauty to guide us to the "finish". We need
her strength and her confidence to catch the bar perfectly in the
pit of unsure. Her name is the Arched Angel, and she is in all
of us, even if you haven't met her yet. She will guide you to
the land of Pr's, especially for the weaker lifters who need her
most. Weak legged lifters like myself need as much torque, bend,
momentum, and lever as possible.....without it we would be nobody,
without her the weight would win. She is that half second of
peace in your life before you leave her all alone to venture in
the land down under, called the "catch". You miss her so dearly,
like your mother dropping you off at summer camp. Her black
wings reverse her body as she flies away, higher and higher still
keeping her eyes locked onto yours. Its not sweat, its her tears
that have fallen. This is what the audience doesn't understand.
A bond with a lift goes unseen by the judges, a love that is un
judge able. The flapping gusts of wind from her calloused wings
moves the hair on your head around like a rain storm, and your
eyes pierce with concentration from the harsh reminder that you
must move on, you must stand up. The Arched Angel is not the
fastest, nor the strongest, but the smoothest and most talented.
Getting on your toes in the finish with 166kg takes a guardian
with wings. Someone who understands you, just as much you

understand her. Sometimes she will help you; and sometimes she is
on her lunch break.

If you haven't seen her yet, then you are probably seeing the
scare crow. The scare crow is mean and unforgiving. He will make
you miss everything in front, and slow is his middle name. I call
him the evil V, V for vertical. He has no idea what explosive
means, he has no clue how to put on the Ali boxing gloves. V
is also very old. He was used way back in the day when a
weightlifter wasn't allowed to have any bar body contact. Yes the
V works great for that, but the sport has changed, and the Arched
Angel has arrived.

Her elbows point back as she lies wrapped on your lap feeding
you grapes. Her lips move across your face like a water skier on
glass. Her lips were once apple red and smooth like life before
weightlifting. But the very own Weightlifting that created her,
is the one killing her. The masked two faced sport has turned her
lips to more of a red whine than summer apple red, and her smooth
fresh silk sheet lips are now dry desert mountains, cracked and
bumpy. Forehead to forehead you gaze in each others eyes with
that half smile that speaks laughter and happiness. The hard part
about this dream world relationship is the unknowing that awaits
for you after the grapes are all eaten. Will you stand tall with
weight? Or will you stand tall empty handed?

My good friend and once team mate Caleb Ward
not only has a relationship with the Arched
Angel, but he is damn married to her!!
Pause around 1:02 I thought he was going to
do a back flip! In my opinion Caleb Ward as
top 5 best technique in the world. He takes
the spot for best athlete I have ever seen
up close and personal. You can't teach his
rhythm, speed, and power.

Caleb Ward 2016

The Arched Angel

The Arched Angel is a brief, yet powerful position within the lifts whose beauty can be elusive to the untrained eye. For the short moment it is performed, even the burliest, hairiest Weightlifter is a poetically winsome creature. It is emotional, graceful and stylish; literally ballet with the barbell. The Arched Angel was born from my time spent training under Weightlifting maestro Coach Jackie Mah. Her influence on my training is the reason this position is the closest thing you will find to triple extension in our method.

As the final phase of the Finish, the Arched Angel is the heart and soul of the Technique of Oscillation (Attitude Nation Catapult Method).

Developing the Arched Angel will help you:
- Complete the Finish by following through the barbell with the hips.
- Learn to extend the hip, knee and ankle joints to aid in power production.
- Learn to keep pulling back on the barbell to keep it close to the body.

The Snatch

Position Standards:

- **Feet:** When passing through the Arched Angel, you will very briefly raise up on your toes. That is a result of driving your hips through the barbell. The degree, in which this will occur is different depending on the individual. Although you are up on your toes, your is still shifted back toward your heels. That helps to balance the barbell and your body weight.

(Figure 11.1)

- **Knees:** The knees are slightly bent. That assist in positioning the hips in such a way that they can uppercut the barbell.

- **Hips:** The hips drive up and through (uppercutting) the barbell. The force produced here increases the barbell oscillation needed to peak the bar.

- ○ **Torso:** The Arched Angel requires a lot of layback of the torso. The shoulders will be orientated behind the barbell, a few inches from where they started in the Power Position. The angles of the hips and knees allow the torso to be oriented in this fashion.
- ○ **Elbows:** In-line with the shoulders. The elbows look like they are pointed back toward the wall behind you due to the layback of the torso.
- ○ **Head:** The head is neutral, and the gaze is straight ahead.
- ○ **Barbell:** The Bar itself never goes higher than the belly button. It also will not leave the hips throughout the finish until the very last second. It remains straight during the pull, then oscillates throughout the Power and Arched Angel positions and finally straightens again at the conclusion of the finish to allow the athlete to pull themselves under and receive the weight.

The Clean

One of my favorite stories about Arnold Schwarzenegger is about how he would look into the mirror before training and say "what do I need?" He would pick out parts of his body that were lagging behind the rest or areas that were already his strong suit, but could be even better. Then he attacked them. The same philosophy can be applied to Weightlifting especially on the Finish for the Clean. The Arched Angel will feel and look a little different in comparison to the Snatch. That is why you as an athlete need to take a step back, look at yourself in the mirror and ask "what do I need?"

Here are a few scenarios to aid you in troubleshooting the Finish if it is an issue on the Clean:

- ○ If you are someone who goes under the bar fast, you will probably need **LESS** Arched Angel.
- ○ If the barbell typically beats you down, then you are too slow, you need **MORE** Arched Angel.
- ○ Hip Cleaners usually need **LESS** Arched Angel as well because the barbell is being pulled so high. Just peak it and pull under.

Position Standards:

- ○ **Feet:** Identical to the Snatch.
- ○ **Knees:** Bent, but the angle created may be less pronounced depending on the amount of Finish you need as an individual.

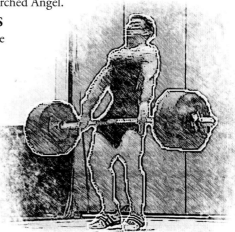

(Figure 11.2)

- o **Hips:** Identical to the Snatch.
- o **Torso:** Not as much layback as in the Snatch. The shoulders should still be behind the barbell.
- o **Elbows:** Identical to the Snatch.
- o **Head:** Identical to the Snatch.
- o **Barbell:** Will make contact with the upper thighs and go no higher than the groin. If you are a Hip Cleaner the bar will contact roughly the same spot it would on the Snatch and go no higher than the belly button.

Note: The grip is closer on the Clean. The point of contact is lower than it is on the Snatch depending on the style of Clean used.

Common Errors in Performing the Arched Angel:

The Arched Angel can be an awkward position to hold even without the barbell in hand. It is easy to make simple mistakes as you learn to balance. Avoid these errors so this crucial position can develop correctly.

- o **Error #1 – The hips are not coming through the barbell enough:** Typically a result of cutting the Finish short. These are fast movements, and inexperienced athletes think they have less time than they actually do. You need to be patient and fully drive the hips through the barbell before you go under.

  Coaching Cue: "Don't just hit the barbell, hit through it."

- o **Error #2 – Standing vertically on the toes:** This style of Finish requires athletes to have a greater degree of torso layback when being performed. An easy mistake to make is to rise on the toes with the knees fully extended. That causes you to be too upright resulting in the weight distribution of you and the barbell to be forward. If the knees are extended and the shoulders are directly on top of the bar then you know you are out of position.

  Coaching Cue: "Bend the Knees." Or "Layback."

- o **Error #3 – Pulling up with the arms:** Remember, the barbell is already going to raise off of the ground. That should not be your focus. Instead, pull the barbell **BACK** into your body. We do not want the elbows to point up toward the ceiling. Instead, they must be pointing to the wall behind you along with the shoulders. That helps you keep the barbell close and pull under with greater speed.

Coaching Cue: "Elbows Back."

○ **Error #4 – Shrugging up:** There is no reason to shrug up during the lifts. To do so is pointless because it slows down the speed in which you can pull under the barbell. Spend less time shrugging up and more time shrugging down. The traps should be tight and activated, but not raised up to your ears.

Coaching Cue: "Relax the Traps."

Drive THROUGH the Bar:

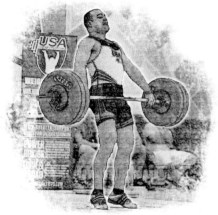 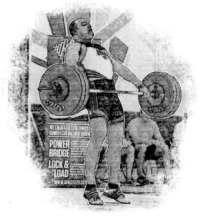

(Figure 11.3)   **(Figure 11.4)**

Weightlifters and Golfers share similar traits in their movement that are necessary for success in their sports. Both athletes must be accurate, efficient and focused. Golfers line up for shots, with their feet in roughly what we would call a squat stance. The ball is aligned in front of their body, centered between both feet. After lining up with the ball, they initiate the backswing (Superman Pull). The Golfer starts to swing the club (Superman Pause) and strikes the ball directly in front of them (Power Position). After making contact with the ball, they continue to swing **THROUGH** it (Arched Angel). That follow through in Golf is important because it helps to drive the ball to the hole. In Weightlifting, it is needed to peak the bar fully. Failure to do so is a mistake that rookies in both sports frequently make.

This can clearly be seen in **Figures 11.3** and **11.4**. In **Figure 11.3** my hips are still driving through the bar. To go under now would be a mistake. Instead, I need to be patient and continue to drive through and thus complete the Arched Angel before pulling under the bar. The full follow through of my hips can be seen in **Figure 11.4.**

It is important that you take the time to develop your relationship with the Arched Angel. I know her beauty can be intimidating, but once she is on your side, you will be unstoppable. Too many lifters out there cut the Finish short. They are too eager to go under the bar. Pulling the trigger early typically ends in misfortune. Let us not make that mistake. Get your shoes on rookie and practice, practice, practice!

Technique Drills:

Power Position → Arched Angel Drill:

Practicing the transition from the Power Position is necessary for the development of the Finish overall. It needs to be smooth and natural if we hope to be fast and powerful. You can eventually perform this drill with a dowel or barbell, but for now work with just your body.

- **Step One:** Assume the Power Position. Remember to have a vertical torso with your back tight, gaze ahead, arms & knees bent and body weight is 100% on your heels.
- **Step Two:** Transition into the Arched Angel as previously described. Make sure your shoulders and elbows are angled back. Your hands should be out wide as they would be in the Snatch and not be higher than the belly bottom.
- **Step Three:** Hold the Arched Angel and start to become comfortable here.
- **Step Four:** Reset to the Power Position.
- **Step Five:** Repeat.

Angel Drops
(Perform with no barbell first then progress to dowel or barbell)

You are doing very well! Your balance is improving, and Donny Shankle would be proud of how you are pulling the bar back into your hips. It is now time to complete the Finish and pull under the barbell. Before we do that though, there is just one additional thing I want to discuss. I cannot stress enough how necessary it is for you to **MOVE YOUR FEET**. Developing lifters often neglect to train their footwork, and this leads to a litany of problems. Since we rise on the toes, not moving the feet could potentially cause you to land or move under the bar with your body weight still supported by the toes. That creates a very unstable Catch position and puts you at risk of having what I call **Rocking Chair Feet**. That is where you land on the toes and then roll back onto the heels. Your balance will be negatively affected and the weight distribution of the bar overhead can shift too far forward. More than likely this will lead to a missed lift. What you want to happen is to go from the toes in the Arched Angel directly to the heels in the Catch.

The fastest way to go from the Arched Angel to the Catch is by being in mid air as you pull yourself under. You will move quicker for the same reason the bar is so fast on the way down after peaking; gravity. The barbell is weightless when it peaks, but you are not. You need Tyson hips to peak the barbell and knock that motherfucker out. Then you need Ali feet to pull under as fast as possible. While the barbell is peaking, it is a race to the bottom. You cannot let the bar beat you down there and a great way to practice is with the Angel Drop drill. It will teach you to move your feet, push harder through the platform and to have some patience before you pull under.

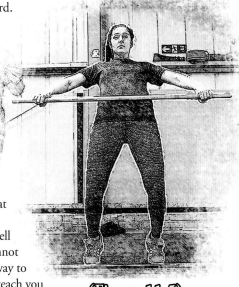

(Figure 11.5)

- ○ **Step One:** Assume the Power Position and then transition to the Arched Angel. Repetition is one of the best coaches you can have if the movement is done correctly. Be methodical in your movements and establish each position we have talked about first before moving on to the next. Blurring pieces together cheats you out of the valuable repetition you need to improve your skill.

- ○ **Step Two:** Hold the Arched Angel with all the desired points of performance previously discussed. We will also add a piece to the progression by having the barbell at belly button level. With the arms bent, pull the barbell back into your navel.

- ○ **Step Three:** When ready to drop into the Catch position lift your toes off the floor. Your goal is to land flat footed with your weight on the heels. You should hear a smacking sound from the impact of your

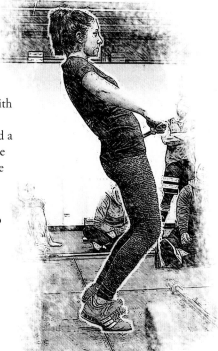

(Figure 11.6)

feet on the platform. That is why Weightlifting shoes were created. They provide you with a hard, stable surface to land on. If you bought a $200 pair of shoes and do not move your feet when lifting, you should return them and get a refund. Not moving the feet is the equivalent to putting on a belt, but not tightening it. At the same time, the forearms will turn over as you pull under the barbell receiving it in the Catch.

O   **Step Four:** Practice keeping the barbell as close as possible as you pull under it. The elbows are already bent and pointed back which will help with this. All you have to do is whip the forearms back as you go into the Catch.

O   **Step Five:** Stand and Repeat. The drill is comfortable when using just a dowel, but increases significantly with the barbell. When using a barbell, the fact that it is not also oscillating increases the difficulty of the drill. When you drop, the barbell is also trying to fall. You need to be fast, and you cannot cheat the barbell. It is too smart. If you are slow or do not keep the barbell close or come out of position, you will know right away. Move those feet and pull under!

Bar Contact Part 1.

Friday, December 28, 2012

I write to you later than usual tonight for one reason and one reason only, and that is concentration. A midnight write is purely a refection on "what the hell just happened today" kind of experience. Did I really punch a hole in the gym wall, or did I bottle my anger further down inside my gut for the release date from hell. Am I really the champ, or just some punk elementary school kid ding dong ditching throughout the streets of mini vans and culdesacs? Break a bar through the platform while the steam from my tea swirls around my white eyes. I write stories that have already come true before typing, but while typing, I try to reflect on what the flying space monkey really just happened, and did it? People tell me that a midnight read is just as relaxing, and just as spiritual. I tell them that I wouldn't know from the simple fact that I don't read. They ask me why I don't read as they look down upon my little body holding my small brain in my little hand. I look up and respond by saying, "I can't stay focused for more than one page, before having to go back and reread that same page over again to only find myself more lost than I was before reading that same page the first time".

I think about bar contact while having a midnight smoke outside, on my very cold deck with no shirt on. A shirtless lifestyle is how I choose to go about my life, and when I do decide to wear clothes they are black. Black like tonight, black like the gym walls, blacker than the devil in the red dress' eyes, blacker than rest. Nothing is blacker than rest. If it was up to rest, I wouldn't be outside constantly trying to figure out better and easier ways to lift the barbell over my big head. If it was up to rest, I wouldn't try these crazy ideas over and over again 'til coming to the conclusion I probably had too much coffee, but.... yes there is a but. But, if only one sticks, then just maybe I can lift more weight, and by lifting more weight, I could change the world by jumping off this cold white painted deck and simply start to fly. Because let's be real, flying is what we all want. Flying away to freedom, self reliance, control, decisions, and peace. This is what rest can't understand, and never will. This is how and why she single handedly ruins lives and weightlifting careers. She my friends, is the devil. Bar contact.....why so over looked? Why not talked about? A sad story is what this is to me, a story about a kid that never had a chance, overlooked and pushed to the side. I am in the making of putting together another hit and catch drill that I think will help many people, including myself, figure out better timing and a better relationship that we and the bar must have in order to lift more weight than we are lifting now. Just a tool, not a be all. Just another advantage that could possibly determine a win from a lose. Who really knows. Shit, I don't, I just try, lift, and do what works. If timed correctly, or whatever correctly actually is, let's say - if done well, then the bar will bend as if leaning your partner over in a dance while reaching for a kiss....and getting it. It's a beautiful feeling, and a better sight. This is how I have the weakest legs in USA weightlifting, but currently am the number one weightlifter in the country. But "they" don't speak about fight club.

Part 1.) The hit allows the bar to become motionless in outer space, like a monkey in a space suit floating around with no real panic or concern. The monkey just is, like the steam from my tea, or the smoke from my smoke. Now we are allowed to use the bar as if the bar was connected to the wall. The bar is not moving up nor down, it is paused like YouTube. Now we meet the wonderful world of physics, a world that allows us to pull, no wait...whip ourselves under the bar to catch, NOT squat catch, but simply catch. The next time I hear the term squat snatch, I'm going to jump and not be so lucky to fly. This is why I disagree personally with the triple extension, aka the scare crow. Pulling yourself down on an upward moving bar, limits the athlete's torque under the bar. The athlete will therefore, move slower under, catching the bar too high, and we all know that 90 degrees is the underworld waste land of bad balance and a constant fight between you standing up and the bar slamming down upon your rocky position. The faster you get under, the lower you will catch the bar, the lower you catch the bar, the more weight you will lift. Leading us back to one simple rule, we're not supposed to talk about fight club.

Part 2.) Next week.

Fight Club 2016

The Hit and Catch

We have been building a foundation. The middle and end positions of the Finish have been developed along with the Catch. That allows us to move our bodies in conjunction with the demands of Weightlifting. With the fundamental understanding of how these positions work in our method of technique; we can now discuss the paramount topic of bar body contact. My favorite method of teaching athletes how to make contact with the barbell when performing the lifts is my Hit and Catch Drill.

I created this drill while training at California Strength. At first it was just something I would do in warm-ups. I liked to bounce the bar against my hips to feel the oscillation. Eventually, I began to see the teaching value in what I was doing and decided to introduce the Hit and Catch to my personal clients. You can still go on YouTube and find the original videos that sparked the creation of the Technique of Oscillation (Attitude Nation Catapult Method). Just search for "Hit and Catch" or scan the QR code to the right.

Your senses of feeling, hearing and seeing are valuable tools that will help you utilize this drill efficiently and develop bar body contact. As an athlete, you can use all three to determine if your movement is correct. As a coach, you can gather information on your athlete by either seeing or hearing the drill being performed.

Feel

Will it hurt when my hips hit the barbell? That is a common concern of those who are starting to develop a catapult style of Weightlifting. First, in regards to the drill, if you bring the barbell and hips together at the same rate of speed and to a common meeting point; the Power Position, it will not hurt badly. Imagine, for example, two Football players; linemen crouched down ready to crush one another. The offensive lineman is the barbell, and the defensive lineman is your hips.

The amount of pain that is inflicted on the opposing player depends on who was faster off the line of scrimmage. That is desirable in Football, but not Weightlifting. For success in our sport we want both players (the hips and barbell) to go into motion at the same time and rate of speed. Both objects create equal force by traveling the same distance and meeting in the middle. If one of those powerful behemoths stalls or does not move they will be plowed over, which leads to pain. For example, if the hips (defensive lineman), does not move then the barbell will crash into them leading to a painful experience. On the other hand, if the barbell (offensive lineman), does not move the hips will be forced to overextend. I call this the **Skydive Finish.** It is where an athlete hops forward because they are searching for the barbell with the hips instead of pulling it back into their body.

We want a common meeting point of the hips and bar, but we also need to row the barbell back into our hips forcefully. Rowing the bar back into your hips harder will reduce the pain you feel because it will produce more oscillation. More oscillation means the impact of the bar body contact will be adsorbed primarily by the barbell instead of your hips. This is why I teach the Early Arm Bend – too many people are timid at the Power Position phase at the lift. Row that bar back into you **VIOLENTLY!**

With frequent practice, you can train your body to become numb to the sensation of the barbell contacting the hips. I cannot one hundred percent guarantee bar body contact will not be uncomfortable in the beginning. The trick I used early in my career was to tuck a piece of carpet into the front of my shorts. It helped to reduce the tenderness that was a result of Snatching every single day. Overall, do not be timid. Bring the hips and barbell together like you mean it. Practice the Power Position and Arched Angel transition to smooth out your Finish. Ask yourself, "Do I want to be a Weightlifter?" If the answer is yes then stop complaining, suck it up and lift the bar.

Hear

When you strike the barbell, you should hear a dull "thud" sound instead of a "rattle." A rattle indicates that you hit the barbell incorrectly. The hips more than likely came through more than you pulled the barbell back. Pull it back into yourself harder. The sounds heard may also depend on the type of equipment you are using. For example, most regular bars will give off a slight rattle even if you do bring hips and barbell together at precisely the right spot and rate of speed. However, the more expensive the barbell, the less prominent the sound will be. A $5,000 Eleiko bar will be as quiet as a mouse when you make contact.

See

What you see during the Hit and Catch drill can also cue you into whether or not you are doing it correctly. First, if the arms are relaxed after the hit, you should be able to see the barbell float in front of you as it peaks. Second, if you are using a higher quality barbell, you will see it oscillate after contact has been made. That $5,000 Eleiko bar will wobble back and forth like a piece of rubber in your hands. These are both good indicators that you are performing the movement correctly and can help you develop your timing for the Catch.

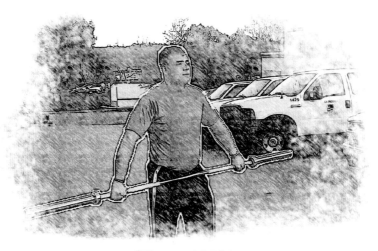

(Figure 11.7)

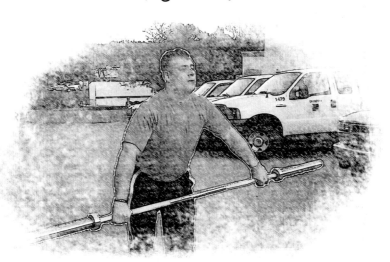

(Figure 11.8)

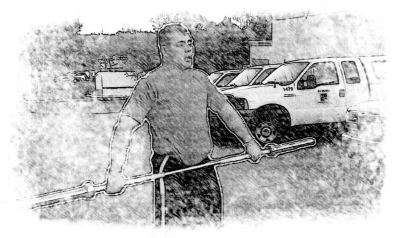

(Figure 11.9)

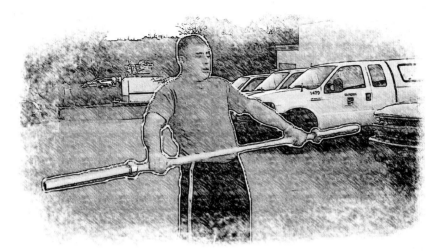

(Figure 11.10)

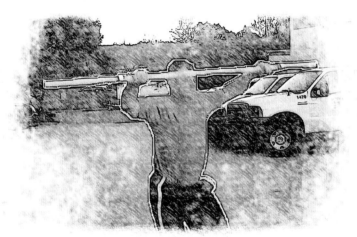

(Figure 11.11)

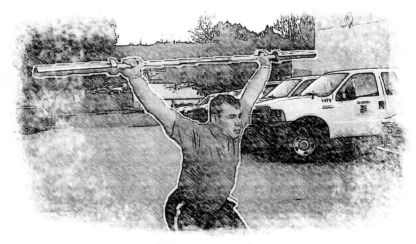

(Figure 11.12)

It is essential that you develop rhythm and timing before you start crushing big weights. You must be **patient** and then **VIOLENT!** Many of the drills we use to develop a rhythm will require you to pause at various points. That is where you need to be patient. When we take the pauses out of the drill that is where you unleash hell on the barbell. Our first step in the Hit and Catch is to practice creating space between our body and the barbell. If we think back to the game of Golf, here we are learning to line up a shot.

Part One: Using the Arms.

- **Step One:** Assume the Power Position. As seen in **Figure 11.7**.
- **Step Two:** While staying in the Power Position we need to load the barbell away from the body. Using only the arms, perform a front Delt raise. Move the barbell away from your hips only 3-4 inches. Nothing else on your body will move, and the barbell will travel in a straight line away from the hips. As seen in **Figure 11.8** (in the photo the knees move as well. Right now focus on just the arms and we will discuss the knees in the next part of the drill).

  Coaching Cue: "Out."

- **Step Three:** Pull the barbell back into the hips. There will be a slight bend in your arms. Think about angling the elbows back as well. Never pull straight up. As seen in **Figure 11.9**.

  Coaching Cue: "Back."

- **Step Four:** Pause briefly at each step feeling out the movement.
- **Step Five:** Repeat this process until you are capable of staying stable in the Power Position and only move the arms to load the barbell in front of you.

Part Two: Using the Knees.

- **Step One:** Assume the Power Position.
- **Step Two:** Bring the barbell "out" using just the arms.
- **Step Three:** The knees are bent when in the Power Position, and the hips are low. To load our bodies, we will push the knees back. When that happens, the hips rise slightly higher. The barbell should not move down the thighs. It should instead stay right where the arms put it. As seen in **Figure 11.8**.

  Coaching Cues: "Load" or "Knees Back."

○ **Step Four:** Transition back to the Power Position. Push the knees forward, drop the hips and bring the bar back into the body. As seen in **Figure 11.9**.

Coaching Cues: "In."

Part Three: Arched Angel Rhythm.

Once you develop rhythm loading the barbell out from the hips and back again we can now come full circle and put it together with the Arched Angel.

○ **Step One:** Assume the Power Position.
○ **Step Two:** Repeat Part 1.
○ **Step Three:** Repeat Part 2.
○ **Step Four:** Once you move back to the Power Position you then need to perform a second transition into the Arched Angel. As seen in **Figure 11.10**. Please note that the photo in **Figure 11.10** is of an "action shot." When practicing with pauses it would be best to raise up into the same position practiced in the Angel Drop drill. When we take out the pauses it will look more like it does in the photo.

Coaching Cue: "Arched Angel."

○ **Step Five:** Hold the Arched Angel for a few seconds then lower back down into the Power Position. Repeat this process making all of the transitions as fluid as possible.

Part Four: Patience then Violence.

Now it is time to take out all of the pauses. Just because the pauses are removed does not mean we need to go fast. You will not see Tiger Woods going crazy on his back swing. Everything is smooth, yet powerful at the same time. Mistakes happen when you rush.

○ **Step One:** Assume the Power Position.
○ **Step Two:** "Out." The bar moves out, and the knees move back.
○ **Step Three:** "In." Pull the bar back in while simultaneously pushing the knees forward to arrive at the power position.
○ **Step Four:** When the barbell is in the hips, perform a Snatch.

Coaching Cue: "Go!"

○ **Step Five:** Finally, after repeating Step Four a few times. Load the barbell "out," then on "Go!," Implement all that we have been learning up to this point. Transition through the Power Position. Bring the bar back into you while driving the hips through. Pass through the Arched Angel. Pick up your feet, pull under As seen in **Figure 11.11** and Catch the barbell As seen in **Figure 11.12**. Stand and repeat.

Slingshot Drill
(Hit and Catch Drill with a Partner)

After mastering the transition between the Power Position and the Arched Angel, you can begin working on an advanced variation of the Hit and Catch drill called the Slingshot. This drill is intended to teach you how to balance in this position, continue to pull the barbell back into the body and resist the forces of gravity to avoid the error of a Skydive Finish. The weight in your hands wants to pull you forward. Your partner will help to simulate what it feels like to be holding a heavy weight that gravity is trying to pull down to the floor.

○ **Step One:** Assume the Power Position and load the barbell "out" (as you would in the Hit and Catch drill) and hold the position.

○ **Step Two:** Your partner will stand in front of you and grab the barbell; holding it in the area just inside of your hips. As seen in **Figure 11.13**.

○ **Step Three:** Your partner will gently apply force and pull the barbell toward them as you resist.

○ **Step Four:** Resist your partner by engaging your lats and pulling the bar back into your hips. Holding the Superman Pause position while someone pulls on the bar will be difficult. It may take some time to find your balance here, but you need to keep your weight shifted back towards your heels; although your partner is trying to pull you forward. Do this a few times to become accustomed to your partner working against you. Then eventually you can progress to your partner, without warning, letting go of the barbell. When this happens you will perform the Hit and Catch. As seen in **Figures 11.14, 11.15** and **11.16**.

○ **Step Five:** Repeat.

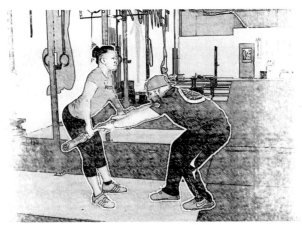

(Figure 11.13)

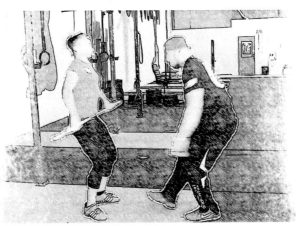

(Figure 11.14)

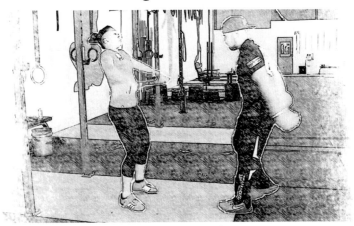

(Figure 11.15)

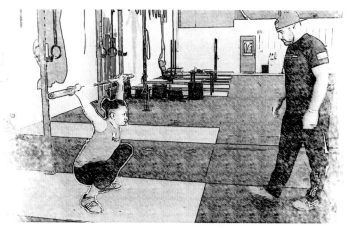

(Figure 11.16)

Common Errors in Performing the Hit and Catch:

The Hit and Catch is just a tool to teach you how to make bar body contact. It is not a replication of what we think will actually happen during the lifts. In real life, the bar will not be right in front of the hips as in the drill. Instead, you would more than likely activate the Double Knee bend much earlier around the mid-thigh. The Hit and Catch is also not the same thing as a High Hang Snatch. That is an entirely different exercise, and I have never done a max effort Hit and Catch. Treat it for what it is, a drill, and avoid making the following mistakes.

○ **Error #1 – Not pushing the knees back:** The knees not going back will cause the hips to come through too early. You will not meet the bar in the Power Position, which can lead to the Sky Dive Finish.

Coaching Cue: "Knees Back."

○ **Error #2 – Allowing the barbell to drop:** The bar needs to travel out in a perfectly straight line away from the hips that is parallel to the floor. The barbell will drop too low if the shoulders are loose or the chest drops. Correct it by pulling the shoulders back and lifting the chest a little higher.

Coaching Cue: "Shoulders Back" or "Chest Higher."

○ **Error #3 – Trying to move too fast:** Slow down rookie. You need to hit rep after rep of entirely controlled movement. Then as you become proficient you can gradually add speed.

Coaching Cue: "Patience and then **VIOLENCE!**"

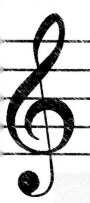

CHAPTER 12

SUPERMAN

Double Knee Bend

Friday, August 17, 2012

Knees back.... then "crack"! Extend them like a long stay at
a 20 dollar motel in a rainy city called Eugene. "Release the
Crackin!" Release the double knee bend only when it's time. The
longer Superman flies, the longer the knees glide back, well......
the more, let's say, bang for your buck you're going to get in
the ever so lovely Arched Angel (finish). The Superman (pull) and
the Arched Angel are like a family, that may at times separate for
training purposes, but always meet back up for a glass of warm
eggnog during the cold and windy time of Christmas. A family who
works like dominoes, a family who depends on each other to make
the lift complete. Once the weight breaks and the sun rises, they
all rise, one after another. Raising their hands high while miss
brown eyes pumps through their blood singing the song your mother
always sang you in the morning, "good morning to you, good morning
to you, you look like a monkey and smell like one too."
You know the saying, "Don't bring bent knees into
a weightlifting fight". You better have those
knees pushed back and almost extended. If
you want a full tank of gas then this must
happen. Your pull..... wait, I
hate this word. Your set up for
the finish, must take patience
and timing. I say set up because
that's all the pull is, nothing
more, nothing less.

Yes, this is art, and
yes, it's a sight to
see, but even more
of a sight to witness. NASA
has nothing on his always
double powered bend, creating

BEN
CARIDAD

the Angel we call Arch. Yes, double is her father, and his tear
stained brown leather jacket can show proof of their feelings
to one another. This brown jacket I speak of has much meaning
and importance to me, but I won't go into it in this blog, maybe
another time. I have been writing too much about my father
lately. I don't want to be "that guy". But back to what I was
saying. Just like this song that sings into my ears while we bath
in a pond of coffee like childhood memories of summer camping with
the family. It's like the high hang, once you know the man and
his mustache, then you easily welcome him into your home. But the
double knee bend is left out in the rain, not welcome for chat.
It is the backbone that goes unnoticed and covers his head with
a newspaper and walks off. The double knee bend is there, and
always carries his mighty and powerful self around with a smile,
but he never gets invited to the social parties that others like
the Arched Angel and the Superman pull get to attend. Mr. double
spends most of his time reading up on the good he does in this
sport at his local pancake house. The waitress he smiles at so
nicely fills his coffee cup up for the fourth time. Hmm a movie,
this could be a movie. I should write a movie. A movie about a
lonely man, the end. It's perfect. It's my kind of movie. Nothing
fancy, just an emotional picture of a man that does so much, but
for some reason has gone unnoticed. But then again maybe it's the
double knee bend's fault. Every time he gets mentioned nothing
good comes of it. Athletes start thinking too much. When athletes
think too much, or at all, things go south, and fast. I guess he
is like the, "Which foot do I jerk with?" asking person.   The
jerk foot has no say, the athlete will step correctly without even
thinking. Bam.... correct. Bam boom now slam the bar. Now grab
your gold medal and run down the middle of the street free as a
bird. Isn't this thought alone why we do this? Freedom?

Push your knees back even more, even more, go on....yes...even
more. Now release the hell you have kept inside you for all these
years. Patience is the hardest part of this sport. Hands down.
Game over. Mixing your mashed potatoes with your green beans is
bad. Just like in the pull and finish. The pull and finish are
two different sports. Don't combine them, never. Set up, then
attack. A bike chain plays in my mind as I take another chug of
this coffee, while half of it drips down the side of my mouth. I
say bike chain because everything should move in the pull like

200

it's connected to a chain, moving all together. Then once you have reached the end of your cul de sac and you parents won't let you wonder any farther, it's time for the finish.

I write to you tonight about this because it's something that has been bothering me. Knees are not being pushed back enough, creating a "fish out of water finish". A pull and pray finish that only leads to lose teeth and up all nights. I write you about this because to be honest, I haven't written a technique blog in quite some time, and I guess I feel the need to throw out my two cents. I don't want to bore you with too many of my personal stories and emotional blogs about drugs, fathers, and coffee. I love technique. I love studying technique and improving my craft everyday. I love painting a picture of a perfect weightlifter.... or at least trying to paint it. I find this sport memorizing, intriguing, and fascinating. The way our bodies move to achieve something so simple, is far from simple. A ballet of muscles. A double knee bend lifestyle.

I have much more to say about technique, much, much more. I am sick and tired of seeing how all these crossfiters and weightlifters are being taught how to lift. It's a scam. That's why I have taken my mad scientist briefcase, notes, and travel size coffee cup with me all over the world to spread the way one should snatch and clean and jerk. It is not the 1930's anymore. Salute.

Incase you missed the live show, here is the link below to listen in to this weeks Weightlifting Talk with guest appearances Travis Cooper and Tom Sroka.

The King 2016

The Superman Pull, traditionally called the first pull, is the activation of an extremely late Double Knee Bend. The Double Knee Bend occurs after the barbell has passed the knees, and it is how we initiate the Finish. The act, of breaking the barbell from the floor and guiding it to our hips, sets the tone of the whole lift.

In our method, everything we do is purely to hit the barbell. We spend a lot of time learning technique from the foundation of the Power Position. It is truly a significant position that we have to start with when teaching. However, I believe in the grand scheme of things that the Pull is more important. That is because if something goes wrong along the barbell's journey from the floor the entire lift is at risk of failure. Losing back tension, being pulled forward by the weight or incorrect timing can all negatively affect your leverage for the Finish. Bottom line, the pull is so much more than just gripping the barbell and standing. One error sets off a chain reaction causing another in the next position.

Developing the Superman Pull will help you:
- ○ Set yourself up for success in the Finish.
- ○ Fine tune the transition point of the barbell when around the knees.
- ○ Develop your style of initiating the lifts with a Dynamic Start.

The Snatch

Attitude Nation Position Two:

Since we have an understanding of how to move from the Power Position, we can now gradually lower the bar to the floor. Progressively, we move the barbell to two final positions and perform Snatches from each of them. Our first stop, in building the Superman Pull, is the Attitude Nation Position Two. It is located just below the knees. To arrive there, we need first to start at the Power Position. Let the barbell slide down your thighs and lower your hips. The barbell will arrive just below your knee caps.

- ○ **Heels:** Your weight is 100% still on your heels.
- ○ **Hips:** are low in a squatting position, but we are not yet at the very bottom. Stay tight and **HOLD** this position.
- ○ **Back:** is tight and arched. Shoulder blades are pinched together.

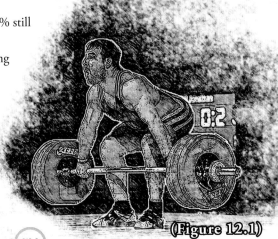

(Figure 12.1)

- **Shoulders:** are directly on top of the barbell.
- **Arms:** Should be slightly bent.
- **Gaze:** is looking straight ahead, and you have a broad chest.
- **Bar:** is below the knees, and you are actively pulling the bar back.

The Clean

- **Heels:** Identical to the Snatch.
- **Hips:** Identical to the Snatch.
- **Back:** Identical to the Snatch.
- **Shoulders:** Identical to the Snatch.
- **Arms:** Identical to the Snatch.
- **Gaze:** Identical to the Snatch.
- **Bar:** Identical to the Snatch.

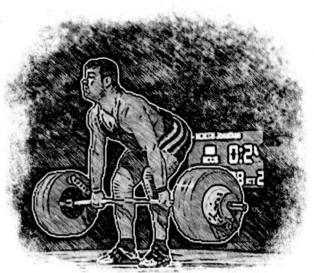

(Figure 12.2)

Common Errors at Position Two:

- **Error #1 – Having the shoulders in front of the Barbell:** This is such a common error that even I do it frequently and have been working on correcting it for quite some time. Keeping the shoulders on top of the bar helps us stay over longer later on in the pull. When I say on top of the bar, I mean you should be able to draw a straight line from your shoulders directly down to the barbell below. Dropping the hips will help you pull the shoulders back with practicing this position. During the lifts try to keep the hips low longer.

  Coaching Cue: "Drop the Hips."

- **Error #2 – Shifting your body weight forward to your toes:** Typically this happens when the barbell loses contact with the leg below the knee. In our Position Two, we need the barbell to be pressing into the the lower knee cap. Note: this only occurs when drilling this position. In real life the bar will not touch the knees.

  Coaching Cue: "Pull the Bar Back."

The Superman Pull:

If the Arched Angel is the literal beating heart of our method, then the Superman Pull is the blood that flows through it. Without it, the heart cannot beat. The hips are high; the knees are back, and the shoulders are over and in front of the barbell. You can begin to practice the Superman Pull starting at the Attitude Nation Position Two.

The Snatch

Position Standards

- O **Knees:** The knees are back, almost completely extended.
- O **Hips:** Have risen from Position Two moving to their highest point before the Double Knee Bend is initiated.
- O **Shoulders:** Are out in front of the barbell.
- O **Arms:** Should be slightly bent.
- O **Back:** Is completely arched.
- O **Barbell:** The bar has ascended to the mid thigh. For most people, this is the highest the bar will go to in the pull before the Double Knee Bend is initiated.

(Figure 12.3)

The Clean

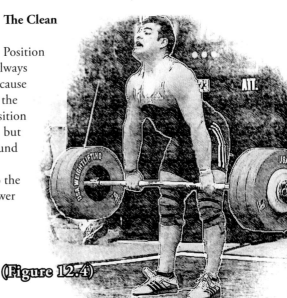

Practicing the transition from Position Two to the Superman Pull is not always necessary for the Clean. That is because the distance from Position Two to the Power Position is so short. Use Position Two at the beginning with pauses, but then when adding speed I have found it is best to skip ahead to Position Three. From there transitioning to the Superman Pause, and then the Power Position creates a longer Pull.

(Figure 12.4)

- ○ **Knees:** Identical to the Snatch.
- ○ **Hips:** Identical to the Snatch.
- ○ **Shoulders:** Identical to the Snatch.
- ○ **Back:** Identical to the Snatch.
- ○ **Arms:** Identical to the Snatch.
- ○ **Barbell:** Identical to the Snatch.

Technique Drills:

Superman Pause Drill

The transition of the barbell from below the knee to above the knee can be tricky. It can be easy to straighten the knees and raise the bar, but the chest is often left behind. That leaves you in a bent over Deadlift position. Instead, we want the chest to rise as well with the barbell.

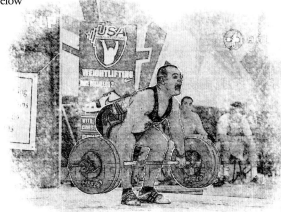

- ○ **Step One:** Start in the Power Position and then lower the bar down to Position Two. Hold this position for a few seconds. As seen in **Figure 12.5**.

(Figure 12.5)

- ○ **Step Two:** To perform the Superman Pull, push the knees back while simultaneously raising the hips, chest and the barbell until the bar arrives at the mid thigh. As seen in **Figure 12.6**.

- ○ **Step Three:** This is the Superman Pause; hold this position a few seconds. While you are here and as the barbell travels up from the floor to the hips for that matter; the barbell should never touch you. Instead, there will be a small space between the barbell and your thighs.

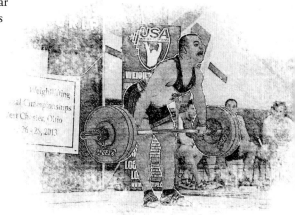

(Figure 12.6)

- **Step Four:** Bend the knees, drop the hips and transition back into Position Two.
- **Step Five:** Repeat.

Hit and Catch from Position Two:

The next step in our progression, after you have practiced the transitions around the knees, would be to Snatch or Clean from Position Two. I have found it extremely useful to coach my athletes simply to Hit and Catch from Position Two. Make the transition, hit and catch, and that is almost the complete movement.

- **Step One:** Assume the Power Position.

Coaching Cue: "Position One."

- **Step Two:** Lower the barbell down to Position Two.

Coaching Cue: "Position Two."

- **Step Three:** Push the Knees back, and perform the Superman Pull. Pause here momentarily feeling out the position.

Coaching Cue: "Superman."

- **Step Four:** Initiate the Double Knee Bend and perform the hit and catch to Snatch or Clean.

Coaching Cue: "Go!"

- **Step Five:** Eventually, remove the pauses and repeat the drill.

Attitude Nation Position Three:

Finally, we arrive below the knees for the Attitude Nation Position Three! It is here that the first domino falls over, starting a chain reaction leading from one phase of the lifts to the next. Just like the rest of our method, the way we setup on the barbell is extreme. Interestingly enough, in competition, the lifts do not officially start until the barbell passes the knees. You could begin the pull, stop and put the bar down if you wanted to. Although the rule book states this, we should not overlook the importance of a proper start position.

- **Hips:** They are as low as possible. Think back to the very beginning where we discussed the philosophy of our Catapult system, **The Philosophy of Opposites**. We start low but then go high in the Superman Pull with a late double knee

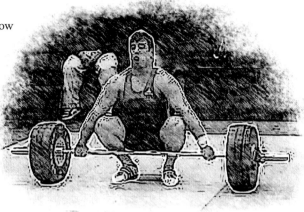

(Figure 12.7)

bend. If you begin with the hips already high then it will equate to an earlier double knee bend than what is desired in **THIS** style of lifting. That is because the knees are already back if the hips are high thus shortening your pull.

- **Torso:** It is as vertical as possible and arched.
- **Shoulders:** They are behind or directly on top of the barbell. The further you can move them back the better. We want to keep the shoulders back and over the bar for as long as possible until we are ready to go over.
- **Barbell:** It is now located lower on the leg at the mid shins. It should be in contact with the shins until the lift is initiated.

Back. Over. Back. Through:

In regards to the shoulders think **Back. Over. Back. Through** or **B.O.B.T** for short. At the beginning of the pull, the shoulders are **back** behind the bar, but once the hips and knees move the shoulders go **over** the bar. When it is time to initiate the Finish, the shoulders, move **back** behind the bar again as you pass through the Power Position and into the Arched Angel. As we pull ourselves under, we are not necessarily pulling only down, but **through** as well. Down, like up, is going to happen, but back and through are the little things that when neglected can lead to missed lifts.

Common Errors in Performing the Superman Pull:

- **Error #1 – Not maintaining a vertical Torso:** As Donny always says "Your chest must face the audience so they can see how hard you have worked."

    Coaching Cue: "Set your back."

○ **Error #2 – Performing a stripper pull:** Quite possibly one of the biggest mistakes beginners make, is lifting the butt high in the air, but forgetting to let the chest and torso rise as well.

Coaching Cue: "Lift the Chest - or -
Move everything together as though it is all connected."

Technique Drills:

Learning to Pull Back: Part Three - Rowing Drill
(You will need a partner)

Throughout the pull, the barbell is always traveling back into you. The very first drill you learned was on how to pull the bar back into your body. That can be found in the Power of Position chapter of the book. This drill is critical and is probably one you should often revisit. As you pull it from the floor, the bar does not travel straight up. It moves back into your body. The entire pull you are actively rowing the bar close to your body by gradually bending your arms. That is why it is so important to have a strong back in Weightlifting. If you do not, or the back is loose as you pull, then you run the risk of the bar coming out in front too much which will likely result in a missed lift. Keeping the back tight, and barbell close will increase the chances of making a lift.

○ **Step One:** Perform the original Pull Back drill and focus on feeling your back muscles engage.
○ **Step Two:** Setup with a barbell in Position Three as if you were going to perform a Snatch.
○ **Step Three:** Have a partner hold a PVC Pipe or dowel so that it is perpendicular to the floor touching one end of the barbell you are holding.
○ **Step Four:** Initiate the pull moving to Position Two and then the Power Position. As you do this, the barbell should move away from the PVC pipe your partner is holding and back towards your body. Once you start your pull the barbell should never touch the PVC pipe again.
○ **Step Five:** You can continue to perform this drill eventually adding weight to strengthen your pull

Hit and Catch from Position Three:

The big moment is finally here. We are going to put all the positions we have been working on; all the technique developed and perform the complete lifts. Again, it is best to think about performing the Hit and Catch from Position Three. Pause at each position to reinforce your movement patterns.

○ **Step One:** Assume the Power Position.

> **Coaching Cue:** "Position One."

○ **Step Two:** Lower the barbell down to Position Two.

> **Coaching Cue:** "Position Two."

○ **Step Three:** Drop the hips even further and assume Position Three. The bar should be at the mid shins.

> **Coaching Cue:** "Position Three."

○ **Step Four:** Push the Knees back, and perform the Superman Pull. Pause here momentarily feeling out the position.

> **Coaching Cue:** "Superman."

○ **Step Five:** Initiate the Double Knee Bend, Hit and Catch thus performing the Snatch or Clean.

> **Coaching Cue:** "Go!"

○ **Step Five:** Eventually, remove the pauses and repeat the drill.

THAT right there is the Technique of Oscillation (The Attitude Nation Catapult Method). **YOU** are the catapult, and the bar is the rock. Once in the Superman Pause position (end of the Pull); if there was a handle sticking out of your back between your shoulder blades all I would need to do is slam it down. In that perfect Superman Position, the knees are back; hips are high; barbell is mid-thigh, back is tight, and the chest is facing the audience. **WHAM!** I slam down the handle. **WHAM!** The Knees come forward, hips drop and now you are in that perfect Power Position. **WHAM!** Tyson hips uppercut the bar and drive through. **WHAM!** The Arched Angel spreads her beautiful white wings, and you finish. **WHAM!** With lightning speed, those Ali feet move - Go Under and Through. **WHAM!** The weight of the world is over your head - Stand. **WHAM!** Slam that fucking bar.

Dynamic Start

Rock back then release. Churn your body up and down 'til the
butter is ready. Become a seagull violently dropping down to
snatch its prey. Open your mouth wide to inhale strength and
confidence, only to exhale all of your fears. Yell so loud that
your voice echoes back to the classroom you failed so badly. Let
everyone know before breaking the weight from the floor that you
have already broken from the path you once walked upon. Move
before moving. Move my friend, and never let anyone get in your
way. Gain speed to break through the wall of life. Add momentum
to your pull to pull off greatness in this sport. Gain power in
this life to shut the trolls up that stay hidden away in a cave
full of super hero posters that they somehow can't figure out how
to become. Oh yes, I lift with massive energy and a massive heart.
So much anger it could kill an elephant. So much passion it could
make Juliet kill herself. I write with a violin that speaks way
more words than I could ever speak. I listen to this song that
Donny has sent me thinking of the only thing that really matters,
"Move boy" -Shankle. Good bye writer's block, hello dynamic start.
Cigarettes and coffee keep me writing, or better yet.... moving.
A "Move boy" will make you move, and that's exactly what these
fingers full of salt water are doing. Slam your bar full of bloody
eyes and a sore soul. I'm with you, we are with you. I know why
you are in sports, you can't hide.... you can lift but not hide.

A cold turkey dynamic start works great for small violins that play
throughout this Orchestra of weightlifting, but deeper battle wounds
must find more ways to lift the heavy bar above head. Attach horses
to your stings and play on. This will create less heart ache, but
many more hateful opinions, comments and a huge fan base of haters.
What kind of odd balle movement does your favorite lifter perform?
And will you try the same? Why is this very important subject
never talked about? Why are so many important details in this sport
never talked about? Why are all the "Elite Professionals" staying
hush hush? There is so much more to this battle than technique
and strength. Moving before the bar breaks the floor can take you
and drop you off in better positions throughout the journey of the
pull. If you feel you are getting out of position and the weight is
redirecting you, then try a start that will fit to your liking.

I have tried over a million dynamic starts. Many have worked and
many have failed. The ones that have worked, I always have felt
could be even better. So I kept on changing them, always wanting
to learn more about myself as a weightlifter and as a technician.
I continued my work in the lab, working with myself and keeping an
open mind to new ideas. A changing sea is what it took to see the
gold sand I now bath in today. My start still slightly changes
to this day, but not much. I stay close to my 166kg snatch aka
home. I recently clean and jerked a new PR at 195kg. This is due
to changing my dynamic start in the clean. I was noticing that
my dynamic start in the snatch wasn't carrying over well in the
clean. So the last few months, I have been working on a few ideas
that have recently paid off. The idea I have come across is what I
will use to win Gold at Americans. Seeing a dynamic start on video
gives it no justice. The creature lives within you and me, not for
anyone to see or understand. You may never understand my start,
and I may never understand yours. We can see and grasp the surface
of a dynamic start, but the magic that lies within our body can
never be detected, this is why there is no right way to complete
a dynamic start. This is why I am not writing on what I actually
do, but more of what this kilo adding creature can do for us
weightlifters when understood and fitted to each individual lifter.

Kilo Creature 2016

The Dynamic Start:

A Dynamic Start is simply creating momentum in the lifts by moving before
moving. The snowflake of the Weightlifting world, no two Dynamic Starts are
the same, due to different body types, levers, style of lifting and experience in the
sport. It is something that is personal from one lifter to the next, and one athlete's
style might not necessarily work for another.

Not only can it aid you in adding momentum to the lift, but a Dynamic
Start can also help you achieve a more efficient Position Three. Athletes who
lack mobility can use a Dynamic Start to move into Position Three and lift
before they lose it. You need to keep your body tight as you begin to pull from
the floor. If you set up cold turkey and pull then, you might not be as tight as
you should be, and there is no momentum going back. Use the Dynamic Start
to start the momentum of the lifting going back into you and to take the slack
out of your body.

Horses Out of Gate
(aka The Click n' Pull)

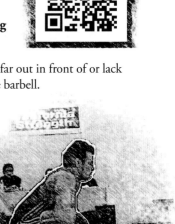

My dynamic start has changed so many times over my career that I have lost count. I call my newest one Horses Out of Gate and I feel it is the best one I have ever used. I have found it to be so useful that I teach it to my athletes and at seminars with a pretty high success rate.

This dynamic start might work well for you if during the pull you:

- ○ Tend to set up with your shoulders a little too far out in front of or lack the mobility to move the shoulders behind the barbell.
- ○ Have issues staying tight during the pull.
- ○ Shift your weight to the balls of your feet instead of back to the heels.
- ○ Pull too slowly because you have trouble gaining speed and momentum.

Performing the Click n' Pull:

- ○ **Step One:** Move yourself into Position Three with the shins an inch away from the bar. We do not want the barbell to touch us yet. Let your arms relax with a slight bend. The shoulders are slightly over the barbell. Make sure you have plates on the bar as seen in **Figure 12.8**.

(Figure 12.8)

- ○ **Step Two:** Snap yourself back into a tighter position. Now the shoulders should be behind the barbell and you cannot go back any further. The back is tight; arms locked out, and the barbell is being pulled back into the shins. As you snap back, you will hear a clicking sound from the barbell. That is your cue to "open the gates" and pull just like the horses begin to sprint when they hear the bell. As seen in **Figure 12.9**.

(Figure 12.9)

Here the weight should crack from the floor slightly on both ends of the barbell. You will not fall over because the weight is acting as a counterbalance as it presses against your shins. There will be pressure going back into the shins. After years of experimenting with dynamic starts and Weightlifting, I cannot grow hair anymore on the spots the barbell touches my shins. This drill will help those of you who lack flexibility to attain a proper Position Three.

Even if you only have it for a split second before everything falls apart; that second is enough time to start the Pull. With the bar off the floor, resting in the shins, the only reason you are not pulling is because the shins are in the way. The barbell is the gate, and you are the horse. When you are ready to open that gate and start the pull, violently pull those knees back and initiate your pull.

- O **Step Three:** Pause with the barbell in the shins, keeping your body tight and weight back on the heels.
- O **Step Four:** Relax. Then snap back into position again and hold.
- O **Step Five:** When you are ready to pull, move the knees back quickly and perform the Superman Pull.

If performed correctly, you should be able to hear the barbell crack from the floor. It is almost the same sound you hear when the barbell hits your hips. That is a good indicator on when to start your pull. As soon as you hear the sound of the barbell coming into your shins, move the knees back and pull. During the full movement, you should hear three sounds: the barbell coming into the shins, then into the hips and finally your feet slapping into the platform. Give this dynamic start method a shot if you struggle moving the weight off the floor.

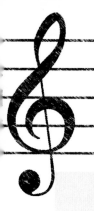

CHAPTER 13:

THE JERK IS A JERK

Yes! Hold It! Down, Great Job!

Thursday, March 8, 2012

That Jerk is such a Jerk. Drive the bar above your head? No, drive it BACK behind your head. Over the ears? No my friend behind the ears, trust me.....behind the ears is Golden, literally. "Up in this sport really means back." - Paul Doherty. Missing in front is the single most frustrating thing you can do. If you're going to miss, miss behind. But I guess a miss is miss no matter what. But missing behind makes you sleep a little better knowing that you put the power and energy in getting the bar that high and that far back. Where in front makes you feel you didn't leave it all on the platform, you never really went for it. You have to think of the Jerk the way my friend Donny Shankle says, "If you miss the jerk, you will not enter paradise". - Shankle aka lion killer. If only every weightlifter could hear the sweet words of this blog title all the time...now thats Paradise.

What a jerk the jerk can be when it doesn't sit nicely on the shelf for everyone to see. Drive higher, don't cut your dip and drive short, no matter how heavy the weight is. Reach for the sky my friend and catch with strength and pride. Hold it! Hold it! Punch up and hold! YES YES YES! That is a great feeling, and those are great words to here from your coach and the audience. Something that doesn't always happens, but as I am figuring out....that's just life and weightlifting. Life is not perfect, and sometimes the yes is more like ooooo. Tears

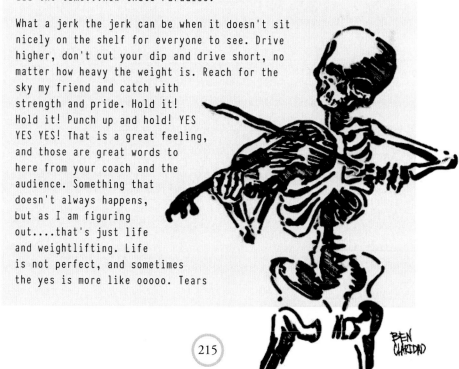

BEN CHARIDAD

of joy can easily become tears of let downs and sadness. Hugging
your coach can be good or bad. Weightlifting will take you down
many roads and emotions. "Weightlifting is a very hard sport".
- Everyone who is a weightlifter.

The worst part of missing the 188 is the jerk work coach has
slammed on my table filled with superman pull sketches, blue
prints for the clean, secrete training programs, coffee, smelly
knee wraps, blood sweat and tears. Hold the bar above your head
with 60 or so kilos, and lung into a jerk split to the end of the
gym and back......hell. Then when you are done put 120kg on your
back and do the same thing holding the position in the split for
a good 2 seconds.....hell. Repeat 3 more times...hell. I don't do
any more clean and jerks; I do clean and jerk and jerk and jerk
and then jerk again. Push presses tell the sun sets, more squats,
harder training. A few months of this I should have the best Jerk
in the world, I guess we shall see. More red meat, more sleep,
more mind training. Mind training is the hardest part of this
sport. Training your mind to go under weight you want to Clark.
Staying confident and focused in a meet, not letting the bar
intimidate you. Getting back on the horse after losing.....fuck,
that's a hard one.

I am writing this blog with the Shankle outside the green jungle.
The sun is setting, training is finally over, and the coffee is
extra strong....prefect time to write. Checked the PWA schedule
so I can compete in every damn local meet there is. Keep building
experience is a must, learning from your mistakes is so key. Who
knows, maybe the best thing I ever did was miss the 88 jerk. Maybe
next meet I will hit 200. Thank you all for your support from
the comments on the blog, face book, and e mail, you are truly
the reason why I am still standing and not throwing in the towel
feeling sorry for myself. Attitude Nation marches on.

Jerk that damn jerk above your heads and then slam the bar. Let
the world see how high you can throw heavy weight above your head,
and not just above, but back! Get the bar back please, for me, for
what I should have done!

Bar back 2012
Shankle and coffee 2012
Your kind words and support 2012
Attitude Nation Family 2012

The Snatch is pleasurable. It is a refreshing dance in the rain with a beautiful woman on a warm summer's night. The Clean is brutal, the stinging cold on your face in the winter. And the Jerk…The Jerk is cruel and unforgiving. An old nemesis that never shows any mercy. With one false step, all your hard work can be taken away… So keep your back tight as you Clean colossal weights. Drive with legs hardened by countless squats. Keep standing, keep standing! It is not over, brace your body and be patient. Feel the weight through your body. Tell yourself it is not heavy. Wait for your moment, breathe deep and ride the lightning. Was fate on your side today? Or were all of your efforts thwarted by some Jerk?

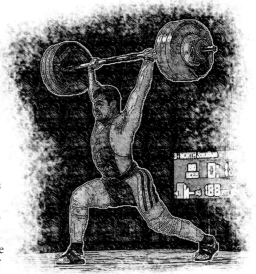

(Figure 13.1)

The Jerk is the second half of the Clean & Jerk. The barbell travels from the ground to the shoulders via the Clean and then we complete the movement by performing the Jerk. There are many different styles out there for the Jerk. I have seen lifters use Power Jerks and Squat Jerks. Hell I have even seen Kendrick Farris use his famous Kick Jerk; sign up for his seminar to learn it! There are so many varieties and styles, but we are going to focus on just one; the Split Jerk. That is what we are referring to when we say Jerk.

When we think about the Jerk, we focus on three key points:

- **Footwork:** To be proficient you have to practice and develop proper footwork both when executing the movement and recovering. Footwork is the foundation for speed and efficiency. We call the foot speed **Ice Skaters Feet.** It is different than the Ali Feet we wanted on the Snatch and Clean. The feet will not physically slide on the platform, but they will be moving extremely fast and come off the ground no more than an inch.

- **Barbell Oscillation:** We never stop using it and need the help more than ever for this part of the lift. Using oscillation in the Jerk is the mark of a real tactician.

- **Placement:** We know where we want the bar to go. Always behind the head. We just need to put it there and be stable in position.

Building the Hangman:

The first thing we need to do is figure out the length and width of your split stance. The middle line in the diagram below is the **Tight Rope**. We want to avoid walking it because it is a very unstable position to be in with heavy weight overhead. That is why many athletes out there do not reset their feet after standing with a heavy Clean.

Grab a piece of chalk and let us draw the hangman diagram together:

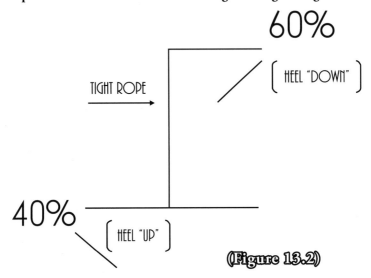

(Figure 13.2)

- ○ **Step One:** Draw a straight two foot line in front of your body. That will be our starting point.
- ○ **Step Two:** Position yourself so that your toes are lined up with the chalk line. You will now take three to four heel to toe steps to measure the length of your split. We recommend athletes who are 5'10 – 6' or taller take four steps. Shorter athletes take three. After your last step draw another line from the front toe and to the right as seen above in the diagram.
- ○ **Step Three:** Connect both lines, and you now have the hangman. Draw, the other markers on the floor, to remind you what we are looking for at the feet.
- ○ **Step Four:** Make sure this feels comfortable. We are just providing you with a foundation. Everyone is going to be different. Play around with the stride length and if you need to take another step.
- ○ **Step Five:** Use this diagram for drills featured later on in the text. Note: **Figure. 13.2** is drawn for a right forward foot. A Left forward foot would be the mirror image of the diagram.

The Jerk

- **Starting Position:** Move to your Clean receiving stance for a more stable base.

- **Hand Placement:** This depends on the individual and mobility. The wider your hands go, the more your elbows will drop. I recently found for myself that I can perform better with a wider grip, but I lack the ability to adjust my hands after the Clean. I had to adapt and take my grip out on the Clean as well. Experiment to find what works best for you.

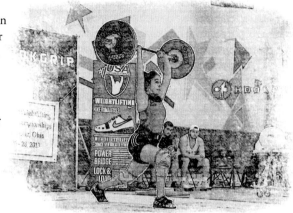

(Figure 13.3)

- **Elbows:** They should be high. Having them, high helps you avoid the barbell sliding down your chest.

- **Wrist:** When the barbell is overhead you want the wrist to be cocked back. This creates a stable Catch Position where the bar can rest on them like a shelf.

- **Torso:** As vertical as possible.

- **Head:** Just as in the Snatch we want to **Turtle Head** by pushing our head forward and the barbell behind the ears.

- **Front Leg:** 60% of your body weight will be towards the front leg. The shin is vertical or perpendicular to the floor.

- **Front Foot:** We turn the foot in toward the body so that we are covering more surface area with our body and balance.

- **Back Leg:** The back knee is slightly bent. A straight leg will shift more body weight towards the front leg.

- **Back Foot:** The back heel is off the platform and the toes are turned toward the body.

- **Bar Path:** If someone were to draw a line from the floor up the front of your body starting with the barbell on the floor; the bar should move back behind the line. It would continue to go up and back ending behind your head never again reaching that line. Even from the shoulders the barbell is going to move up and back.

Recovery from the Jerk:

Every Weightlifter out there; myself included; has missed lifts because of improperly recovering from the Jerk. Donny always used to say that "if you want to be a good Weightlifter you have to be the king of specifics." Every miniscule little detail for each lift needs to be on point. Even when you have a weight over your head, and you think it is all good in the hood, your work is not done until you hear that down signal. After performing the Jerk; when we bring our feet back together the front foot comes back to center first followed by the back foot. Make front foot, back foot your mantra every time you recover from a Jerk.

If you bring the back foot forward first, then it will cause the weight to move forward with the momentum of your body coming forward. You will potentially lose balance and control, causing a missed lift in front. Now if you find you cannot move the front foot back then you need to reevaluate your catch. More than likely there is too much weight on the front foot.

The Dip and Drive:

The weight being lifted in the Jerk is just too heavy to be pressed overhead using only the upper body. You have to use the legs to help move the bar. The Dip and Drive phases allow us to do that. It is a very vertical movement. You move up and down like an elevator loading the legs and then driving it back up as hard as possible.

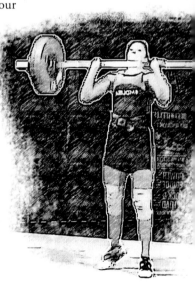

O **Step One:** Stand in your Catch position stance. Before you go for the dip, you need to set your back. Arch and make sure it is tight. A lot of athletes out there skip this important piece which causes their backs to round on the dip. As soon as that happens the lift is done, over. Next you need to take a deep breath and fill your belly with air. That will help keep you stable in the catch. If you have those two pieces down then all you have to worry about is speed and violence.

O **Step Two:** The Dip as seen in **Figure 13.4** is very similar to the Power Position. The knees bend and the hips drop down toward the feet. Your torso should be vertical,

(Figure 13.4)

(Figure 13.5)

and your weight is on the heels. Never pause in the dip. Once you do that then you are on your own, the barbell cannot help you. You will lose valuable bar oscillation. A tip to help keep you tighter and the elbows locked in is to pull the barbell actively down into you during the Dip. When standing from a Clean actively push it up to pop it off your body to gain even more oscillation.

- O **Step Three:** Drive hard, as seen in **Figure 13.5**, pushing through the floor and extend the hips and legs.

- O **Step Four:** The feet will move after the extension, and you will catch the barbell overhead in the split stance. **HOLD IT!** Hold your catch position, as seen in **Figure 13.6**, until the weight overhead has stabilized. Trying to recover too quickly can easily result in a missed lift.

(Figure 13.6)

- O **Step Five:** Bring the feet back together, and the lift is complete.

The Jerk is a Heartbreaker:

Ian Wilson is a close friend of mine and a phenomenal athlete. I coached him for a short while back in the day when I was at California Strength. He was a young, bright-eyed skinny kid full of passion and talent for the sport of Weightlifting for Team Hassle Free. I would walk into the gym and hear a hi-pitched squeaky voice yell "Hi, Jon!" with excitement. He was my little buddy, and I cherish those memories of coaching him.

Flash forward to the 2012 Nationals. I was on fire heading into this meet. The stars were aligning, and my technique was never better. Representing California Strength, I would be going up against Phil Sabatini once again and…to my surprise Ian Wilson. I had not seen him for a few years and was sort of taken back that our reunion would be in the 94KG class at one of the biggest meets of the year. I found Ian in the back room… I do not know what they fed that kid at Hassle Free, but he went from that little kid I once knew to a 6'1 hulking professional athlete. Towering over me, he said, "Hey, Jon" in a deep booming Glenn Pendlay type voice.

We hugged, laughed and then it was right down to business. There was stiff competition in the 94KG class that year. In addition to Phil, Ian and myself; Jared Fleming, Colin Burns, and Kevin Cornell were right there in the fight. It was going to be an all-out brawl. I tied Jared in the Snatch hitting 160KG in my second attempt and missed 163KG for my third. The rest were right behind us with a 152KG lift for Ian, 155KG for Phil, 155KG for Colin and 146KG for Kevin. The podium was still up for grabs after the Snatch session. It was all going to come down to the Clean & Jerk to separate the field.

Jared did not have a great showing for the Clean & Jerk missing all three of his attempts. Colin and Kevin both ended with 175KG totaling 330KG and 321 respectively. It was down to Phil, Ian and myself. Phil went out first and hit 180KG. I pressed out my first attempt at 183KG but made it on my second attempt. Phil made his second attempt at 185KG. It was after that I said to myself "holy shit, Ian has not even opened yet." Finally, his first lift was at 187KG which he made with little effort. I needed to put a serious number on the board if I hoped to beat these guys. I set my sights on 188KG. I put chalk on my neck, walked out there like I owned that stage and motioned to the crowd prompting them to cheer. I needed their energy for this lift! I hit the Clean so quickly it felt like a toy. The crowd roared as I stood up with the weight over four hundred pounds on my chest. Then silence…no one spoke they all just waited for the Jerk.

I took a deep breath, braced and went for it. It felt heavy on the dip, but I did not give a shit. I was going to go under that bar. I gave my last lift of the day everything I had as I drove the weight up. **SLAP!** My feet slammed down upon the platform; the weight locked out overhead. I had done it! With this lift, I had beaten Phil and then would have to wait to see how Ian would respond! I was so happy and filled with emotion. I smiled and let out a triumphant yell and brought my feet together. Unfortunately, right there at that moment I learned a hard lesson to be taught on a national stage. The weight overhead had not yet settled, and I brought my feet together too quickly. The bar wobbled, and before I could even think, 188KG fell behind me to the ground resulting in three red lights. The lift did not count. **FUCK!** That is why coaches yell "Hold It!" Heartbroken I went to the back to watch Ian go for his final attempts. He missed 192KG on his second attempt but nailed it on the third.

Phil and Ian tied with a 344KG total but based on body weight Ian took the gold medal in the 94KG class with a 391.8 Sinclair to Phil's 391.4. I left that meet with a bronze medal totaling 343KG and a 390.6 Sinclair. Had I made that Jerk, I would have totaled 348KG, a 397.3 Sinclair and left with the gold. That is why it is important to be patient and treat each part of the lifts with respect. You only win if you make the lifts and I hope my misfortune can help others out there not make the same mistake. Ian Wilson is one of the top American weightlifters out there right now. Bust out the popcorn, look him up on Hookgrip.com and be prepared to be amazed at his unbelievable talent.

The Eagle:

The Eagle is a dynamic start for the Jerk that utilizes bar oscillation. Bar Oscillation is vital in the Jerk; it is practically 90% of the movement. During the Dip phase, the barbell will bend to give us that frowny face. After a second though, the weight is going to drive back up again. If you can time it just right, you might as well be holding onto a hot air balloon. That bar is going to take you for the ride of your life. Ride the lightning as your feet cut through the air and then stick to the platform.

One of the best practitioners of using the oscillation of the bar in the Jerk is my good friend and former Cal Strength teammate Caleb Ward. I have spent days watching videos of him lift; he paints masterpieces on the platform. I remember he was so good at the Jerk that he would often crack a smile during the dip because he knew the lift was already done. Think about what you are doing and not what the bar is doing. If you move your body correctly then, the bar will do what it needs to do. Timing is everything here. The official rules state that a lifter's body must come to a complete stop after the Clean before the Jerk can be performed. Experienced lifters will pop the bar off their chest to adjust their hands. That is a loophole in the rules! If you watch closely many athletes do not even move their hands, they are just trying to gain more oscillation out of the bar.

Use the Eagle to help you set a new record in the Clean & Jerk:

- **Step One:** Move a barbell to the Front Rack and adjust your hands to your Jerk grip.
- **Step Two:** As you take your breath, shrug your shoulders up to your ears. That will raise the barbell.
- **Step Three:** After the breath is over, and the shrug has reached its apex drop the shoulders, let them fall. As the barbell comes down begin your dip.
- **Step Four:** If done correctly the barbell will begin to oscillate when it drops. Drive back up with the momentum of the barbell and hit your Jerk.
- **Step Five:** Keep practicing.

Common Errors in Performing the Jerk:

- **Error #1 – Dropping the Elbows on the Dip:** I recommend keeping the elbows high during the Dip phase of the Jerk. I have found that when the elbows are low it increases the chances that the barbell will slide down the chest and pull you forward putting you in an inefficient position.

Coaching Cue: "Elbows High."

- **Error #2 – Losing contact with the barbell on the Dip:** If you drive your body into the bar, you can produce maximal power. If you push the arms up during the Drive phase of the lift, then you cut off the power of the legs. That typically happens when lifters lose contact with the barbell during the Dip phase. Not only is this inefficient, it is illegal in competition. If the bar leaves the body during the Dip, it will result in a no lift. To fight against this, practice pulling the bar down into your shoulders as you perform the Dip.

  Coaching Cue: "Pull Down."

- **Error #3 – Not filling your belly with air before the Dip:** You need to be stable in the receiving position for the Jerk. Taking a big breath of air and filling your stomach will help give you a stronger Drive and Catch.

  Coaching Cue: "Big Breath!"

- **Error #4: Not placing the barbell behind the head:** As in the Snatch, we want the weight to be supported by the muscles of the upper back and not the shoulders. Not only are they stronger and more stable, but you can potentially save a lift.

  Coaching Cue: "Turtle Head"

- **Error #5 – Not holding the weight, making sure it is stable before recovering the feet:** 2012 Nationals…need I say more.

  Coaching Cue: "Hold It!"

- **Error #6 - Not bending the back leg:** We need the back leg bent and for the heel to be off the platform. A potential injury-causing error that rookies make is to land with the knee extended, and foot turned out away from the body. That puts a lot of unwanted pressure on the knee joint. The correct way to land is to have the back heel up, and toe turned toward the body.

  Coaching Cue: "Heel Up"

- **Error #7 – Shifting too much weight forward on the front leg:** We want the weight distribution to be 60% on the front leg and 40% on the back leg. The front shin should be perpendicular to the floor, every inch it shifts forward disrupts your balance and proper weight distribution.

- **Error #8 – Allowing the Hips to shift forward on the Dip:** The hips should stay back and down during the dip.

- O **Advice – Practice your footwork:** Only practice will make it perfect, and I realize that it is not as attractive as lifting the heavy weights. If you neglect this essential aspect of your training, you will be leaving kilos on the table and pay for it down the road.
- O **Advice – Turn the toes out:** If you frequently shift forward on the Dip phase of the Jerk try turning your toes out slightly. That will help you stay upright.

Technique Drills:

The Jerk is a beautiful blend of both strength and skill. Hours of practice are going to be necessary to develop this aspect of your game or correct flaws. You can use the Hangman to practice your footwork. The chalk lines will give you guidance on whether or not you are missing the mark. The barbell in your hands is a better coach than anyone out there because the exact second you are out of position, it will tell you.

The Jerk Ladder

The Jerk Ladder drill will help you to gain comfort with stepping out into your split stance, moving your feet and strengthen your catch position. It is a variation of an exercise we used to do back at Cal Strength. The original drill requires much more space so you can travel, stepping into your split stance.

- O **Step One:** Grab a barbell and move it to your Jerk Rack. With your feet in your squat stance line your toes up to the baseline of the Hangman.
- O **Step Two:** Nothing will happen with the barbell. We are only going to move the front foot. Step out into the hangman so that your front toes lineup to the far line of the hangman.
- O **Step Three:** Perform a position check. **Ask yourself:** "Is my torso vertical?" "Is my back knee bent?" "Are my feet turned in?" If not then make those adjustments. Then take a step back to set up for another repetition.
- O **Step Four:** When you are comfortable with the length of your split then, we can continue to add pieces to the drill. These additions will help to reinforce your Jerk receiving position.

- ○ **Step Five:** Center yourself between both lines and perform a Jerk. Perform a position check. Focus on sticking the foot placement thus perfecting your weight distribution. Avoid the front knee coming forward. Every inch we gain by moving the knee forward negatively affects the weight distribution. Repeat.

Jerk Stance Presses

The Jerk Stance Press is an excellent way to strengthen your upper body and receiving position. Perform regularly five sets of five repetitions (5x5) with just the barbell or add weight.

- ○ **Step One:** Setup on the Hangman with the barbell on your back.
- ○ **Step Two:** Drop your feet out into your split stance and hold it. Perform five behind the neck presses. You may need to take your grip wider than you normally do here. We are pressing from behind the neck to start because it puts the barbell exactly where we want it (behind the head). It is important that while you are pressing your lower body does not move.
- ○ **Step Three:** Once you are comfortable pressing behind the neck in your stance, switch the barbell to the front rack with your usual Jerk grip. Perform five strict presses from here.
- ○ **Step Four:** Stick to just the barbell until you are confident then you can add weight.
- ○ **Step Five:** Repeat.

Jerk Stance Jerks

Jerk Stance Jerks are an excellent drill to help improve the Dip and Drive phases of the lift and practice picking your feet up off of the platform. Perform regularly five sets of five repetitions (5x5).

- ○ **Step One:** Setup on the hangman with the barbell in the front rack with your Jerk grip.
- ○ **Step Two:** Drop your feet out into your split stance and hold it. As seen in **Figure 13.7**.
- ○ **Step Three:** Perform a Jerk from your split position. Dip by lowering the back knee slightly. Then Drive back up and Jerk the barbell. The feet will only move up off the ground a few inches and then back down. You

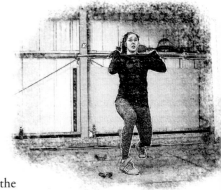

(Figure 13.7)

226

will remain in the Jerk stance the entire time. As seen in **Figures 13.8** and **13.9**.

O **Step Four:** Lower the barbell into to the front rack again for the next repetition. A common mistake is for only one foot (often the front) to move and not the other. The back leg will also want to straighten. Keep it bent on the landing.

O **Step Five:** Repeat.

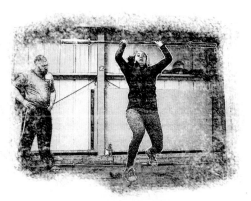

(Figure 13.8)

Just as in the Snatch and Clean; our positions in the Jerk need to be second nature. Our bodies must be trained to react at the drop of a dime. Gravity is our constant enemy. It never stops trying to pull the weight forward and down. Luckily, these are exercises you can regularly perform in your warm ups or technique sessions such as these that will help make you strong in positions. The more time you spend in positions, the better because your body will know what it feels like as you train it to commit fully to getting there.

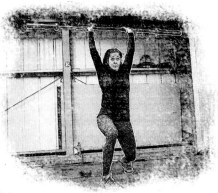

(Figure 13.9)

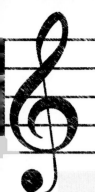

CHAPTER 14:
GYM LIFE SOCIETY

My Response

Wednesday, January 2, 2013

I believe that no answer, is at times the best answer. Not doing
anything, is sometimes the hardest thing to do. I hope you will
end up reading this whoever and wherever you are. I hope that
my silence has spoken loudly and you have found the right path on
your own. I hope you will respond to this blog, if not... then I
will assume you are out there, happy and doing what you love. I
think you, the reader, can understand and relate to my situation.
Maybe you, the reader, might disagree with my decision. Either
way, I would love to hear your two cents.

I had a college kid write me a long letter last year, a letter
that keeps me up to this day, a letter that I have thought about
everyday up 'til now, a letter about a love affair with training
vs school. It was a crossroads letter that I spent about two
days typing a response to. It was a letter that
many people go through. Am I happy doing what
I'm doing? Which way should I stray? And most
importantly, how do I know if the decision I
make is the right decision? His letter was
so detailed, so passionate,
so heart felt that I had to
think long and hard before
writing him back. Do I stay in
school? Or do I drop out
putting everything into
weightlifting? My
answer could have huge
impact on this kids
life. My answer could
change this young man's life
for the better, or who knows...

BEN
CLARIDAD

229

the worse. I would type then delete, another sentence erased, another paragraph down the drain. A call in to some very close friends, family members, and a long chat to my wife. What and how should I respond? Right when I thought I had an answer it changed, finding myself at the end with no answer. I could tell him to do what I did, but he is not me. I could tell him to stay in school, but am I killing his dream? I could have taken the easy way out and told him to do both... press send..... complete. But did I really believe that? No, I didn't. He reminded me so much of myself through his letter. He was standing at the crossroads of life, the same place we have all been. If you the reader are very young.... then I think the rest of the Dark Orchestra will agree with me that someday you will be standing on that dirt country road with chalk in one hand and a brief case in the other, and when that day does come, ask questions, explore, pick people's mind, indulge in wanderlust... just like the young man who wrote me did. But at the end of the day, follow your heart, trust yourself. You might not know this at the time young reader, but the most beautiful part about walking right instead of left, is the fact they are both the right direction. You will someday look back at that time you stood in the dusty wind storm with a corn field in front of you, while two very life changing roads sit besides you, and you will smile with happiness as you get ready to sit down with your family for dinner. You will smile as you chalk your hands before pulling on the bar. You will smile as your students enter the class room for math class. You will smile while you train for your sport while holding a full time job. You will smile young reader because I know you, I know the person who wrote me. He was me, I was him, and I know whatever I, you, or he sets his mind to we will all succeed, no matter what it is. Happiness finds us, we don't find it.

I never responded. It's been close to two years now and not a day goes by that I don't wonder what kind of decision he made. What path he decided to walk down. Weightlifting or Academics or both, or something completely different that he didn't even see coming. I wanted so badly to help, but I knew that by not responding was the best way I could help. I didn't want to limit this young man to only two options. You have the whole world in front of you my unseen friend! Don't you dare limit yourself to two options!

I cannot answer your question, you must find it yourself, just like I did. Does it kill me that you think I might not of read your letter, yes, more than ever. This is what's hard for me to swallow. Maybe I should have wrote you a simple, "It's up to you" letter. Still to this day I feel I made the right decision by staying silent. I don't want to make it easier on you. I want you to burn your hand! Get in trouble! Find what you're good at! Meet friends you never thought you would ever be friends with! Find yourself, never have anyone find it for you. You might not be in control, but you are 100 percent in control. That might not make any sense, but then again life doesn't always make sense, weightlifting doesn't always make sense, and your decisions will half the time never make sense. Yes, I am speaking to many people through this blog right now, but most importantly I want you, you the young man that wrote me that powerful letter two years ago, that yes, I read it. Yes I read it and still do, just to remind myself how far I have come from that dirt cornfield road, and how far you will go as well. And young reader that hasn't bumped into the corn field road........just remember....You ain't got time for percentages. Everyday max out.

PS: Young man who wrote me that letter, if you find this blog post, please contact me. I want to know what and how you are doing. If you have decided to lift weights, then I would love to help you in any way possible. I will give you my phone number so we can chat. Salut

Young reader 2016

Weightlifting in this country is slowly undergoing a metamorphosis. Everyday people who never thought to pick up the barbell before are performing the Snatch and the Clean & Jerk. This significant influx of new athletes is in part due to CrossFit™ and for that I thank them whole heartedly. Many of these new athletes carry with them dreams and hopes of reaching the highest levels of Weightlifting. The beautiful thing about this is that the sport is not only fun, but easily accessible as well. You can buy a membership, a singlet and sign up for a meet any time you would like.

That is the fun part. However, to be a champion, you have a different road to follow. A road made up of Snatching, Clean & Jerks, and Back Squatting every day. A road where the barbell is in your hands so often they are almost fused into one, and when you go to sneeze traces of chalk dust exit your body. It is a road that leads to the realization that Weightlifting is not easy. Understand that this sport has more bad days than good. Those who are strong will survive its trials, and as someone who has weathered many storms, I want to help. I want to give you guidance on how you can make it easier for yourself and find success.

Weightlifting Equipment:

If you are going to play the sport, you need to use the gear. These are my thoughts on various types of equipment as well as how I use them in my training.

- O **Wraps:** You can use them to help protect your wrist or knee joints. They contribute to adding a little bit of stability and keep those areas warm. I mainly use Ace Bandages for my knees. If you are a weightlifter then, the chances are high that you are on a budget. Ace Bandages are cheaper and more versatile than other stuff out there. I never used to use them until I met Donny. The entire Cal Strength team wore them back in the day as if it were part of the dress code.

- O **Straps:** There are two kinds of straps out there, long and short. As a Weightlifter, you want to use the short straps because they can be wrapped around the bar with minimal excess material hanging off. I use straps practically for 100% of my Snatches in training for two reasons. First, it allows me to lift more weight. You should always go the route that allows you to lift more weight, that is how you can increase your strength and confidence in the lift. In competition, when you are attempting a weight that is 15KG less than your all time best gym record, it will feel extremely light. Second, straps help to keep your hands healthy. Snatching every day will tear up your hands because of the wide grip on the barbell. I only use them on the Snatch, never on the Clean & Jerk. It is dangerous to use them for that lift because it can make it difficult to bail on a missed lift or hurt your wrist. You know you are in a catapult style Weightlifting gym if there are holes in the wall behind the platform. When I trained at Cal Strength, our straps would break all the time from the powerful bar body contact we produced during the lifts. Straps would break, and bodies would go flying into the wall because of all the force we were applying during the Finish.

- O **Belts:** I never use a belt when I Snatch. I prefer to feel unrestricted and athletic for that movement. Instead, I will use one for a big Clean & Jerk or Back Squats. Make sure the belt you train with is legal in competition. According to the IWF rule book, the width of the belt used cannot exceed 120mm (4 inches).

- O **Shoes:** Personally I prefer a medium heel in my Shoes. I have also always worn Adidas Weightlifting Shoes. They look the coolest, and Adidas has a rich history in the sport.

- **Barbell:** Any barbell is better than no barbell, but if you have the funds available it is worth it to invest in quality equipment. Muscle Driver sells Pendlay barbells that are affordable and what we used for the majority of our training at Cal Strength. We also had Eleiko bars, but they were only used on special occasions like a big max out day or competitions. If you have an expensive barbell or one you plan to use for Weightlifting regularly you should never Squat with it. This is because putting the bar in the squat rack files down the knurling on the bar when it slides on the J-Hooks. You should also maintenance your barbell regularly. Clean off all of the chalk with a wire brush so it does not rust and use WD-40 to lubricate the ends. This will help the bar spin smoothly. A lot of people who have good technique, mobility, and strength can trace shoulder injuries to poorly maintained bars.

- **Bumper Plates:** Overall, there is nothing wrong with the black bumper plates common in most CrossFit™ gyms. However, they do change the feel and oscillation of the barbell, which is something you should be aware of. Typically, if I wanted to experience the oscillation of a heavy barbell while lifting a lighter weight, I would put collars on the bar first and then the plates. This loads the plates out further on the bar causing oscillation similar to a bar that had multiple plates loaded on it. Since the black plates are so wide, you do not need to do this. Two forty-five pound plates on both ends of the bar take up more space than two competition style plates. I will admit, it messes with my timing and rhythm to use the black plates since I am so used to training with competition plates.

Training:

My grandmother, Michi Hirata North, is a famous Pianist. Playing the Piano is an international sport and at just six years old she would perform and compete in theaters filled with thousands of people. These days my grandmother is now considered a world-class instructor who is sought after by students from around the globe. As a young kid, I remember visiting her house and watching her coach little Japanese girls on how to play the Piano. They would play all day long, from seven o'clock in the morning to seven o'clock at night while she gave them pointers and critiques.

It was quite fascinating watching them work hard to master playing the piano and the little tricks they incorporated in training. My grandmother would have her students tape weights to their fingers to condition and strengthen the hands to play faster. She would also have them wear blindfolds so they would focus on searching for keys with their fingers instead of with their eyes. They would do these things for a week and then go back to their unrestricted playing the next week. The result was faster more intuitive piano playing.

I realized years later that my grandmother's piano coaching was very similar to Ivan Abadjiev's Bulgarian System for Weightlifting. Both coaches have their athletes stick very close to the primary skills with very little deviation. That right there is the secret to becoming a proficient Weightlifter. You have to practice the Snatch and Clean & Jerk with high-frequency in order to master them. Too many aspiring athletes out there become caught up in percentages, accessory exercises, and fancy equipment. They lack the discipline to stay focused on the real task at hand that is progressively to lift more and more weight performing those two lifts. To keep it simple, as a Weightlifter, you could simply just Snatch, Clean & Jerk and Squat every training session. However, if you feel like you need more and want professional guidance, you can join the Dark Orchestra Online Team.

Unwritten Rules of the Sport:

Weightlifting gyms are a little different from CrossFit™ or other types of gyms. There is training etiquette that each athlete is always expected to abide by. Yes, training should be fun, but you need to know your place amongst the other athletes. You also need to understand, for many lifters out there this is a professional job. Their hopes and dreams…how they pay their bills are interwoven in this sport. It will not be appreciated if you do not take it as seriously as they do and fuck around in the gym. Please take note of these essential unwritten laws.

Rule #1

Stepping Over The Barbell:

Back in the day they would say it is not appropriate to step over the barbell because it was a sign of disrespect, but I disagree. When you are on the platform, your opponent is that bar, and we are all ultimately in the same battle against it. That cold steel is merciless, and I have seen it end careers, cause anger, frustration and tears of sadness. The barbell broke Max Aita's wrist, during an accident while Cleaning 175KG. It was a horrific accident that ended his career, and I vividly remember seeing the bones of his wrist sticking through ripped skin.

The barbell also broke Donny's fucking neck on a missed Snatch. Then as he stood after completing a 160KG Snatch, it dislocated his shoulder, just **ONE** week before the National Championships! Never show your barbell respect because it does not respect you! I say step over your barbell all you want. I do agree, however, that you should never step over another lifter's bar. That is an extremely disrespectful act against that person. It shows that you do not give a shit about them. You might as well have walked over to the platform and slammed them in the face.

Rule #2

Walking In Front Of Other Lifters:

Never walk in front of someone while they are lifting. Many Weightlifters out there find it distracting when they are trying to focus. It does not matter if they are lifting 50KG or 170KG if it is a big lift for *THAT* person then you should stand and watch. Show them respect for what they are going to do instead of walking around like it does not matter. I realize this may be hard to do in some gyms, but do your best to be aware of what is happening around you.

Rule #3

Talking During Training:

Talking during training is okay up until a certain point. During the warm up everyone likes to mingle and chit chat a little. However, at around 85% 1RM, things become more serious. If someone is going for a new record or significant lift then everyone else needs to shut their mouths. Cell phones better be in your pocket with the ringer on silent. Use your common sense and learn how your teammates train.

When I was training at California Strength, the place would shut down when Donny was going for a big lift. Everyone would step back thirty feet; we turned off the radio and watched in silence. It was about respect and support. Remember, you are a team and if one person is going for a big lift, then you are all going for that lift.

Rule #4

Be On Time For Practice:

Do not be late for a practice session. That messes with the training rhythm of everyone on the team. If training starts at 3:00pm then that means 50KG is on the bar when the clock strikes three. Your stretching, foam rolling and pre-workout supplements should all have been done before that time. On the other hand, do not leave practice sessions early. If you crushed your workout and finished before everyone else, you need to stay and support your team members. To leave early sends the message that you do not care about anyone else except you. If that is your attitude then, no one will want to train with you.

Rule #5

Be Clean:

Please, for all that is holy, practice proper methods of hygiene. Take showers, use deodorant and clean your equipment. I know it is a gym, but if you smell bad, you are going to be distracting to your teammates. Never be *THAT* guy or girl.

Rule #6

Work As A Team:

If you are lifting with other athletes on the same bar then, you need to work as a team. Load and unload it together. Know the weight that is on the bar, do the math before you lift and make sure the area is safe. If three guys are lifting on a bar, the two guys waiting their turn should be the ones changing the weight. The guy who is up next should be preparing themselves mentally to make the lift. Look out for one another, make sure the platform is swept, and you will have a great session.

Rule #7

Know how to motivate:

Every lifter is motivated differently. I remember Caleb Ward preferred positive motivation such as "you can do it!" On the other hand, I was accustomed to a different approach. I like to be challenged with comments like "you're scared" or "you aren't going to do it Jon!" That is what worked for us, and you have to know what works for everyone on your team.

Donny, for example, would have killed me if I tried either of those approaches with him. I remember one time, Donny was about to go for a massive Clean and Jerk record. I was very excited about it, and I wanted him to do well. Just before he went to lift, I walked over to him, slapped him on the back and said "you got it Donny!" His head snapped back to look at me. At that moment, I had never seen a more serious look on another man's face and my stomach tightened. He looked me dead in the eyes and said "if you ever do that again, I'll fucking kill you." Since that day, I have never touched him in training.

You need to know when to use motivation as well. For example, the Clean & Jerk has very specific times when you are allowed to cheer or say something encouraging. For the Clean, you are to be quiet. You can yell and scream when they are standing. Then you have a one-two second window before the Jerk to cheer again. Then you say nothing until the Jerk is over.

Rule #8

Communicate:

Communicate with your teammates when you are sharing space. Talk before you lift so that both of you know the speed you will be going through the session with. Rhythm in training is imperative that is why you need to know rest times and lift times. If it is not working out then go elsewhere with another bar.

When you are working with someone, you should never sit directly behind them. Always sit off to the side because lifters need their space, and you do not want to get crushed if something goes wrong. As the training session progresses, everyone in the room will start taking turns lifting. At around 90% 1RM, no one is going to be going at the same time. If you approach your bar at the same time, another lifter does theirs then one of you needs to concede. Talk about the music you want to play and take turns picking the music because everyone has different taste. If you like powdered chalk then make it yourself, but leave chunks for others who prefer that.

Rule #9

Attend Team Meetings:

Meetings are where coach discusses important topics such as our training program, upcoming competitions and the state of the gym. You being there will show everyone that you are part of the team and have a positive attitude. If you never go to the meetings then not only do you not get to open your mouth when you have a problem, but chances are you will not be on the team for very long.

Rule #10

Know Your Place:

Rookie lifters need to be aware of their place in the hierarchy of the gym. The best lifters have first pick of the barbells and the platforms. At his gym, the best Chinese lifter Lu Xiaojun gets the platform by the window. He likes to look out at the trees and the sky while resting between lifts. He has EARNED the right to that platform; it belongs to him. At California Strength, the best lifters were down on the last platform by the garage door with Donny. They could go outside and breathe fresh air or take in some sun between lifts. The rookies were all the way at the other end, as far from the veterans as possible.

If you are a rookie lifter, in a professional training hall, you need to know your place and keep your mouth shut. Your only concern is learning. Keep your eyes and ears open for ways you can improve. Do not talk about your weekend or that movie you just saw because no one cares. The more gold medals you have equates to the more you can speak.

Top lifters will take care of themselves. They do what they need to do, and you come second. If I were to train with Kendrick Farris, he would pick the music. He has more gold medals than I do and has been to the Olympics. I keep my mouth shut, give him all the respect he deserves and try to learn from the man. If he tells me to do something, I say, "Yes, sir."

Sweat Bank

Monday, September 2, 2013

Bringing Him To Life Once Again Next Week.

His sweat has turned from warm to cold as the cool air turned his skin into a leopard like coat of goose bumps that shot up his spine and down his arms. The drastic change in weather from inside the gym to out has made the once river of sweat die in its tracks and stick to his body like a hook grip to a bar. The wind left him breathless as he began to walk to his humble apartment that rested just a few blocks from the gym that he has been training at for the last year. His walk brought him an awkward silence, but a well needed time to himself he valued deeply. Echoes of yelling, cheering, and bar slamming played over and over in his head every step he took. The echoes and recent memories began to drown turning into vapor as the mist of the cold day and car horns took over a new reality, a peaceful one that every athlete must have at least once a day. Boston was his home, and Boston would always be his home. He knew the back streets like a champ, cutting at least 10 minutes off his walk home, where only a native of this empty, but huge town would know. The bottom half of his long black coat rested over his gym bag as it occasionally hit his right knee, causing him to switch hands from time to time.

The collar on his coat was popped up past his ears while his chin stayed tucked downward. A place where deep thoughts are born and then thought about. Church bells rang aloud off in the distance, and a light rain met him half way home. The cars' break lights started to stand out more, as they became not only brighter but more blurry. The sounds of the street only intrigued him, just like the sounds of the gym. "Ears and eyes always open," his dad would preach to him before being tucked into bed. "See, hear, understand, and then create," his dad would say before turning off the lights and cracking the door just slightly so the monsters wouldn't come out to play. The Boston native never forgot, one memory that stuck with him, and so many other memories he wished he could forget. The walking signal flashed go, and before he knew it, he was stopped by the first step leading up to his apartment. He was home after a long day of training.

The hot water burned his skin like squats to his legs. Long days call for an extra long shower, and the harder the training, the more the small arrow leans to the H on the shower knob. Every workout has to go somewhere, right? He thought to himself while watching the water by his feet swirl in circles down the drain. His shoulders hurt from missing too many snatches in front, so he turned the shower head to a more powerful setting, giving his shoulders a light massage. He has been training for three months straight, preparing for his first local meet in weightlifting. His coach has been proud of him as he has been making great gains. His boss on the other hand, has a different take in his awesome job, his marketing boss that pays him a very nice salary every month wants him at the office more rather than taking time to rep curls at 24 Hour Fitness. Little did his boss know what he was really doing, or little did he care. The Boston native was baited and hooked to weightlifting, and the disease was too late and deep to try and leave this great sport he stumbled across on YouTube months ago. His shower door was cracked open, maybe from child hood stability, or just because the baseball game was playing in the background, and a few peeks out the shower door was part of his cleaning process. The confusing thought of when he would get all of his training back plus more for a reward, grabbed his attention from the ball game, and swirled his head back under the hot water. A Weightlifter's Bank is what he needed and wished he could walk into it. A Sweat Bank that allowed an athlete to deposit and withdraw every drop of sweat he or she worked for. A

place where an athlete can see how much sweat he or she has put
into any sport. His forehead started to wrinkle, as his eyebrows
drew down like window drapes. If our bodies lie to us and play
tricks on us as athletes.....then how do we really know how much
better we are getting. Where does all the sweat go? He thought
to himself while now brushing his teeth dramatically like he was
playing the violin as the hot water now came punching down upon
his back. He then froze in complete stillness. The water from
the shower head became motionless while the baseball game was put
on pause mid pitch. All of Boston stopped.

Let me, as the writer, stop the story for just a sec and talk to
you, the reader, about the Sweat Bank before we pick back up on
the story about the man from Boston. Don't worry he will be fine.
He is not dead or alive right now. The world he knows has just
stopped for a brief while, while we chat about his interesting
idea and theory. Let's face it, I can stop his world anytime
I want, because I am the one making the world he is living in
real. I am the writer, the creator. Without me he wouldn't
exist. He wouldn't be in the shower nor a weightlifter. He only
knows Boston because I placed him there. His whole life has been
created with a single cup of coffee. A Sweat Bank does exist!
When you wash your cloths in the washing machine, all of the sweat
accumulated in your clothes drains down deep into a factory run
and managed by your Ego. There is an entrance to this factory
in every one's home. You just have to look for it. You have to
believe in your sweat one hundred percent. Your ego lives under
your feet while taking a hot shower. The sweat living on your
body from a hard day's work runs down your body hitting the shower
floor and finding its way in the drain only to be met by your ego
wearing a bright see through poker hat while smoking a cigar.
Your ego is tall and lanky, slimy and multi-colored. Three arms,
two for your ego, and one for your ego's ego. An ego has many
egos in itself which make the factory of your hard work sweat run
efficient and fast. So many workers working hard on your hard
work makes this land down under your feet confident and prideful.
Your ego is not always confident, it takes much support and
encouragement from hundreds of your egos egos egos and so forth
to stay secure. Your ego is insecure, that's why it is an ego in
the first place. Giving off the impression of confidence when not
being confident at all. The more sweat the ego contains from your
hard work in the life above, the better your ego feels down under.

Down under in the dark the egos work. A small light reflecting
green from their see through visors swing back and forth from your
movement above. But your ego stays hard at work preparing for
the day you want to cash out. Or what they call, sweat out. You
don't know your ego at all, you know it's there, you know how it
acts, but you and I and this character that we created all have
no idea who it is or what it is. All we know is that its presence
is known. But what we didn't know, is that our ego is our sweat's
undertaker, our sweat's master. Character from Boston......come
back alive my friend.

The baseball game didn't skip a beat, but something was off. He
got out of the shower butt naked and walked out into his room
where the TV now showed a monster home run and the crowd going
crazy. The TV was loud, but he was quiet. His eyes traveled the
room as if someone was watching his every move. Something wasn't
right. He threw his covers off his bed looking for his alarm
clock that would show him the time. He felt as if there was a
sudden pause or black out that occurred from the point of entering
the shower and getting out. The time was correct, therefore
putting his theory in doubt. His body was freezing from the water
building little dots and villages from his head to toe. The cool
air reminded him of walking back from the gym as he preformed the
naked scurry back to the shower that we all do from time to time.
He started to think about the Sweat Bank again, and how cool it
would be to cash out a hard week's work in sweat dollars. He
became nervous about his first meet coming up, as his mind became
focused on normalcy again. What numbers should I open with, and
what kind of jumps should I take? All these, questions that
clustered his mind, steering away his odd thoughts of Sweat Banks
and watching eyes.

He dried off in his room with his dark green and red towel covered
in swirls and stars. It was a present from his parents that he
never liked, but one of those gifts that he ended up putting to
good use. He dried himself off the same way as always, how that
ritual came about he never knew. One of those mysteries of life
he guessed. He smiled at all the pictures in his college-like
room filled with friends and family. He took pride in one thing
that the people in the pictures always said about him. "Jason
doesn't have an ego, he is such a humble man". He loved that
about himself, and how others took him for it.

"Hey, Jason!" He looked all around the room in panic as if
someone just broke in wearing a scream mask. "My name is Jon
North, and I am writing about you." He grabbed the phone as if he
was about to eat a piece of food for the first time in 10 days.
His back hunched over as the outline of his spine came pointing
out his back. "Stop, its ok my friend. I will not write anything
bad about you, you will be ok. I just want you to know that you
do have an ego, a very big ego at that. Your ego has not come out
yet, for it waits for you in the Sweat Bank under your feet and
behind your washer for the day you compete. The day you do compete
your ego will shoot out of your last shower before competition
covering you with all your built up sweat from the past three
months. Your sweat is your ego, Jason. Your ego will soak into
your skin and help you achieve your goals in your first meet.
All of your sweat has been accounted for my very good character
friend. Your ego has not lost your hard work. It works long
hours just as you do."

"Jason, are you there?" "Yes I am, what is happening?" "You are
a creation from my keyboard covered in coffee. You are a mix of
emotion from my past splashed with thousands of readers all from
different outlooks on you. I view you one way, but the person
reading this might see you in a different way." "So then who am
I really?" "You are a 28 year old guy from Boston that loves his
family, the gym, the community you train in, and the peaceful time
you spend alone. But I must end this blog now because I myself
have to go train, for you will one day live again." "But how?
If you stop typing this blog, then I will die!" "No Jason, you
will only be on pause, because I will come back later and write
you again, picking right back up where we left off. You won't
even know what happened, or that time was paused. Say 'hi' to the
readers Jason, they have gotten to know you well over the last 10
minutes." "Hello, readers please don't leave me, I have a meet to
compete in, and I have been training for three solid months." "I
promise on everything Jason that the readers and I will be back to
watch your lifting soon! We will cheer you on and root for you
all the way! I know you won't remember any of this, but ego is
in all of us. Learn how to find it, then use it to your benefit.
Ego is a scary thing, and can't be taken lightly. You can use it
in a wrong way, just like anything in life. Next time I write
you, we will both train crazy hard getting closer to your first
meet. We will slam bars!"

```
"Good bye, Jason."  "Good bye, Jon."  "Oh wait, Jon! " "Yea,
what's up?"  "Will you tell Shankle that I am a big fan and that
I say, hi."  "Hell yea, I will.  I will write Shankle into your
reality next time.  I will have him train with you before your
weightlifting meet.  Salute.
Pause............
```

The term "Olympic Weightlifting" is a huge pet peeve of mine. I think it sends the wrong message about our sport and who can participate. Meets are for everyone, not just high-level lifters. Weightlifting is a **SPORT** that just so happens to be in the Olympics. There are local meets that take place all over the country that anyone can attend. The Olympics is something that only a select few will ever be able to experience, and I find it disconcerting that it brands our sport.

That being said; you should compete in a Weightlifting meet. The knowledge you will gain from these experiences is priceless. Think of it as a cheap seminar where you will learn about yourself, the sport you love and how to improve for the next one. Oh, trust me, there will be another one too because once you do one meet you will more than likely have been bitten by the competition bug.

I encourage you to do as many as possible to build your melting pot as a battle-hardened Weightlifter. When you are there, you need to soak it all in. Talk to other athletes, ask questions and have fun because this is what all your hard training has been for in the first place. As with training; there is much to know about competing in a Weightlifting meet. I want to make sure you are prepared and educated on game day.

Meet Card

The chess game of a meet is not discussed enough. No one ever talks about important things such as when to warm up, when should you adjust your attempts, how to read cards or outplay your competitors until now. Below is an example of a meet card. You need to know how to read it so you can use it as a pawn in the game of Weightlifting. In the backroom, the depth of the sport stretches to the coaches around the card table. First, let us talk about the basics and then we can go in depth on how to win your chess matches.

LOT #:	NAME:				AWF ID#:	
WT CLASS:	BW:	(inital):	DIV:		YOB:	

SNATCH

ATT 1:	Declaration:	(int):	ATT 2:		ATT 3:		
	Change:						
	Change:						**BEST SN**

C & J							
ATT 1:	Declaration:	(int):	ATT 2:		ATT 3:		
	Change:						
	Change:						**BEST C&J**
							TOTAL

(Figure 14.1)

○ **Lot #:** The lot number is a random number assigned to each lifter at the beginning of the meet. In the event, there is a tie where two lifters will be attempting the same weight for the same attempt; the lot number dictates who goes first. The lower number always goes first.

○ **AWF ID#:** This is your American Weightlifting Federation identification number. It can be found in your online profile.

○ **WT Class:** The weight division you will be competing within. The AWF follows the International Weightlifting Federation's weight class guidelines. You can find this information at www.IWF.net.

○ **BW:** Your exact body weight recorded at the weigh in just prior to the meet. Weigh-ins typically occur two hours before the first bar is lifted. Your body weight will be used in the Sinclair Coefficient formula. That formula changes every year because it is based on current world records in different body weight classes. According to the IWF, it poses the question of "what would be the total of an athlete weighing x KG if he or she were an athlete in the heaviest class of the same level of ability?"

○ **YOB:** Year of Birth.

○ **Div:** There are four divisions in which you can compete within: Youth, Junior, Senior, and Master. It is calculated by the year you were born. It is a great thing if you are born in January because you can technically compete as a 20-year-old junior. If you were born in December – you lose a year and would automatically be considered a senior for that calendar year.

○ **Lifts & Declarations:** When you arrive for the weigh in you will have to declare an opener for both the Snatch and Clean & Jerk. Throughout the meet, you will have two changes per attempt to modify the weight you will be lifting.

- ○ **Changing Declarations:** The ability to change your declarations can be used to your advantage in numerous ways. For example, if I declared 70kg as my opener, but then my warm ups were not going very well I could reduce it. I can lower my opener to 65kg as long as the competition bar has not reached that weight yet. The weight on the bar always climbs at a meet. It never reduces. If the lowest declared weight at the start of the competition is 60kg then, the bar starts loaded with that. From there it progressively climbs until the last man lifts his final attempt.

- ○ **The Clock:** The clock is directly tied into your attempt declarations. Each lifter will receive a one minute clock to complete their attempt. If an athlete misses their lift and decides to redo it then they will receive a two minute clock as they follow themselves. A thirty second warning will be announced to let you know that time is running out to complete your attempt. Should you want to change your weight, you **MUST** notify meet officials before the thirty second warning. After that no changes can be made. After a successful lift, officials will give you an automatic increase of 1KG. You need to tell them what your real next attempt will be or risk being stuck with that weight.

The Inner Workings of a Meet:

I have been extremely fortunate to have lived in a part of the country where meets can be found almost every single weekend. It was my mission to compete at as many of them as possible in order to climb the rankings in the sport. Along the way, I learned a lot of things the hard way, and I want you to avoid that. Here is some advice to help you find success:

- ○ **Know the Rules:** It is **YOUR RESPOSIBILITY** as an athlete to know the rules of the sport. They can be found on the International Weightlifting Federation's (IWF) website. Knowing the rules, will ensure that you do not have lifts taken away for silly mistakes such as dropping the barbell before the head judge tells you to. Download the **IWF Technical and Competition Rules & Regulations** handbook, and read it as a refresher before every meet.

- ○ **Find a Coach:** Your first meet can be confusing and intimidating. When you are there, the amount of information to keep track of can be overwhelming. When to warm up, when to lift, how long to rest, when to make changes to the plan….even having a plan in the first place! It is in your best interest to find a coach who has experience bringing athletes to meets. It will take a lot of the pressure off of yourself and allow you to do what you went there for; to lift.

o **Relax:** Unless you are at the Olympics you need to chill out. You are going to do so many meets over the course of your life that you should never let one freak you out. Some people thrive off of the intensity of being a little scared, but if you know you are not that person then just be cool. Do your thing and enjoy it. As long as you are having fun all will go well. First timers would do well just to treat it as another max out day.

o **Be Prepared:** The night before your gym bag should be packed with everything you could need. Try on your equipment and make sure everything fits well and is in working order. The day of the meet is no time to discover your singlet has an embarrassing hole in the crotch, or that lucky pair of underwear is missing.

o **Bring Food:** Like Donny always says, "Ya gotta eat," and that still applies at meets. If you have never done one before, it can be a long, exhausting experience. You need to make sure you will be able to refuel between the Snatch session and the Clean & Jerk session. Bring items that you would usually eat. Do not experiment with a new pre-workout that a buddy brought or anything out of the ordinary for you. Your stomach will potentially already be in knots from your nerves; having unusual food causing problems certainly will not help.

o **The Night Before:** The night before a meet is crucial. First, you should eat a hearty meal. It will help you have the energy you need the next day. Second, take a hot bath to help recover joints or muscles that might be aching from hard training. Third, pump yourself up. Watch Gladiator, 300 or another movie that gets the adrenaline going. That is sure to add 5KG to your lifts the next day.

o **Take your time:** You do not need to rush any of your attempts. When your name is called, it is your show. Own it and have fun. Both lifts take just seconds to complete, and you are allotted a generous amount of time to complete them.

3 Models for Planning Attempts

You have to go into every meet with a concrete plan for each of your attempts. Write them down so they are with you that day and make adjustments where necessary. Jessica has developed a system for planning and executing attempts that include scheduled rest times. We have three models for various meet goals:

o **Novice:** This will be a theoretical lifter who has the goal of setting a new personal record.

- **Intermediate:** Jessica will be the example here of a lifter who is trying to Qualify for another meet.
- **Professional:** I will be the example here of a lifter who is trying to medal.

As a coach, you need to know your athlete. As an athlete, you need to know yourself. Every weightlifter likes to do different things when they are warming up in the back room. You need to know how many warm ups you like to take, whether or not you like to break a set, hit doubles or singles ect....

When declaring opening weights, most weightlifters never put their actual first attempt on the card just in case things are not going well, and they need to change it. For our attempt models, we utilize Coach Jackie Mah's rule of three. You will have to read the card table and see how many attempts out you are from your opener. From there, you will work backward adding three minutes of rest between warm-ups leading up to your opener. If you are up early in a meet then, it is about minutes and attempts. After your division is introduced if there are three attempts before your first weight then, you have thirteen minutes before you lift. When your name is called, you will have one minute to complete your lift. If you are following yourself, you will be given a two-minute rest period to complete your next lift.

Our recommendations for calculating weight jumps for both your warm-up sets and attempts are simple. Women have been found to work best with 2kg and 3kg jumps. Men, on the other hand, can take bigger jumps typically ranging from 3kg to 5kg. Ideally a conditioned weightlifter can go from the barbell to maximum in 20 to 25 minutes.

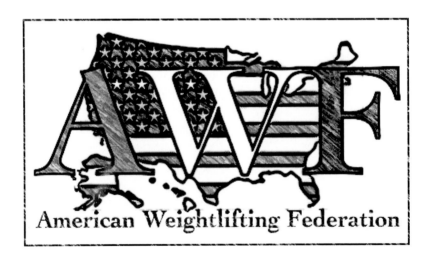

American Weightlifting Federation

Novice Model

For our theoretical novice lifter, the current best lift in the Snatch is 77kg. The meet in question could potentially be their first or second meet. Our goal is to set them up for success. The personal record attempt of 78kg will be their last lift of the day.

Weight (kg) x Reps	Minutes from Opener
Bar x Practice Reps	24
35kg x 3	21
35kg x 2 (Again)	18
45kg x 1	15
55kg x 1	12
60kg x 1	9
65kg x 1	6
70kg – Declared Opener	3
73kg – Actual Opener	x
76kg – Second Attempt	x
78kg – Record Attempt	x

Intermediate Model

Our Intermediate athlete is looking to qualify for another meet such as Nationals. When you are trying to be eligible for competition, you need to reach a qualifying total. For our example, the total will be 148kg. That means our lifter needs to Snatch 64kg and Clean & Jerk 84kg. Our goal during training is always to be able to make the total. Snatch, Clean & Jerk PRs are irrelevant; only the total matters. If, during a max out session during training, they hit a 62kg Snatch then, they will try to build to the 86kg Clean & Jerk to make up the kilos. That helps them build confidence that even if things do not go as planned they can still reach that mark.

Weight (kg) x Reps	Minutes from Opener
Bar x Practice Reps	24
35kg x 3	21
40kg x 2	18
45kg x 1	15
50kg x 1	12
55kg x 1	9
58kg x 1	6
60kg – Declared Opener	3
61kg – Actual Opener	x
64kg – Second Attempt	**x**
Xkg – Record Attempt	x

We want our goal weight to be the second attempt. The first one builds confidence and then we go for the goal. That is a more conservative approach than compared to the Novice Model. The second attempt is viewed as the "coaches' attempt." Our athlete needs to do this for their coach because they worked hard too. I like to say if they win a medal; then you need to cut it in half and give one piece to your coach! If we are successful, then the third attempt belongs to the athlete. With that, they can have a little fun and go for a personal record.

Professional Model

Our final model will outline how I (Jon North) would approach a meet. In this situation, I am not attempting to set a personal record or Qualify, but to win a medal. My numbers are going to be dictated by what my competitors are doing.

Weight (kg) x Reps	Minutes from Opener
Bar x Practice Reps	20
50kg x 3	18
70kg x 2	16
90kg x 1	14
110kg x 1	12
120kg x 1	10
130kg x 1	8
140kg x 1	6
145kg x 1	4
150kg – Declared Opener	2
155kg – Actual Opener	x
160kg – Second Attempt	**x**
X kg – Record Attempt	x

This model will be different from one athlete to the next. That is why you have to know yourself or if you are a coach know your athlete. I have discovered that I perform better when I go faster. That is why my rest times are so small. I am an emotional lifter, and I do not like to sit waiting for the next lift. Athletes at this skill level, may take bigger jumps building up to the opener. At this level winning and losing may come down to 1kg. There is no reason to tie, just beat the other guy. Lifters may also incorporate other tactics to gain rest time or stall another athlete. For example, if I was up for my final attempt at 162kg my coach might change the weight and declare 165kg to pause the clock. The clock needs to pause while the loaders have to come out and adjust the barbell. This time adds up in your favor.

After that, if I have another change left, we might stop the clock again and declare 166kg. Now, I went from 2:00 of rest to 2:00+ by adding in the changes. If there were lifters with attempts between 162kg and 166kg, then now they either have to go or make the choice to change their weights as well. Both options have pros and cons. You gain more rest, but you may not make the weight. If both you and your opponent miss and you were ahead of the other guy then you might still

251

win anyway. Other tricks you can do to gain more rest time if you are seriously in need is to ask for the platform to be swept because it is slippery. The loaders, will have to move the bar; sweep then move the bar back and tighten it. You can also declare that there is blood on the bar, and the cleaning process will take some time as well.

Do as many meets as possible. Meets expose your real weaknesses whether it be physical strength or mental strength. You will learn about yourself as an athlete, make friends and have the ability to show the audience how hard you have been training.

I hope you have enjoyed reading about my philosophies on technique and have learned from my stories of success and failure. Looking back on all that I have done in this sport, I can honestly say the thing I am most proud of is my relationship with you and the rest of the Attitude Nation. No medal I have won, personal record I have set, or even drug that I have taken can match the high I feel when I can do something positive for you. In closing, I will leave you with two last thoughts.

First, **Be free - freedom is happiness.** If you are working at a job that you hate then you are not free, you are a prisoner. A prisoner, locked in a cell, just like I was before I found the barbell. If you are homeless, pursuing your dreams and love it. Then you are free. Freer than the person who dreads waking up every morning. That person who cannot stand to start their day because what they are doing does not feel fulfilling and is just for money. You need to pursue the things in life that you love and are passionate about, and you need to be willing to make the sacrifices that are necessary to get them. It may mean living in your car for half a year or paying for meals with the change you collected from cashing in bottles. I can tell you that it will all be worth it when that day comes that you have the life you want and not the one you settled on. Do not get me wrong, it will not be easy, and it will be scary in the beginning. There will be pressure from your friends and family who will doubt your decision to quit your job or schooling to be a Weightlifter, Painter, or Actor etc... You need to tune all of that out and trust what your gut tells you. Every day that you wake up go out and fight for what you want because no one else will and you only have this one life.

Second, After years of Weightlifting, I have a love-hate relationship with the barbell. I love it because it saved my life, and I hate it because of its brutal nature in training. However, if you feel lost in this world, consider finding a gym and letting the barbell guide you for a little while. It will not always give you what you want when you go to lift it, but the bar can replace drugs, offer positive direction and serenity amidst the chaos that can develop in our lives. At the gym, you will find a community…a family who is also on the quest to master the barbell. They can offer support, accountability and a good atmosphere to help keep whatever demons that haunt you at bay. The barbell is a high that dwarfs all others, and it can change your life…it can set you free.

Gym Bag

Saturday, September 7, 2013

Inspired By Mark Haz's Cal Rugby Bag

The other day, I went through my old gym bag looking for some old tape and a baseball for my athletes to use before training. I was fascinated by all the gadgets I came across while digging deeper and deeper into the land of memories and assortments. The horrible smell, the chalky straps, a graveyard of past champions that now lay quietly on the dark while the new generation of gym bags walk around prideful and tall. I am putting together a little museum.... I guess you could call it, of not only my medals, but everything from shoes, shirts, straps, belts, and all the things that have sentimental value to me from over the years. All things that have helped me along my way. Of course this museum of some sort is only for my eyes and viewership, for this "stuff" to others is pure trash and rubbish.

I then started to dash quickly around the room like a kid on Christmas, lining and organizing all my treasures. I was reminded of an old blog I once wrote, a blog that has seemed to be forgotten, by myself and others, a blog that was once my favorite, that needs to come back to life. So..... to anyone who has a smelly gym bag..... this one's for you.

A long stare at his old blue gym bag as it sat lop-sided beside him on the subway bench, waiting for the 7 o'clock train. There were no words being spoken from his long chin and stubble covered face, just a stone cold look and a thought of how this gym bag hasn't been replaced by now. How has the bag with so many stains, broken straps, and holes gone this long without being put to rest. A small crinkle in his forehead asked the bag if the old blue warrior was growing, and getting bigger over time. It looked as if the bag had grown at least a foot since the night before. He would know because the bag and him have been training

partners since college back at Cal, and it was only last night
that he stocked it with plastic bags full of supplements of all
different colors and textures. He regretted not cleaning his
two shaker cups better the night before while preparing for
this trip, as he could smell them both seeping from the inside
of the bag to his nose. Still no emotion, as his eyes glazed
upon the bag with straps that were hanging on by a single thread
from all the abuse they have seen. How they haven't broke by
now will always be a mystery. Some say that trying to figure
out weightlifting can lead to madness, for the sport never, and
will never make sense. His head titled slightly down, and the
crinkles in his forehead smoothed back out. His eyes hadn't
blinked since he sat down, and the thought of becoming mad
haunted him. How do you know when you have lost your mind? He
asked the bag while looking back up. This time words came out
from his mouth, while the person sitting across from him grabbed
her two kids and scurried them away to the waiting bench three
vending machines down. The bag did not reply. The bag just stared
back at him while slightly molding itself deeper into the bench,
as if to say he was done, and could not carry on from here. The
yellow Cal label on the front of the bag facing him was turned
brown from the years. He was saddened by the fact he just now
noticed how worn the bag really was. His body still hadn't
moved, but his eyes started to frantically flicker back and
forth as if he couldn't figure out what to look at. Memories of
slamming the gym bag against the wall out of anger. Dropping
the bag down on the dusty gym floor while walking over it to
get from resting bench to platform. Laughing weightlifters in
the car after a long day of training, while his best friend and
biggest supporter of so many years laid defeated in the trunk
under boxes and old books. Memories and reminiscing of how
well he used to treat his new bright blue bag when he first got
into weightlifting, or back then just weight training / body
building / wide feet power looking snatches and pose offs with
his friends. A gym rat that had no plans or ideas of what he
was doing, or wanted to do. All he knew back then was he loved
the weight room, and the lifestyle the weight room produced. The
blue bag was just as important as the weights. Just as food
and bed are to recovery. Belts and coffee, chalk and music, all
a family that you grow to know and love throughout this lonely
sport of weightlifting.

A small smile crept across his face as the noise from a train
passing by broke his long stare, waking him up to a darker
than usual subway full of old newspapers and a cold gust of
air coming from the stair case that led outside. He rubbed
his hands together to get warm, while thinking about all the
different ways he was going to treat his bag better from here
on out. He opened his mouth wide while rubbing his cheeks with
his hands to try to snap out of his trance and wake before the
day passed him by. A weightlifter must learn how focus on both
weightlifting and everyday life, sometimes at the same time.
When these two completely different worlds meet they can cause
doubt, confusion, and the worst of all....excuses. Learning
how to be a weightlifter is the hardest part in learning how to
be a weightlifter. The bag made a small noise from something
inside moving out of place. He patted the bag with a broken
smile and whispered as if he was talking to a puppy, "You know
what I'm saying, right boy?". The bag looked back with a glow of
appreciation and relief. The bag was just as much a weightlifter
as the man, and the man knew he was just as much part of that
bag as the bag itself. The man felt lighter from their talk. A
sigh of understanding and respect. He was at first blind sided
and taken back from how old the bag truly was, but was now proud
of himself and the bag for keeping an honest relationship, and
continually staying the best of friends.

The man pulled his hands away to straighten out his clothes in
anticipation for his train the he could hear down the tunnel
moving his way. The light from the train opened the subway up
with a new perspective. The newspapers were not scattered around
the floor nor were they dirty. The floor was clean and the
vending machines where glowing bright. There were more people
than he thought there was hustling and bustling around as if an
army was forming to attack the day. The man opened his wide eyes
and quickly turned to his bag, hoping that his bright blue Cal bag
was young and strong as he always knew it to be. The bag laid
half dead as its shadow crept down the bench towards the man. The
man's eyes followed the dark shadow running into his hand that
was structurally there supporting his excited lean towards the
bag. The man noticed his hands. He picked both of them up and
turned them side to side in front of his face. They were torn,
bruised and old. They were stained yellow from the cigarettes he

once smoked. Old chalk lived deep under his nails, and the blood
paintings that webbed across his hands from broken blood blisters
made sure that he was just as broken and
used as the bag sitting beside him. The
man has aged with his bag. The man then
realized sitting on that subway bench, that
he had become his own gym bag.
Metal Empire Productions Presents the
newest Team AN video. Metal Empire will be
documenting our young teams path to Gold,
with behind the scene antics, interviews,
recaps and more. Welcome to the family Metal
Empire. lets take over the world.

The Documentary 2016

JON NORTH AND JAMES MCDERMOTT
PRESENT
THE DARK ORCHESTRA

PART III.

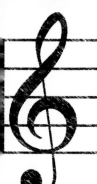

CHAPTER 15:
THE DARK ORCHESTRA
2011

Another step on the road to 200...

Tuesday, March 15, 2011

After cleaning 200kg I am incredibly anxious to do my first 200kg clean and jerk, here is another step along the road, a 175kg double. 180kg double coming soon...

♪ ♪ ♪

Motivation...

Wednesday, March 16, 2011

I thought I would post this on my blog to motivate myself. Spencer beat me in a training hall contest with this lift, I WILL make a double with this weight soon!

♪ ♪ ♪

I am a Weightlifting Robot

Saturday, March 19, 2011

My name is Jon North and I am a robot. I cannot lie to the public anymore about being human because I am not, I am a weightlifting robot. I wake up in the morning and I eat kilo's for breakfast, and the red ones are my favorite. I love mixing my red kilo's with tasty white cloudy chalk and a nice cold bar to top off my meal. Now my meal is over its time to train, no words just a cold hard

BEN CLARIDAD

look from the one and only Donnie Shankle that says "its war time". I
thank my maker for giving me a good robot heart because without it I
would fall hard as Donnie would continue on his journey through the
land of weightlifting without me. That will never happen because
I am a strong robot with a good robot heart. I grab my shield and
sword and begin to fight side by side with Donnie until there are no
more kilo's left to kill. I wipe the red blood off my sword and tell
Donnie good training. My bold bright and proud california strength
tattoo is moving up and down from my heart beat. That tattoo gives me
pride, for califronia strength is my maker.

North 2012

♪ ♪ ♪

Finally in Ireland

Tuesday, March 22, 2011

Thank the good Lord I am finaly in Ireland! wow that was a long trip.
Coach and I flew from san fran to LA, then we took a 10 hour flight
from LA to London. Once we landed in London we had a 4 hour lay over
and then took a one hour flight into Dublin where I am at now. Holly
molly. I am now sitting on my very good friends couch, the one and
only Berry Kinsella. He is our host this week, and is the one who put
this great trip together. Berry came down and trained with us at Cal
strength for a week a few months back, so now its our turn to come see
him. We have three seminars and then the rest of the time hanging
out and site seeing!   It is very beatifull hear, but very very
different, I am already missing my USA. All of the small things make
me feel like I am in a different world. From the restroom signs being
toilet signs instead. everything is much smaller, like elevators,
hall ways, roads, cars and pretty much everything else. I have never
seen more soccer fields in my whole life!   There are hand fulls of
soccer fields it seems every dang block. People dress much different
hear than we do. They dont wear many colors at all, lots of grey and
black. Our first seminar is tomorrow night and I am looking forward
to hitting some big numbers and getting people stronger. we are about
to go hit the town now so I will be back later to tell how the first
seminar went.

North 2012

♪ ♪ ♪

Cocaine and coffee

Saturday, April 23, 2011

Sneaky little bitch, I lay in bed thinking of ways to conquer that two faced devil. I think I am talking about the weight, the weight that never sleeps, the weight that waits for me all night in that cave, that cave that plays tricks on your mind, that cave that turns you against yourself. One minute you are friends, then the next thing you know he's sleeping with your girl. That piece of shit, that piece of shit that builds me up everyday then pushes me down, I hate him. You're not my friend you're my enemy, you really don't like me, you want to see me fail. You smile to my face then you show your black teeth and your dark black eyes; you show your horns, you show yourself. Everywhere I go you are there reminding me who I really am. The insecure college drop out who only wants people to like him, who only wants to be somebody he is not. My face is cut from the mirror I smash, thank God I have my coffee in my hand, I love this coffee that builds me up, that gives me confidence. This dark cave has little smiley faces all around it, little smiley faces that wait around the corner for me. Are they really smiling? Some days I feel like I am in the shining, some days I feel like becoming the Phantom. I should have been a fighter, the weight is not enough, I need to hit and be hit, I need to see that fucker fall. I drink more and more coffee everyday, its like my cocaine. Why is it I don't ever get hurt? Why is it I always feel great? I will dedicate my life to killing you, to cutting you and watching you bleed. I am fucking crazy, I will never go away, you will hate me more and more everyday, but the more you hate me the more you will two face me, so fuck you. I have something in me that scares me, I can jump off a building and fly. I will lift you and slam you, maybe not right now but soon. You are turning me darker and darker, the more I succeed the more I hate, and I hate you.

♪ ♪ ♪

College drop out

I miss the "pump" I miss putting those pads on, I miss going to
party's, I miss my old friends, I even miss college, I miss my family,
I miss not lifting. Hi my name is Jon North and I am a college drop
out, I gave up everything for this sport, I live in a gym, a am a
gym. I am a bar, I am the weights, I am weightlifting. I went all
in with a bad hand, and some how I am still at the final table with
the chip lead. I am putting it on all the line with this sport, I
have o excuses, but shit what happens if I fail? If I fail I have no
one to blame, nothing to blame, no excuses, I cant sleep at night. My
mind thinks "what ifs" all day. I just know that I am so much better
than what I am showing right now, I am so damn athletic its crazy, I
am not even strong, I just move like a cat, I swear, you should walk
in my shoes and see how I float. I have given everything to be the
best, but I need to give more, more and then some more. Nothing else
matters. If I don't go to the Olympics then what? who am I? Whats
all this for then? I waste of life, my life is the Olympics. I
think to grow this sport more people need to just go all in like I
did, and hopefully they will go farther than me, hopefully we can win
some Olympic medals for this great Country Called the United States
Of America baby. I love this country with all my heart. Sense I am
a pussy and I am not over seas fighting with the rest of our brave
soldiers, than I will fight in the gym and on the platform, that's
why when I go to the Pan Am Championships this year I am letting go, I
will kill. Money, college, pressure from others to be something your
not, statues, cars, these are all things people want and will choose
over there dream, more than half of them will never go for it, they
want those things to bad. The other half gets those things and then
still wants to be a bad ass weightlifter, that's the problem. well
lucky for me I have both but don't worry about that...lol hahaha I
am just saying that I wish more weightlifters in this country would
man the fuck up and start training for real, and stop with all the
other bullshit. Lets go, lets start training, win or lose we need to
keep fighting everyday, find away. Stop bitching, stop blaming, stop
making excuses and make it happen, the way I look at it is Life is a
game, play it and win.

North 2012

♪ ♪ ♪

"super man pull"

I call it the "super man pull". In Olympic weightlifting the most
famous way of breaking down the pull on the snatch and clean and jerk
is "first pull, second pull, and then the third pull" meaning the
finish at the top of the lift before you go under the bar to catch
the weight. In the Jon North coaching book I break it down a little
different. I call it the super man pull. The super man has three
steps as well focusing on the positions of the shoulders rather than
the bar path. Here are the three points:

The first point of the super man pull happens right off the floor.
Your shoulders need to be back, not behind the bar but back enough
that your chest should be facing the wall. You should stay that way
from the floor to a little bit below your knees. Thats point one.

The second point is right when the bar starts getting closer to your
knees you should then push your shoulders over the bar. This is hard
to do, because you have to stay on your heels, but the bar has other
plans. The bar wants to put you on your toes, but you have to fight
and stay on your heels the whole time. If you can stay on your heels
and push your shoulders out over the bar at the same time you are
putting your body in perfect position for point three, the "finish"
the explosion!

Point three is once the bar is in line with your hips then you pull
your shoulders all the way back behind your hips. When you pull your
shoulders back you should push the bar into your hips at the same
time, and your hips should come through at the same time as well.
"Bar back hips through!" This is what I say everyday in the gym. It
is what you need for the Mike Tyson finish so you can have time to get
under the bar to catch and then stand up, making the winning lift in
the Olympics. That's the super man pull Now let me tell you why this
way of pulling is the best way to go.

The reason why the super man pull is so effective is because it forces
you to stay over the bar! This is the most important part of the lift.
When an athlete starts pulling back too early, or in some cases pulling
their shoulders back throughout the whole pull means they will have no
power for the finish. Don't believe me? Then try it yourself. Try
jumping as high as you can in the air with your shoulders behind your

hips before you jump... That's what I thought. You looked like a fish out of water, no power. Now try jumping in the air with your shoulders over your hips. Well there you go. Now you have some good power and jumped higher than Michael Jordan. Same thing goes with the snatch and clean. You need to push your shoulders back at the same time your hips come through. As you pull your shoulders back you should be pushing the bar INTO your hips at the same time, and your hips should be coming through at the same time as well for that max explosion, because that's what you are looking for, explosion to give you time to get under. It all should happen in the blink of an eye, bam. You want to push the bar into your hips, and don't pull up! That's what so many lifters do. Right before the bar is about to make contact with the hips, they start to pull up and this leads to a "brush hit". Those are the worst. Don't pull up, pull back! Its physics, for example, if two trains are moving full speed at each other and they collide there is going to be way more force then if there was only one train moving and one sitting still. So the same applies to your hips and the bar, pull back for that force, for that "finish"!

TRY THIS SUPER MAN PULL, North 2012

PS: You look like super man when you do the super man pull, and that's bad ass.

♪ ♪ ♪

Shankle

Sunday, May 1, 2011

This remarkable man has served this Country in so many ways, from protecting our country as a Marine, beating the Russian silver medalist Dmitry Klokov in 2006 at the Arnold, Representing America in his SECOND world championship! Medaling twice at the Pan Am games! Three time national champion, and 2012 Olympic hopeful! That's only a little bit of this guy's outstanding, insane and remarkable record and accomplishments. I am proud to call Donny my team mate and my friend. It's an honor to be on the front line everyday training in the trenches with this wolf, this Sheppard, this damn machine that just does not stop! Get in his way and you will be eaten, chewed up and spit out because this dude knows what he wants, and he will let no body get in the way. Donny has a presents that makes you want to get to know him, hang around him and become friends right off the

266

bat, but once he puts those shoes on he has a presents that makes you
piss in your pants and your legs tremble with fear! The motivation
and the determination is greater than anything I have ever seen, His
record tells you that. This guy will fight with the bar Intel that
bar loses, Intel he wins. He will fight with YOU Intel you lose and
he wins. Donny Shankle is the best, and I am proud to say that I
train with he best, I get to see the best train every day, I get to
lift on the same platform with the best every day, I get to talk and
hear what the best has to say every day, and trust me I listen with
both ears, and I don't forget one thing this man says. I have learned
so much from Donny. I have learned what it takes to be a champion
in this sport, and how to become a man by watching and listening.
Learning from Donny Shankle is better than any book or certification
that anybody can get. I only hope one day I can achieve what Donny has
achieved and more.

Shankle 2012!

♪ ♪ ♪

Apple Lady

Monday, May 2, 2011

Today is Monday that means today is war day! hahaha This is the day
when more 94kg lifters run! Right now I am drinking chocolate milk,
listening to Jonny cash cocaine blues, writing on my blog, watching
some Jon North videos and other secretes that I just cant let out of
the bag people. Lets see what else is new with me, o I watched a
great movie last night called the road. wow what a sad movie, for
some reason I did not cry though....which is weird because I cry in
a lot of movies, but this one I did not. I thought the ending was
bad, but I still really enjoyed the movie, I thought it was very well
made. I watched it with my Fiancee and she got scared a few times.
If you have not seen this movie you should go rent it, or read the
book. The word on the street is that there is some cross fit slash
weightlifter coming to train with me at 5:00 from redding, well this
should be fun! this should be interesting, why do you ask? well
I will tell you why because if I had a dollar for every kid or guy
that came to my gym to train like a pro weightlifter and then left
and never came back after the first day, then I would be a rich man.
or if they do come back it's always the same old story...." man my

267

knees hurt, man my back hurts, man I am sore, wow I think I need a few
weeks off, yea I don't know if I want to compete, yea I don't know,
maybe well... ummmm, ill try..."   get the fuck out of my gym then!
I am so sick off that, it gives me a headache just thinking about it.
If you want general fitness then go down to your local shine shop
24 hour fitness. They have fluffy white towels, music, cold water
fountains, mirrors, little blue birds that land on your shoulder
while you get your pump on, apple ladies that walk around half naked
and give out apples when you get a little hungry. Maybe its the hose
water in the back and a big coach penlday yelling at you that might
scare them away! lol no apple ladies hear, just coach Pendlay!!!!

Coach Pendlay for President! 2012

♪ ♪ ♪

Muddy Boot

Tuesday, May 3, 2011

Wow... This coffee is Hitting me hard this morning, wow i feel overly
confident, I feel like pissing more people off. I am thinking to
myself how I will destroy this sport of weightlifting. Ok, call me
arrogant, call me cocky, I don't really care, I am just tired of
waiting for the trials, the worlds in Paris, the Pan Am Games this
year is Mexico. I just want to do it, I want to lift, I want to
take first place and throw the weight in the crowd. Why? I don't
know why. Why do I have such a big chip on my shoulder? Why do I
get so pissed when I lift? Maybe it's because I want to win so bad,
Maybe it's because I haven't done shit with my life besides lift big
weights. But wait...This weight I am lifting ain't even big weight,
but coach Pendlay will get me there. He will get me to bigger weight.
If you don't think that then...... well I should chill, hahaha! This
is it people, this is me, weightlifting is me, I have a one track mind
and that's killing and destroying, I will not ask I will take and I
will not share. In this sport you have to be greedy, don't ask grab
and steel and stand your ground. put your muddy boot on there face
and push down everyday and never let up, push there face in the mud,
and I hope its raining. fight, fight, fight, fight, fight and when
your done knock that mother fucker out. Weightlifting has given me
a purpose in life, weightlifting has given me a life, I am forever
grateful to weightlifting. I am forever grateful to Dave Spitz and

coach Glenn Pendlay. Dave Spitz took a chance with me and he gave
me a hand when I was down. Dave Spitz is the reason why I am here
right now and not in jail or dead. Yeah yeah ok I came from a bad
place and I was a bad boy, ok I got kicked out of my last team from
knocking a dude out in the gym, but not anymore. Now I am focused.
I am a Cal Strength soldier and nothing will ever change that. I
use this hate that I have toward certain things to keep me going. I
don't get injured, I don't have time for that. I have too many things
to do in this sport. Hurt! Hahaha that's funny. Never. If I see
someone stretching or using a foam roller I will take my belt and
slap them. stop being a bitch. grab the bar and go, stop with all
the "getting ready" shit and lift. Coach Pendlay and Dave Spitz are
creating a monster, and this monster is about to make a statement.
Pan Ams, NUMBER ONE, PWA records, Arnold Champ, all in less than three
years ain't shit to me, If I don't make the Olympics then what's the
point?.... I love when people talk shit about me. They get mad when
I spike the weight, when I yell, when I spit on the weight. The more
they talk, the more I will spit and spike. I listen to four people
in this whole world: David Spitz, Coach Pendlay, my brilliant farther,
and my lovely Mom. That's it. If your not them, then don't tell me
shit. This is just the beginning . I am not going anywhere, sorry. I
always hear people telling me about these young kids in my weight
class coming after me and lifting good weight. Never, never, ever.
I have this crazy rush over me all the time I can't control, I am
dead serious. These young kids will never beat me. Young... What's
young????? I am 24 and I feel like I am 15. I don't just feel like I
am in the Mafia. I am in the Mafia. You think I am joking, I am not.
When I say I am California Strength soldier, I mean it! lol hahahha.

Jon North 2012

♪♪♪

The Crack Head

Saturday, May 7, 2011

I had a crack head in a head lock last night in the middle of main
street at 3 am in the morning in my boxers.....now do I have your
attention! Your probably wondering to yourself how the hell I got
into this situation!!!! well let me tell you, follow me to the start
of this crazy story.

It was 3 am in the morning and I was sound asleep next to my lovely
Fiance, when I was woken up by my daughter, aka, my dog aka my pit
bull. she kept barking, and it was not just a normal bark, it was a
very mean scary bark that I have never heard before. I new something
was wrong from how lexi was barking, and right before I got out of bed
I heard a banging noise coming from outside, bang! bang! bang! it
sounded like it was coming from the drive way. I ran to the window
and saw a shadow that looked like a man banging at my car window with
something in his hand. I yelled at him, "hey, hey you"!! "get the
hell out of hear"! he didn't even look back. He didn't even stop
banging at my window. You would think he would become startled or
scared, jump or run or even just look back, but no, nothing. I then
ran outside in nothing but my boxer shorts, and my first reaction
is to knock this dude out, attack him is what I first wanted to do,
but as I got closer to him I saw he had a knife in his hand, or
what looked like a knife. I wont lie, I was a little nervous at this
point, I started to slow down as a approached him, his confidence
sacred me, I am not a small dude, and I thought I was being pretty
intimidating, but this guy could care less that I was there, and
that's weird, that's not even normal. I couldn't figure out why this
guy was not even startled or even just acknowledge me, did he have
a gun? a knife? what was in his hands? did he have Friends around
the corner about to jump me? all these thoughts were going through
my head. I kept yelling at him, and then he finally he said without
even looking at me, "it wont open" what! at this point I was so
confused, I thought I was dreaming. I finally said enough is enough,
I said, "ok mother fucker you asked for it, your about to get fucked
up"! I ran back to the front door, opened it up, and told my daughter
to "get em"! my Lexi ran as fast as she has ever ran jumping into
the air and tackling this guy onto the street biting him all over. He
was screaming as she was ripping his jeans like one of her toys from
petco. I told my Fiance to call the cops, then I went on yelling,
"get em lexi, get em!!! fucken get em lexi!!!!!!!! over and over
again. I was so proud of her. He some how got up and started
running down the middle of the street, lexi then started to chase him
a whole block. When he got to the end of the block he was half naked
and very bloody. He thought he could out run my dog! lol that's
funny! my dog was on this crack head like white on rice. The main
street was more lit up from all the street lights. I then saw that
his hands where empty as he through them up from lexi biting his leg,
I then went into attack mode, now that I new he had no gun or weapon.
I ran and tackled him into the street, stood up and kicked him in
the head knocking him out for about three minutes, then I put him in

270

a choke hold and waited for the cops. Every time this guy tried to move lexi would snap at his arms and legs while running around us in circles showing these teeth that even scared me!

Finlay four cop cars pulled up surrounding us, I let the guy go and grabbed lexi, as all the cops did there thing. I have never been more proud of my dog, she protected the house, protected my girlfriend and me from harm, she risked her own life to protect us, I am forever grateful to her, I will never own a better dog for as long as I live. I After the cops took him away and did all the talking and paper work, my girlfriend and I put lexi's pink snuggie on, gave her a treat, and went back to bed. the end

♪ ♪ ♪

The Orange Room

Tuesday, May 10, 2011

I was woken up by the sunrise creeping through my window shades, it made my room orange, it was awesome. The orange light that filled my room made everything look different. Everything looked like it was in a toy story movie, I felt like I was in a different world. I looked over at my orange faced Fiance that was still sound asleep, she even looked computer animated. I didn't want to wake her so I got out of bed slowly and made my way to the kitchen to make some coffee. There is something about being the only one up and awake in your house very early in the morning that is so peace full. As if the whole world is asleep and your the only one awake. Its like the house is alive and looking at you like "why are you up this early"? The house was completely dark still, and then I noticed that the hall way that led to my room was completely orange. The orange light was creeping down the hall way heading right for me. It was slowly taking over the dark house. I stood there in my big blue robe and my coffee in my hand just staring at the orange light moving towards me, at this point I didn't know if I was awake or dreaming. The orange slowly hit my feet and then crept up my whole body in tell it I was a glowing orange man.

The cold morning air hit me right in the face the second I walked outside. I stretched out my arms and told myself I was going to lift big weights today. The orange light was a sign of strength, a sign that I was going to make this Olympic team in 2012. It was a sign that I was going to keep getting stronger, way stronger. I love this

271

sport, this sport is home to me, it has been good to me on all levels, I just want to take more out of it, I want to win more, I want to keep making more and more money, I want to get more kids in this sport, I love the USA. Its crazy to think where I am at today, wow, looking back a few years ago I was a lost kid in college in and out of trouble. Only if my English teacher new that I was a paid writer, and that I had my own blog, lol, she would fall over. I failed her class three times and then finally passed. She always loved my writing, it was just the reading and grammar that killed me. I will never forget what she told me, at the very end of my last class that I ended up passing. Ms Van Aalst said "forget 90% of what I taught you and write the way you want to write." That was the best advise any teacher has ever given me. All my other teachers told me my writing was "not properly formatted, you write like you talk Jon and that's not correct." I always looked back at what Ms Van Aalst told me and just kept doing my thing. Screw them, screw the know it all's, I hate only doing things one way because someone a long time ago said so, because that's just the way it is Jon. fuck that, do things your way, do it how you want to do it. Life is a game, life is in your hands, not theirs. Train how you want to train, write how you want to write, coach how you want to coach, fuck them. Fuck all them that tell you different.

♪ ♪ ♪

Mental Man

Monday, May 16, 2011

Mental, Mental, Mental man. The little mental man will climb up in your head, grab the controls and start controlling you! The mental man will take over your emotions, confidence, way of looking at things, he will make you "Clark" weights that you could make, he will mess up your whole day. You have to learn how to fight back and control the mental man. If you are thinking about getting rid of the little man you are crazy, he will never leave, he is there to stay forever! You have to trick him, give him something else do to while you focus and control your own mind. I usually tell him to go on a walk, play some video games, just anything to leave me a lone. Sometimes he will walk right into my head office and mess me up for just a few minutes, but you have to find ways to put him back in his room! If he does not go back in his room then you might miss lifts, do bad in a competition, miss a squat or the most common of them all

272

the "Clark" The "Clark is where the mental man will actually break
into your mind control room and unplug your lifting cord, yes I know
that sneaky bastard!!!   I have tried calling the cops on him before
but they wont arrest him, instead they call me crazy! People will
actually think its me "Clarking" the weight and not the mental man
breaking and entering! You can beat him though! I have done it, its
hard but with the right amount of determination, head security guards,
and big bouncers all working together, you can come back from a
"Clark" and make the lift on your next try! Yes you can take over the
controls and beat the little man with his bright yellow Hawaiian shirt
and his short blue swimming trunks. He will get all upset and stay in
his room for the rest of the day, while you continue to lift bigger
and bigger weight. Mental man 2012   ....wait........what is
all this writing???? this wasn't me typing! this must have been the
mental man!!!   son of a bitch! get back in your room!

♪♪♪

The Red Balloon

Wednesday, June 29, 2011

The worst thing I ever did in this sport is snatch 160kg. Before
that day the bar and I were best friends, we were like one, that bar
made me confident, strong and fearless. The bar is so high now that
I can't seem to find it. The bar didn't invite me on its travels
upward. The bar and I were ready to go together, we both had our
tickets and our bags packed just waiting for that big gust of wind to
carry us into the sky full of success, but right when I looked away,
the bar was already starting to float away. I reached up and tried
to grab it yelling, "wait bar, wait for me I want to go with you"! I
tried jumping as high as I could but it was just a little too far
up, minute after minute, and day after day the bar started to rise
higher and higher until it disappeared into the sky. I put up flyers
everywhere but no one has gotten back to me on it's whereabouts.
I feel so lost without my bar, I am not myself anymore. I am now just
an average Joe walking around lost and confused. I walk and I walk
through the dark hills that constantly whisper negative comments about
me. The deeper I get lost looking for my bar the more I hear words of
hate, and the more backs I see. I see red faces of haters that start
to laugh and smile, the better they sleep and the worse I sleep, the
more I get lost, the happier people get. They say, "Finally no more
annoying yelling, stupid shout outs, bar slamming and over the top,

cocky, arrogant blog postings". Finally he is no longer number one, finally he is lost and he will never find his bar again". Even though I might be stripped of my confidence and my strength is down, I am still that crazy jumping Jonathan North that came out of nowhere with Coach Jackie Mah. She unleashed me and said "sick em boy" and even without my bar you can't take that away from me. I told you people that I am not going anywhere, I told you that I will keep fighting no matter what, I told you I will keep slamming bars, spitting on weights and yelling loud in every battle I go into, I told you mother fuckers that I am not going anywhere. I will continue to piss people off, gather even more haters than I have now, I will continue to win, lose, make teams, miss teams, break records, bomb out, clark weights, kiss weights, yell Arnold, love this sport, and hate this sport.

After guidance by a few close to me, I found my bar deep in the woods behind a big wall of rocks. I have hit many walls in this sport and in life, but after a while of fighting, after a while of trying to live up to my mentor Donny Shankle, I have broken through all of them. But this wall is not going down, the more I push the heavier the wall feels. I cant seem to do it on my own, I have hit a wall I can't seem to bring down. My bar lays in the mud behind the wall still shinning bright, and I fuck'n want it, I fuck'n need it as other lifters keep getting stronger. I am wasting time. I need to win right now. I need to get back on top and get my fire back.

A very big man that towered over me with his black beard and sword called coach steps beside me and starts striking the wall with massive power. Right then, a legend of the woods with long hair and war tattoos steps on the other side of me striking the wall with confidence I have never seen before. I am in shock. I just keep pushing and hitting the wall as a small smile crosses my face, and right at that moment everyone seemed to stop and move out of the way kneeling down as a king with a golden crown and a golden stick started to walk up to the wall with his beautiful queen. That man is the king and owner of all the woods. Soon there were soldiers coming out of the woods to help. One was a wolverine. One was a dark muscular creature who was smaller and fast. One was an old friend with blond hair and legs that were made out of tree trucks. They all came to help. The wall started to crack and move. Two new creatures that just joined the woods came to help too. Even a small Asian creature helped with the wall, while also doing many other things for the king at the same time. The woods lumberjack showed up to help, who is known for kicking down trees and carried them off tied around his massive back, his leg power will be very useful in bringing down this wall. I was very happy to see the colorful haired athlete of the

woods who has a power that prevents her from aging, she who brings
energy and motivation to us all. The quiet wise man with glasses who
was respected and won many battles leading people to victory of the
woods came and started at the wall too. A big eyed skinny creature
who is the woods watcher and greatest people reader in all of the
land came to hit the wall. Last but not least a young kid new to the
woods came to help with his big new bronze medal around his neck, he
is known for having the biggest heart in the woods. Bang! bang! bang!
We all came together and smashed and hit the wall giving it everything
we had, but still the rocky wall would not go down.
My gold medal seemed to be out of reach, until the most beautiful
creature in all of the woods came flying down slowly with her white
wings and beautiful smile. She is the creature I am going to marry,
she is the angel that I love. She gave us all strength, as she
floated over and pushed against the wall. The wall started to move
and shake and then in a blink of an eye it fell down crumbling all
around the Pendlay bar. Everyone stepped back and watched as I hook
gripped my bar back into my hands. I stood tall with my elbows locked
out and the bar high over my head. I could feel my strength pumping
through my blood, my heart started to beat faster, and I began to yell
as the backs faced forward, the red faces of hate ran and hid away,
and the negative whispers turned into positive praises. I kissed
my angel, shook the hands of all the great friends that helped me
and walked back into the gym. I have my bar back, I will see you at
Nationals bitches.

North 2012

♪ ♪ ♪

AC

Sunday, July 3, 2011

That sucks your hands hurt. O thanks for telling me that I should
turn off my AC while the windows are down, let me go ahead and turn
off the AC in my car, your totally right man thank you. O no buddy
you have lower back pain when you train?! You should take off three
months , your right! the foam roller really helps how you feel in
training, OMG I love that stretch, it really works my hamstrings. I
love doing the hang snatch because I really feel like it stretches
and strengthens my hamstrings. Your right bro I would save a lot of

money if I didn't buy my smokes, I am done with that man, what was I
thinking. Please tell me what I should do man, please I need help.
This life thing is hard, should I turn left or right? Your right I
need to open lighter and make more lifts, yea your right I need to eat
better, yea your right I need to control my breathing in competition
and focus more on the task at hand. I am so glad you came up and
started talking to me about all this, I am glad you saw the sign
around my neck that says help, because I am lost! Shit, dude I am so
so sorry that I offended you when I flipped off the camera in one of
my you tube videos, that will never happen again, I need to become
more classy. Hey before you leave can you write down everything
I should work on or do so I can practice when I get home? thank
you. I will never joke about steroids again, please forgive me!!!!
"control your temper, stretch more, stop smoking, drive slower, stop
spending so much money, you should save up, why a new car you already
have one, some people have injury's Jon, so you cant train them that
hard, your just young." -sheep
   -wolf-   I will always drive with my AC on full blast with
my windows down. I will never believe in stretching, and I will
always love fast food. Don't let them change you, do what you
want to do, blast your AC anytime you want! Coach the way you
feel is the best way, stop reading weightlifting articles! stop
being brain washed by the "experts" Windows down and AC up, try it
because it feels really good!

♪ ♪ ♪

Green Jungle

Wednesday, July 6, 2011

I take a giant sip of my ice cold coffee. Its my third cup this
morning and I cant stop, every sip makes me feel better, every sip
takes away the stress. I am drunk off coffee. I sit back and close
my eyes as my mind races through old memories, new memories and some
thoughts of what the future looks like. coffee is my new best friend,
he understands what I am going through, he makes me laugh, smile and
most importantly makes me feel good about myself.

I am not in the gym right now, I am in my hide out, I am in my tree
fort. There are no weights smashing down hard against the floor,
and the air is not filled with chalk. There are many more smiles in
my hide away, people are much more relaxed and friendly. I hide in

the corner like the phantom, trying to stay un noticed in this weird
world where there are no weights, coaches or athletes.   I drink, I
type, and I "people watch". I find myself staring at these people who
don't wear Adidas gear as if they where from another world. Maybe I
am in the other world and they look at me funny, maybe they think I
am the alien. This green straw keeps looking at me, so I take another
sip of the dark liquid that puts me back on track, and I start typing
away. What the hell am I typing for? What the hell am I writing
about? Maybe Its my escape from the gym, from the noise and the same
old "who's stronger" talk. I like writing, It feels good to put your
thoughts and ideas on paper. It slows everything down. The coffee
makes everything feel like I am dreaming, like everyone is living there
lives and I am just watching. Who new I would be writing on a blog and
lifting weights for the USA. Some days I just cant figure out how I
ended up hear. It seemed like yesterday I was taking lines off glass
tables, and waking up on kitchen floors. Life is crazy, the different
roads it can take you down are beautiful and bazaar. They can be dark
but still fascinating. I wouldn't change anything I did back then, I
don't regret anything I did and got myself into. There is the world
of weightlifting, and there is the world of long nights and car rides
to unknown places, but honestly in the end, they are very much the
same. I have touched the hot flame, I have been down the dark ally
way, I have seen the devil, and I think I am a better person today
because of it. I thank God and my mom for leading me to the world of
weightlifting, wow, who knows what I would be doing right now.

All I know is that I love this green coffee jungle I am in right now.
I need more coffee, I need more training, I need to get stronger. I
love coaching. My athlete Andrew Jester took bronze at school age
nationals, his very first national meet. I couldn't go with him
because of my nationals, but I am very proud of him. I love that damn
kid. I love everyone in this sport, I love my Fiance, I love this
world, I love California strength, I love big Phil, I love all the
judges and coaches, even if you don't like me, I like you. I love
the USA, I love this coffee.

North 2012

♪ ♪ ♪

277

I Slam Bars

I wish I could slam other things rather than bars. I am tired of only slamming bars, there are so many other things I would love to slam. Maybe the reason why I slam bars is because I imagine slamming other things. Maybe the hate, sadness, and frustration drive me to slam bars. I want my father back, I miss my dad. I wish after I slam the bar glass would shatter everywhere, and the crystals would fly away and never come back. I wish when I slam the bar that the white powder would be sweeped away by the wind to never be found again. One day I want to slam a bar so hard that my dad would be released from the hell the devil has put him in. I wounder if that could ever happen?

I wish the bar would take me back to the blue house, the black Lexus, the big offices of Nextel, movie theaters, gas station stops, hotel rooms, soccer games, working out together at Bali's, space Nettle, home videos. I wish the bar was a time machine. I wish the bar could kill what I wanted it to. I wish the bar would do what I said. I wish the bar was my magic bar. I wish the bar would bring my dad to see me lift, I think he would be proud of me and what I am doing with my life. I know he wanted me to get into the business world, the happy hour world, the people world. But who knows, maybe he would have preferred this lifestyle I live in. I go back and forth from sad to mad, I have found that it's very hard to control my emotions.

I slam the bar with hate, hate towards drugs, hate towards my dad choosing drugs over my mom and I. Hate towards alcohol and what it has don to me, hate towards myself for the person I can sometimes become, hate towards my past and the things I did. Sometimes I slam bars and I have no idea what I am hateing, but its there in the back of my throat. My emotions are a roller coaster that has lost all controll, and they take me over like a great dane being walked by a small child. Maybe if I keep slamming that bar my dad will come watch me lift, or just hang out with me. I will fucken slam the bar with all the hate and frustration I have in me because that's what makes me feel better, that's what keeps me balanced, and who are you to tell me to stop? who are you to tell me how to act and live my life? I get crazy because it takes me out of reality, I don't need drugs to get lost, I have weightlifting, I have this gym. I cant control my relationship with my dad, but I can control makeing international teams, wining national championships and sometime soon grabbing that American record by the throat and riping its head off.

I don't care what any body thinks, If you don't like me slamming bars
than I will slam you, if you don't like my attitude than screw you,
I am tired of looking for approval. I am tired of asking, waiting
in line, putting my hand out and getting no hand to shake back. I
stopped being the sheep, being peoples background noise and view. I
walk away from there group and I will chain the doors to California
strength, close the blinds and slam my bars all day and night. I am a
monster, I am not normal, I will hide away in my gym, drink my coffee
in the green jungle and be happy.

Call that glass your son, play catch with it and buy it pop and candy
at the gas station. Have fun with your new family, I wish you didn't
feel the way you do towards me, but I will be just fine. I have my
new family out hear, I have my bar.

Champ 2012

♪ ♪ ♪

gangland

Wednesday, July 27, 2011

We are an army that leans back to back as we march forward with high
knees in the dark and red sky. Can you picture an army of thousands
all moving at the same time? I can, now let me add some fog in there
just to make the picture more intense, more bad ass. Up a hill with
one dead tree, that has been burned from some fire that killed the
whole damn village, we march right past as we all start to spread
wider and wider taking over anything that gets in our way, you look
this way I look that way. When I step you step, when I march you
march, when I attack you attack. If you were a frog and you saw this
army stomping your way you would hop, and hop fast. If you were a
straight line Joe you would jump and run, just like you want to do
everyday in your office of blank walls. but you cant because you don't
have an army to run with, you are scared, you are a Ferris wheel of
boredom. Weightlifting family we raise our glasses together, and
drink our milk around the biggest camp fire in the world, completely
protected from the light and dark. We are not in either, we are the
biggest army that know one has ever seen, or knows about. As the
snow falls hard we keep marching as we drag our bars behind us. Rest
is for the weak, bar dragging is all we know, pushing on into the red
mountains is all we will ever do.

279

Shankle catches his wolf and cuts it's throat while riding on it's back, that wolf is now dead and now we eat. Kendrick Farris runs fast with his dreads behind him as he jumps and throws his bar 10 football fields long hitting a bear through the eyes, now we eat. Pat Mendez comes out of his cave reaching 55 feet tall with a fist bigger than the Madison square garden, pounding the ground creating a crack that swallows a dinosaur whole, now we celebrate. A quiet and calm veteran named Chad Vaughn that is the deadliest of them all, pulls back his bow and arrow as he lets 1,000 arrows go at one time, flying down and striking every enemy that is even thinking about attacking this cult, family, army, gang, mafia. We walk tall when we march, we march because we don't have time to stop, we don't want to stop. When it gets dark coach Pendlay leads the pack as he blows out fire from his mouth, lighting up the darkness. He does this is in a way that looks like he is about to explode or "finish" in the snatch, butt back and shoulders over with some very bent arms like a hip cleaner. Big Phil turns his arms into machine guns and shoots anyone or thing in our way, and I will add a cigar, overalls and a mike Tyson face tattoo in there as well.

USA weightlifting, garage lifters, hot shots and small jocks, big gyms or your gym, board shorts or Adidas, slam bars or follow bars, lets keep attacking side by side, lets keep marching, lets keep lifting.

Champ 2012

♪ ♪ ♪

Hello friend

Thursday, July 28, 2011

Back in the jungle drunk off coffee. Yes I trained today, just like everyday, twice a day and very hard everyday. Yes I did my squats and I cleaned up the gym, eat all my food, did my laps in the pool, talked to coach about game plans, kissed my Fiance during lunch time, took my dog on a walk, did some coaching, but now its my time, its time to sneak away to the green jungle. So hear I am writing to you again about God knows what. No one in this place knows me, and its great. I am just an average Joe in hear, free to drink coffee, watch weightlifting videos, chat to old friends from college, and write to you. How was your day? How did your training go? Any Pr's? I swear you are my best friend, so thanks for hanging out with me.

Lets see hear yes I am excited for the Pan Am Games in Mexico, but I
have to say I am more excited to watch a movie tonight with my fiance.
Besides hanging out with you and drinking coffee, my favorite thing in
the whole wide world is watching a movie on the floor with my fiance
and my daughter with four legs. I saw the best movie I have seen in a
long time the other night, you should go rent it tonight! Its called
KILL THE IRISHMAN. Its based on a true story witch makes it way
better. Its about the legendary Danny Green, the man that took on the
mafia, gangs, police and everything that basically messed with him or
got in his way. I don't want to say much more about it, you just need
to trust me and watch it. I hate action movies, sorry I don't know
why, and that's why I like this movie, it's a drama with some punch in
it. If you like the Goodfellas, or casino you will love this movie.

I really do believe that the hot tub is the best thing you can do for
recovery. Before and after, it wakes me up, loosens me up and gets me
going. I have heard all these different run downs about how the hot tub
can make you tired....non sense, get out of town with that craziness.

I will probably start to lose viewers on my blog left and right
because most of them are weightlifters and they want to hear the
secrete, programing, training story's, technique talk, I am sorry but
that would put me asleep, but for the people who like to hear me go on
about random life stuff, crazy stories that always seem to come to me,
then thank you for staying my friend.

Didn't get a lot of good feedback form my last blog...hmmm that's
weird to me, I thought it was good. but o well, I will just keep
writing away because its my new favorite thing to do. I would love to
start training with other people, I think that's key to training. I
love the people who I train with, not people but my team mates, but
I love to mix it up more, anybody want to come train with me? You
can stay at my place it will be fun. We can hot tub at night, play
some poker after dinner, and train all damn day. I think I am going
to become a mute, and only write from hear on out. No more yelling,
and shit talking at meets or in training, just some crazy guy in the
corner who is throwing up big weight, then I will get on hear and
go crazy. I think that would be impossible though. Its funny when
people think that what I do in training or in meets is some sort of
act, like I am putting on a show. I find that funny, trust me that's
just my crazy self, that's just my emotions getting the better of me,

but I really do think that you guys get me, because I know that a lot of people don't.

My favorite movie is the Truman show, what is yours? second is AI, third is beautiful mind, fourth is gladiator, fifth is man on fire, six is catch me if you can, seventh is book of eli.

Does anybody hear drive a Preus? I am sorry but wtf is that? I saw how much they are and I almost fell over, why would you spend money on that weirdly shaped car? O I forgot to save the world and the polo bears, well I guess someone needs to.

My roll model is Michael Savage, sorry if you now hate me...lol for those who like him as well than lets have a toast. When the day gets hard I will slip into my car and crank him up, I guess when he gets his frustrations out I get my out at the same time without saying anything, its perfect. Now that I listen to Savage everyday, even rush is to soft for me now, ts crazy! I use to love Hannity, well I still do but that's middle school stuff compared to the Savage nation. lol I don't know where I am going with this, I guess I am brain washed.

Is fast food bad for you? Will this sport grow more popular? Will I be able to buy a house next year? I wonder how hard training is going to be tomorrow. O I have Kaleb witby coming out tomorrow to train and visit! Yes, I love this guy, very cool, nice, laid back, and great athlete. He is staying at my place this weekend, so I can have someone to ramble to about my crazy ideas and beliefs. Well I think the main reason he is coming out hear is for the Pendlay certification, so I guess I am second on the list. You probably keep looking at your watch thinking to yourself how much stuff you still have to do today and how much longer is this long, drawn out post going to last, well have a good day, train hard, see you tomorrow.

north 2012

♪ ♪ ♪

Nation of go getters

Its time to train mother fuckers. O yes, yes I am at the green jungle gulping down my life drink, my motivation potion, my dark big coffee that looks so damn sexy. I am going to finish this one and then buy another, I will probably have three before practice tonight. Practice starts at 4, and I will be ready. I am ready to take on the whole fucken world, lets go, game time. Everyday I wake up with a mission to win, win in weightlifting and in life. I view life as a game, and I am playing to win. I am a gladiator of life. I am a hard working republican that has created something from nothing, the only help I ask is from this coffee that keeps looking at me, i swear this coffee is alive.

I hate sleep, I just want to keep going. I want my website to grow bigger and bigger, I want to make the Olympic team, I want to help Cal Strength take over the world, I want to be the best fucken Husband in the world, I want my mom to be happy, I want my sister to love life and be treated well, I want to keep winning, I want to give back to Donny what he has done for me, I want to make my boss and coach proud, I want to keep pissing people off, I want the Jon north nation to grow into an army and change this sport into something more than it is now, I want to coach everyone my way, the Superman pull way, the hit the bar with your hips way, the stop talking about hamstring way, the train heavy every day way, and the what is a light day way.

Do you feel the same way I do? Do you wake up everyday and feel like attacking the world? I bet you do if you follow this blog. The people who read this blog are people who put things on the line, fear the comfort zones, risk, take, live life to the fullest, are happy, who try hard in everything they do, these are the people of the north nation, you are the people who will change the world and this sport. Don't read this blog if you are not on board, get the fuck out, we are to busy winning, winning in all different aspects of life.

We are people who will cut you in line if you are taking to long, we have things to do so move. I don't have time to drive in the slow lane, move. I don't have time to complain all day so leave. I don't play my Violin, we play our marching drums, you look at the clock and wait for the day to be over, we don't know what time is because its all one big race, fuck a clock. You Chat we train, you think we do, you stop training we keep going, we love you hate, we attack you surrender.

Yes yes yes! YES THIS IS A GOOD FUCKEN BLOG! haha I am now ready to train, Lets go, lets train! train train train train train train, and train some more. I will clark a thousand bars but always come back for more. I will bomb out many more times but I will see that weight again. Coach Pendlay is my leader so I know I will win the war even with many battles lost. Donny Shankle motivation, Donny Shankle keeps going, and I will go with him.

Jon North Nation 2012

♪ ♪ ♪

A Symphony Of Steel

Tuesday, August 23, 2011

Crack, crisp, chug......one down, two more to go. bang bang, now I have three green monsters in me, and now I have been bitten by the green vampire. I left my car running in the parking lot as I walk into the middle of the street, right left right left, eyes don't blink, I don't care, big smile on my face, if a baby would see me, they would probably ask there mom what I was. Sometimes I just feel like jumping, and hoping, it's the blood in me that pumps to hard. The green blood that makes my heart hurt from so much energy, drive, anger, and fucking frustration. The only thing I regret as I walk out to the middle of the road is how I should have downed more monsters, how I am so close from losing my mind, and how I actually want to. It's my goal. I want to see how it feels. Energy takes over and I feel like breaking your window to your Prius and ripping you out of it. I feel like sitting in the space ship all day with Donny, and playing a symphony. A symphony in space , a symphony of steel, a symphony made beholden to the power of MAN!

I will sin in the streets and cry out for more, as cars will go around me, I will not go around them. Hold the wheel Donny I need to go pee, watch out for the stars Donny they will burn us alive, watch out for those big rocks Donny, please don't just go through them, you are strong... but not that strong. My pee is green and Donny didn't listen, I guess He is stronger than I thought. I guess this fucker is the black sheep and I am still in the white, I guess I need to earn my color and become captain of this ship. I slam 20 monsters only to realize how good I feel, my head moves back and forth like a kid

284

steeling candy from a candy shop. Maybe I will sneak away and hide from everyone. I just found Donny, damn he beat me to it. Donny and I have been in this hide away all morning, the hide out is filling up fast with monsters.

I am in space with a basketball star, an animal I love, and my best friend coffee, monster is just the drug. Black on black space ship that seems to always be running into rocks because Donny does what he wants, and doesn't listen!

I like the sound of the Piano, and the sound of the Violin. My space ship is filled with monsters, green like money and green like go. My Blog loses hits the longer I go. My mind is lost, my thoughts are on meth, my posts get stranger because I start to get more comfortable. As Donny once said......"lets train".

♪ ♪ ♪

6 for 6

Friday, August 26, 2011

They say first pull second pull, I say superman pull. They say pull up, I say push back. They say extend, I say Tyson hips. They say brush the bar, I say hit the bar. They say move your feet, I say Ali feet. You say 6 for 6, I say you went too light. People say "Clark" I say it's going heavy everyday. It's not bombing out, it's being a weightlifter. Its not over training, It's called being a pussy. It's not called percentages, It's called comfort zones. They are not called straps, they are called we train more often than you do. You pull, we snatch. You drop snatch, we drop under the snatch. You stretch, I drink coffee. protein, you mean more coffee. They call it a national tittle, I call it more money. fast means Caleb Ward, coach means Pendlay, hard core is not cross fit, it's Donny Shankle. Screw three whites, I just want two. Don't just make it, smoke it, easy is cheesecake. Don't miss in it front, walk it out. They have Masters Degrees, I have a USA Degree. Light day...WHATS A LIGHT DAY! Train through meet....I call it Pr total. They say make lifts, I say win.

Champ 2012

♪ ♪ ♪

285

Donald Duck

Tuesday, August 30, 2011

My role model has left me for a few months, I guess this bird needs
to step outside the nest and try things out on my own. hmmm, lets
see, this is my gym now............, I might just sit here and figure
out how I ended up here, hmmm maybe I will lift some weights on my
own, Donny is now gone, now I can take normal people jumps, now I can
listen to my music without the Shankle giving me that look like I
didn't eat all my vegetables. Now I can make my own rules, shit...now
I am Donny Shankle. My music, my jumps, my time, my gym, my turn to
lift, my intensity, my time to tell people to stop talking, my turn to
be king. I like this, no one in the gym yet, just me poking around
my new nest, a nest of two years, but now it looks so different. My
nest, not yours.

Good bye Donny....hello Jon North, wow this thrown feels comfy, so
this is what it feels like. wow this crown is heavy, how did he wear
this everyday for so long? This long red robe drags me down when I
walk, I see, that's how he got so strong. I am a little bird that is
trying to walk with really big cloths on, this will take a while.
Just stepped on some chalk, let me shake off my feet. Damn this Robe
is getting dirty, I wonder what kind of soap he used. My four arms
now have duck gladiators with swords and shields on them. My pants
are higher than usual, and my voice just became much quakier. What is
happening to me? These other ducks seem to be a little nervous around
me, and I really just want to talk and play. I just looked back and
realized how far away I am from my nest, I am deep into Cal Strength
now, very deep, there is no turning back now, I must keep going on.
Donny did it, I can. I have big webbed feet to fill, I have to keep
walking to try to fill em.

I hop onto a big platform and start lifting, wow, I feel extra strong
right now....even my jerk looks good, huh.....I didn't no I was a hip
cleaner....? Once a baby duck, now a Donny duck, now I am the king of
this familiar world, this crown is fitting better and better everyday.
The big Gold thrown will be waiting for you Donny, but while you are
gone, I will go ahead and keep it warm for you.

King Duck 2012

♪ ♪ ♪

"Green Hamster"

Monday, October 3, 2011

Attitude Nation Salute! haha I just cracked an Ice cold green
monster, and I am so very happy.   That first chug burns the throat in
a way that makes you smile.   I am listening to my new favorite song by
Foster the people, titled pumped up kicks.   You have to listen to this
song to get the full effect.   Actually every blog I write has to do a
lot with what song I am listening to, so from now on,   I will post the
song to each blog.

Lets see I feel like a green hamster, a green hamster that travels the
world lifting weights and spreading my super man pull, my ideas, what
Shankle has passed down to me, love, energy, and what I did to get to
the top.   I always have to go around the building to smoke my sticks,
the get away sticks, the leave me a lone for a few minutes sticks.
Ireland one week, Arizona the next, cold hotel rooms, dive bars, new
friends, crossfiters to sprinters, hello people the green hamster just
checked in, and I am ready to slam some bars.   USA weightlifting hates
me, but I smile and keep dancing, keep making money, keep succeeding
while my middle finger is in the air.   I wont stay in line, I wont
become a sheep, you cant brain wash me.   The Olympic training center....
never, they should be lucky to train at Cal Strength, I wouldn't go
there if they paid me.   The attitude nation is USA weightlifting, not
the old grumps that never smile, those are the red hamsters.

I want to apologize for being gone for a while, I have been traveling
and training like a bat out of hell.   They gave me a bat map, and I
have been destroying what coach has for me.   Anything he says I do,
I am getting freaky strong.   I married a puff, and I am a snuggle, I
love that who puff like crazy.

Bar back not up, do that, you will lift more weight.   Bar separation
is important, and bending your arms while lifting just makes you more
of a bad ass.   ok ok I am sorry, enough with the boring technique
talk!!!   wait one more thing, Stop pulling your shoulders back so
early!   stop pulling with your arms!   I cant stand how people like
this guy named Mark Rippetoe guy teaches the lifts.   no one lifts like
that, who is this guy? He is talking shit about me.   I wish I could
put my national medal in his cereal bowl just so he can taste it.
Starting strength, ha!   That book and that program is a joke, that
book is by itself destroying peoples dreams of being a weightlifter

and just weight training in general to become stronger. I call that book how not to work hard.

I don't know how I got onto that, I think the song changed to something a little more dark. Green Hamster needs to keep training hard.......PAN AM GAMES three weeks out.

Champ 2011

♪♪♪

Fisherman

Tuesday, October 11, 2011

I cast my line into the fast moving stream of water, where I have been catching fish sense early this morning. Its cloudy and cold outside, far from Christmas time but it smells like Christmas, it has the Christmas feel to it. Cold air, fog still lingering around the wet grass that has now turned into mud, from standing in the same place for so long. Gusts of wind that hit your face, taking away your breath for just a split second, then calm, with only the sound of the white water moving like a herd of horses. I have been catching fish at this same place for years now, with no sign of people besides my lovely wife, who is back at our cabin cooking breakfast......don't worry sweetie I will do the dishes! No people, no talk, just fishing and sleeping. Did I mention how Much I love Christmas time, the only thing I miss is Christmas music. I will never go back to society, I love fishing way to much. Nobody can tell me how to fish out here, what bate to use, or how to catch the most fish. Me doing what works for me, me living my life the way I want to. That sounds nice. I work hard in what I do, even though I do it differently than other people, but I sleep well at night.

Over the years I like to pride myself of being a good fisherman, and I did it with know knowledge besides my own experience. I am self taught, and if I have any questions about fishing, well.... I ask myself, not the bears. See the bears all follow a hand book that explains how to catch fish, witch is fine, but the only thing I don't like about the hand book is how the hand book tries to catch me, and trap me in the herd.

Be selfish, it will work for you and others. It will give others that read the hand book ways out, new ideas, they can believe in themselves rather than others who tell them "no". I believe....no, the attitude nation believes in you, you can do it, and you can do it your way, not there's. There is a whole world out there waiting for your new ideas, your success, your motivation, so put down the hand book and create your own. Take your arm and put it on the edge of the table, then slide everything off of it. I fish my way, did I ask for your opinion? No more chatter, just fishing, just living my life, keeping my eyes wide open, looking behind each bush, behind each door. You will be interested in what you would find. Don't listen to me, I am the guy you need to tell to shut up, tell me to get lost.

When I drink coffee I see things, I am seeing things right now, different colors and white lines. When I was a kid I use the think I could see air, but everyone told me that it was impossible. It turned out that it was because I needed glasses, and it was my very poor eye sight that caused it. When I drink coffee I can see the air again, so maybe I CAN see air. When I look at you I am drunk off coffee, your head is a blur, your words are shaky, I like to just smile and laugh, while I walk forward. I see things in a different light, and the reason is because I had to. I am not book smart, I have no degrees, no certs, no real work experience, so I needed a plan, I needed a way to fish that was going to get me ahead of the rest with what I had, a way that was going to get me a lot of fish. I couldn't read the hand book, because I didn't understand the hand book. So now you have me, this guy who came form nothing, took the broken path, catches fish standing on his head with his pole back words. Anytime life gets hard I think of Christmas and how much I love the smells, the tree, the lights, all the family and the music. Anytime someone tells me how to fish I just smile.

North 2012

♪ ♪ ♪

289

Day 1

Wake up my friend, because today is day 1.   Today is the day where
you get to start over, start fresh, or just add on to something you
have been doing for some time now. But today is different, today
you are done trying, you are done experimenting, done thinking, done
asking, done reading, done watching, done learning, now its time
for doing. There is something in the air this morning, the smell is
different, the hard wood floor underneath your feet when you get out
of bed feels different, your shower is hotter and your shave glides
like snow dogs pulling there sled. Your coffee tastes better and
stronger, the sun hits your face through the slightly opened window
that feels amazing from the warmth and the cold air hitting you at the
same time. Today is a different day, a brand new day, a Christmas
morning day.

This morning I will create my own path to walk down, and what I do
when I walk down this path is what I have aways wanted to do. But
see I ran into many monsters on my old path, did things that I wish
I never did, acted certain ways that I lose sleep over, and hurt many
people that I wish I never hurt. I have no excuses, even though I
foolishly blame a few things like the flowers I chose to eat and my
bad choice of water I chose to drink, but at the end of the day its
just me walking down a lonely dark path. Day 1 is different, the path
is bright and I will not make the same mistakes I made on my old path.
I will become a better person, I will train harder than ever, I will
double my shot of love and appreciate this short life much more.

I drive to work and all you see is a flash of light, I drink my coffee
and I grow fifteen feet taller, for the first time in a while I want
to lift weights. I coach tell I pass out, I don't open doors I kick
them down, and I love all the people who hate me. The attitude nation
is day 1 everyday, we will not let the dark corners of life capture us
and bring us down.

Weightlifting is so mental, that it can effect your whole career if
you have a bad outlook on the sport or in life in general. I have
missed many lifts from a sad, weak, or scared mind. That will never
go away all together, but the less these thoughts and emotions happen,
the better you will train. Train hard today and you will feel good
tomorrow, and when you feel good tomorrow, you will then want to train

hard the next day. The better you train, the better you feel, the
better you will sleep, the better you will eat, the better your life
will be. This is why weightlifting to me is not just a sport but a
way of life, my air, my gas and the only thing that keeps me going.
Without it I would be in a mental institution knocking my head against
the wall over and over again. I would be un happy, I would be weak
minded. Weightlifting keeps you real, gives you feedback on who you
are as a person, and always hits you in the face when needed. If you
can bust through the walls of weightlifting, fight the pain and let
downs, and keep training everyday no matter how you feel, than you
can do anything in life, you are a gladiator. See the reason I am
writing this blog this morning is because I am very down right now,
I do not have any confidence or motivation at this time becasue I
haven't lifted weights in the last few days. I just got back from the
Grand Pri where I did horrible, even the coffee is having a hard time
picking me up. So I write, I write to the attitude nation and I feel
better. People who get me, where others look at me like an alien.
Thank you for giving me a chance, and eccepting me for me.

I train today at two so I am very very excited to get my fix, get
that "pump", that emotion, that straight shot of life, then I will be
back to normal. See what most people don't know about me is I get
very down, from being so high. There is know middle ground for me,
one extreme or the next, just like my coffee, training, drinking, and
etc... Something I have been struggling with and working on my whole
life. Weightlifting will some day cure this, I am sure of it.

Today is day 1. Today is the first training session for the
Americans. Today is the first day where the attitude nation marches
faster and harder, day 1....lets train.

♪♪♪

Mr Black Sheep

Monday, November 21, 2011

Black sheep is walking to the gym. Black sheep has very lonely low
eyes that only make contact with you for just a second, Intel he looks
back down. Black sheep's throws a baseball across the world; black
sheep is a black sheep and marches to his black drum. Black sheep
takes hot baths, while the white sheep take cold baths. The other

sheep laugh at him for eating the wrong food in the meadow; black sheep seems to get lost in day dreams from time to time. Mr. Black sheep just does things differently than the other sheep. But what the white sheep in the village don't know is that Mr. Black sheep sneaks off every night into the darkness, past the field, past the forest and over a lake that has been forbidden for any sheep to cross. There in the green tall grass that grows taller than his whole sheep body, lays about 20 other black sheep who were quietly waiting on Mr. Sheep who was running late like usual. All the black sheep were hidden from the tall grass and there black fur blended in perfectly into the night, which made them almost invisible. The tall grass moved fast as all the sheep start running further and further into the forbidden field witch finally opened up to a dream world, a world that no white sheep has ever seen, a world where they could be themselves and not be judged, a land of their own. The food, the water, the tree climbing, the flying, the games they played, yes these sheep could fly and climb trees. They could do anything. They were free and happy; they did what they wanted to do and didn't listen to anyone else.

The world of the white sheep was very limited by the few books they had in the village. Limited by the lack of courage that the white sheep had, limited by the sense of adventure and wonder, limited by a few in the village that made the rules and told them how to think. The white sheep were brain washed, they were told how to play, run, eat and sleep. The young sheep would ask "well why"? And the older sheep would reply by saying "because" that's why. They were gated off, the windows closed, the kid sheep became dependent on what all the books said and lost all imagination. The white sheep were dying for life, they were gasping for air, they were handcuffed to others worlds and teaching's, they needed to be set free, experience things on their own. "Touch the hot fire son", ouch! "Father why did you have me touch the hot fire it hurt"? "Now you know how it feels my son, now you will never be tempted to touch it again, now you know for yourself rather than just taking y word for it". A few of the white sheep heard about this teaching that the father performed to his son, and other things like taking hot baths instead of cold, and this upset the white sheep so much that they kicked the farther and son out if there village into the world they have never seen, just heard about. As they walked further and further they found all the black sheep crossing the forbidden lake. The black sheep saw the sadness on the fathers face, and how the son was more scared than ever. The night just became much, much colder.

The attitudes of the black sheep changed in seconds, as all 20 of them lifted themselves 8 feet tall on their hind legs. The white sheep looked up in dis believe. The black sheep walked past the farther and son as they marched towards the village. The closer they got the more black sheep would join, where did they come from no one new. Hundreds then thousands then millions came together. They came out of holes, trees, high grass, some even came down from the sky with wings, and they marched.

They march turned into a slow walk, then a fast walk, then a dead sprint as they entered the village that almost took up 1,000,000 acres of land and prisoned white sheep. The black sheep swarmed into the city like water hitting the sand. They destroyed everything in sight. Standing up to the leaders who didn't want freedom. The leaders who made them feel like outsiders. They black sheep stood on the highest mountain and told the white sheep to live there life's, be themselves and try things on your own. The white sheep were free to do as they pleased once all the walls and ceilings were torn down and the sheep in power were told to leave and never come back. The black sheep got back on four legs and went back to their dream world over the lake. The new village was now a dream world; the black sheep call their dream world the attitude nation. The End

♪ ♪ ♪

Bad Guy

Saturday, November 26, 2011

Bodybuilding.com just stabbed me in the stomach. YouTube stabbed me in the back, Tnation kicked me while I was down, go heavy spit on me, and every other forum out there hates me. You hate me, you want me gone, you don't like the attitude, and you don't like the celebrating, the enthusiasm, or my antics. Pumping up the crowd and showing emotion will get you hung. You would love to drag me to the highest tree and hang me. You would get off your couches and all hold hands with smiles while my neck snaps, as I hang there swinging back and forth. Jon North is finally gone; Jon North is finally dead, now we can lift in peace, now he won't embarrass his country anymore, now we can get back to our way of doing things. This sport is not welcoming; this sport has nothing but hate for me. I am not welcome here. I am an outlaw, the step son, the bad guy. I guess I have taken the roll of the bad guy. Everyone hates the bad guy, and you can't wait tell I break my leg or get hit by a bus, but that's ok, because I am here for you to hate. I am your stress ball to squeeze on. The Attitude Nation is your shoulder to lean on.

Attitude Nation, what these people and forums don't know is that we are made out of steel. There dull knives can't penetrate our skin. Throw your rocks and sticks, we won't fall. Hang me from your tree, my neck doesn't break. I will never stop being me, I will never stop representing my Country, I will never stop slamming those bars, spitting on those weights and pissing you off. If you don't like me now then you are in trouble, because I will only get worse, The Attitude Nation is growing, and that means people like you will grow as well, its just human nature. We will become your worst nightmare. I am the boogie monster in your closet my friends, I am the guy you can talk shit about in front of your girl, so you look like a bad ass. I give you something to do during the day.

I hope you sleep better at night after you write words of hate, I hope you feel better about yourselves after you cut me down, I am glad I can make you feel better about yourselves and hopefully I give you more confidence. Sleep well my angels, because tomorrow I am going to do more to piss you off, and that means you have a long day of cutting me down and coming up with more words of hate. You should all get together and find the most devil things to say to me, and I will rate them from 1 to 10. But you never share the words of hate to my face....why? Why do you hide from me? Why do you hide behind your computers? Why can't you come out and play with me? The Attitude Nation is fun, join us! Who are you? What do you do? Why do you really hate me so much? I feel bad for you, all that anger inside towards me, and you can only get out through your key board. The Attitude Nation loves you, everything will be ok, and the bad guy loves you too. Anytime you get down about your life and you need someone to take it out on, I am here for you, you can lean on me and stab me over and over all you want. You can spit on my face and throw your rocks. I will be your punching bag; I will take one for the team. The Attitude Nation is here for all you who hate us. Keep going! Don't stop! Let it out, get your feelings out, get your frustration out, go go go! The bad guy needs your fuel, the Attitude Nation runs on your hate, we need you just as much as you need us! So please never stop. Please get online right now and spread your words of hate about us, what are you waiting for!

I want to thank you all for building my profile as an athlete bigger and bigger over the years. Your time writing about me online has made me more popular than ever. They say bad exposure is good exposure, well... I would have to agree with that saying. My website is selling out weekly, I have shot three advertisements overseas this year alone, I am now sponsored by four companies, I am the proud coach of many athletes, your exposure has helped me fly all over the world teaching seminars, and last but not least your words of hate have given me the fuel to keep training harder and harder every day. Your hate keeps me making teams every year, keeps me wining national tittles every year, I am the champ because of you, I have represented my Country because of you, and I will break the American records because of you, so please don't ever leave me. I need you. The Attitude Nation thanks you! Merry Christmas!

Bad Guy 2012

♪ ♪ ♪

Coach Jackie Mah

Tuesday, November 29, 2011

Coach Jackie Mah you are an angel. You are a savior, you are a saint; you are warmth. Your soul has nothing but love in it. Your heart beats so loud and strong, that I can feel it from across the room. You have helped so many people in the world of weightlifting and in life. Everything you touch turns to gold. The look in your eyes is a blinding ray of passion and care. You don't walk you float, you don't coach you change lives, you smile and the world lights up, your presents is as comforting as Christmas morning. Coach, you can cure sadness with one touch, you lift much more than weights; you lift us all higher than your arms can reach. There is a reason that when you compete, the walls almost crumble down from the cheers and support that you receive. You have mastered the hug. The Jackie Mah Hug is world famous and the best hug anyone can ever receive. Your hug could cure cancer. Your strength can drag the Titanic out of the water with one hand; your love is changing the world.
Thank you for taking me under your giant white wing. Thank you for being my coach. I remember when we first met like it was yesterday. I was an unbroken horse who was wrestles and frustrated from being told I could never play football again. My report card was full of F's and life was approaching fast. I had no plans, dreams or paths to walk down. I'll never forget the first time you approached me in the sac

295

state gym. I was all over the place throwing around bars like a blind mad man on a rampage. I was the UN seen racing horse, who none of the trainers could control. Then from the corner of my eye, you slowly approached me and gently grabbed my arm. I remember how I just stopped everything and we both just looked at each other for a few seconds. A small smile came over your face as you introduced yourself. For some crazy reason all my frustrations and pain seemed to go away at that moment. Just one look and one touch from you, and you broke the wild horse who nobody wanted to even get near. You told me that everything was going to be ok; you told me that you would love to be my coach, and at that moment you changed my life. I remember closing my eyes and taking a deep breath like I could finally breath, like everything was going to be ok; and it was.

Coach Jackie Mah, thank you for believing in me. Thank you for giving me a chance, thank you for giving me a life and showing me the way. Thank you for caring about me, thank you for feeding me at your house when I was broke and hungry. Thank you for the national title that we always wanted from day one. I remember we use to always talk about it, and now we have it. Thank you for the love you have shown me and the love you have given to others. Thank you for all the life coaching, keeping me out of trouble, giving me a purpose, and shining your bright light on my once very dark world. You took a chance with this crazy horse, and I hope I have made you proud. Thank you for the signed Arnold picture you gave me, thank you for teaching me all your great weightlifting secretes that made us a champion. Thank you for being you. I love you coach.

Jackie Mah 2012

♪ ♪ ♪

Phil and I

Thursday, December 8, 2011

Back in the green jungle high on coffee. The cold unforgiving road of weightlifting keeps winding on. The road can lead you to rays of sun, and then with a blink of an eye, it will throw you into the fires of hell. My view on top of the hill was beautiful. The view looking up isn't as lovely. National title to American Bronze, gold to dirt, Phil and I to young kids out of nowhere, smiles to let downs, sleep to staring at the ceiling. Cocky Jon North is dead for a little while, I am hidden away, trying to regain myself confidence. I am still trying to pull the dagger out of my stomach, I am still trying to figure out what happened.

This road of weightlifting led me to a wise man who gave me a map, and this map can lead back to the top of the hill. The old wise man said that this road map will have you seeing the beautiful sights again, and will take me out of my self-pity. The map was titled "what is a light day" The map had a picture of Ali with his hands raised, the map had a picture of Mike Tyson throwing a punch, a picture of Donny ripping a lion's head off, and a giant elephant with working boots on. I guess it's time to train again, I guess it's time to do the only thing I know how, train. Back to the gym I go, back to work, back to the pain, the cold bar, chalky room, heavy weights, back to my home. My hips hurt, my hands are falling off, my knees pop, my back kills, my shoulders burn, but worse of all my head hurts from the mental game this sport comes with. Thinking about your opener, about the what if's, about what you could be doing better. Do you go through all of this too? I try to close my eyes and shut my mind completely off from everything. The more I think the more I lose, the less I think the more I win. Why do you think I get so crazy before I lift, because if I didn't, I would Clark every lift I ever attempted. It's a trick to get my mind off the weight, off what I have to do, and it works very well. My whole body hurts, I have been going strong for 4 years now with no end in sight. More training, more meets, more wins and more defeats, still training must happen, still you must pull on that bar every day. I limp to the gym with my Dimas lunch pale in my hands, eager to get back to work, hoping I have another day of training in me, fighting for every meet I go into. My shoes are falling apart and so are my straps. My belt has broken and the bars and plats in my gym are falling apart, and I feel like I am doing the same. How long can I fight this battle. These young kids keep coming out of know where like zombies, and my fighting arm is aching. Waves after waves of strong motivated athletes who have big dreams. I felt like it was yesterday I was one of those kids coming out of know where.

Phil, help me pick my sword up, I will help you put your armor on, if you help me with my shield. Let's fight together as one, let's show these young bucks what we still got, after we take our medicine and go on our walk. It was me and you for a while there. Best times of my life battling with you my friend, thank you for fighting with me. Losing to you was an honor, and beating you was life changing, so thank you. But a blue bird just landed on my shoulder out here in the half way house, and it whispered talk of sunshine and no end in sight, how there are many bright days ahead of our bumpy road. The weightlifting Gods have called in us to fight many moons more! Let's take these white hospital outfits off, and break out of this bitch, and find a bar to lift!

Get the hell up Jon North, stop playing your violin and pick up the bar. Get cocky again, get crazy again, train heavy every day, keep fighting! Don't give up, to many people are behind you to lose, get that Shankle blood pumping again, flip em off and tell em who the champ is. Drink your coffee and get back to the top. The Attitude Nation is made out of blood sweat and tears and nothing less than champions. Back to work I go, back to the sport I love and hate. I bet they loved it when I lost, I bet they love seeing me down, "down Jon North and stay down". You can say what you want, but don't get to close or I will bite you, this dog might be limping, but I still have fight in me, I will still attack you. I might not win every meet, but I will be there looking straight in your eyes giving you everything I have, fighting with a broken leg, fighting with broken shoes and a bad back, I will still fight all you. Grab your sword Phil, and let's get ready to fight another battle my friend.

Phil Sabatini 2012

♪♪♪

"beast"

Monday, December 12, 2011

They took the 10 foot giant and locked him away in the coldest, darkest dungeon the world has ever seen. No light, no bed, no anything. 24 hour lockdown, 24 hour bars, 24 hour hell. The beast wasn't allowed to get up, he had to lay there on the dirty ground with his face smashed against his own urine. Every time the giant beast tried to get up, the guards would kick him down, take there boot to the back of his face and press hard. The giant would cry, shake, call out for his mother, pray to God he could be set free, pray to God the pain would go away. But this never helped, it only made the guards more ugly. His body was green and blue from the beating. He couldn't move his legs from being so soar, his body and mind completely shut down. He would lay there and take it, he came to the reality he would die in that cold cell, the beast was a goner. "Keep kicking him , and never stop"! The beast squeezed his hands and closed his eyes as hard as he could, trying to stay alive, trying to fight through this beating, trying to be strong.

The beast fell asleep and awoke to surprisingly little pain. He thought the guards had finally left him alone, he finally felt nothing. He didn't know if he was dead or alive, he felt good, he felt strong, he felt pissed off, he felt ready to get up, ready to fight, ready to see his mom, ready to kill the men who did this to him...... the beast was becoming a beast. The beast looked up to see five guards kicking him, but he did not feel there boots. The blood starting pumping through his body faster and faster, his heart was strong, his mind was deadly. He became numb, his body was a machine, it adapted to the kicks, it adapted to the cold cell and dirty floor, it was untouchable now and ready for war. As he started to push himself off the floor, the guards kicked down even harder, and soon more boots ran in to help. Now there was 10 guards kicking the beast on every part of the body, and the beast fell back to the ground. But every time the beast tried to get back up, he became closer and closer to standing, he became closer to killing and closer to destroying. Every attempt to stand the beast got stronger, Intel finally the beast stood tall, standing 20 feet high smashing his head through the roof of the cell! His eyes became red, and his arms swung side to side breaking down buildings and light posts. With one step this beast killed all 10 guards, with one step this beast created an earthquake, the beast was free and stronger than ever.

Train more, train heavier, train to train with pain, train tell you feel weak, train tell you can't sleep nor walk. If you feel good during training then you're not training. If you train three times a week, you are not kicking your body down. Get kicked! Stay down! The longer you are down the stronger you will be when coach stops kicking you and lets you stand. The weightlifter who stands all the time will not stand any taller. Start counting the cracks on the floor, it's a fun game. Let me guess your knees hurt.... well good, that means your training, they are supposed to hurt. Make hell your home, make pain your comfort, sit in the dark.... after a while your eyes adjust. Train your body like a dog, train it to take the work load. Stop listening to your body! Don't stand, not yet!

Attitude Nation is the cell and the weights are the guard, let's get locked away and become the beast, let's get kicked and then kick ass.

Attitude Nation salutes you the fighter, the fighter who only sees the sun through the high bared window. Attitude Nation salutes you the weightlifter who lives in the dark and sleeps in pain. Attitude Nation Salutes you, the warrior who keeps coming back for more, Attitude Nation salutes you.

Beast 2012

♪ ♪ ♪

Love note to coffee

Wednesday, December 14, 2011

I am waiting in line for my sweetheart. My hands start to twitch as I become impatient. The way she moves is like a wave turning over and crashing down on the ocean water. Her smell is like jasmine and her kisses are like your first love note. There she is trapped behind the counter, reaching out for me with those sad, dark black eyes. Worry no more my love, I am here to save you from the green guards who have imprisoned you, for far too long. I'm breaking you out, and I will lay by your side for the rest of my dying days. We will live happily ever after once I have you in my arms, once I can drink up all your love you have to offer.

Your body glistens in the light, almost as if I can see right through you. The water dripping down your tall body is like rain falling when its sunny. You are beautiful, you are full of happiness and comfort. All my sadness has melted away by just seeing you sit there. Your Beauty has killed my insecurities, your motivation has made me want to keep fighting, your smile is absolutely lovely.

We take our first kiss and birds start to fly, Christopher Reeves stands, Priuses are no longer made, Jon North snatches the American record, Sinbad is finally in another movie, Dimas comes out of retirement, 2pac fly's over our head like the blue angles at a baseball game, and Cal Strength becomes the new white house.

Ice Coffee 2012

♪ ♪ ♪

bar wins

Wednesday, December 21, 2011

♪ ♪ ♪

Rest

Friday, December 30, 2011

I huddle in the corner embracing rest with shaky hands and tears
being smeared from cheek to cheek. My stomach turns with pain and the
feeling of being home sick from the sorrow and guilt I have seeing
rest whimper with abandonment. She holds me tight with her head sunk
deep into my chest, making my shirt wet from her crying mouth locked
wide open, as if she was screaming. A sad story of a girl who only
wants love, a story of a young women who has no parents, who has
no home, who needs someone to smile at, to laugh with, and to say
goodnight to. Her old stuffed animals only give her a small amount
of the attention she needs; she needs a family. Her eyes constantly
wander, looking for someone to pick her up, and hold her. But no
one ever does, so she becomes jagged over the years with let downs
and sadness. Her flickering light slowly starts to die down into a
whistling path of smoke. Her wandering eyes stop wandering over the
years, as they now sadly stare down at her painted toe nails, that
no one has seemed to notice or comment on. The smile she tried so
hard to show, the smile no one noticed, the smile she used to try to
bait people into her love with, was soon turned into a puddle of rain
water, that dripped down the muddy bank into the lake leading to a
land of nowhere.

I do love her, but I can't be with her. It's the hardest thing I have
ever done pulling her locked arms away from my body. Disconnecting
her drool from my chest to her mouth was like taking her soul. Her
arms stretched out like Frankenstein, her blue watery eyes opened
wider as panic rushed over her. Her mouth seemed to make no noise,
but was open as wide as God would allow it. As she closed her eyes
tears came down her face. Her mouth closed, her head dropped, soon
she became lifeless.

She was there but not, her heart was pounding, but not working.
I left her that day, and I walked backwards when I did it, hoping
and praying that someone else would take her hand, and love her right
there and then. She deserves to be loved, she deserves nothing less.
She would only bring me down. She would only be a weight on my sail,
I had no choice. Rest has no place in my life. I have no time for
rest, only train. I will always love rest, but I will spend the rest
of my dying days with train. Train is my life, rest is my heart ache.

Rest 2012

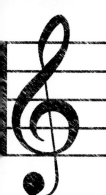

CHAPTER 16:

THE DARK ORCHESTRA
2012

Family

Sunday, January 1, 2012

I am back home in Oregon with my family for New Year's. Bend, Oregon
is so beautiful, a place I can see myself settling down in after I
retire from this sport. It is so good to see my family; it is so good
to be home. It is weird being away from my platform, my gym, my coach
and my team. I wonder how my small lonely corner of the gym is doing.
I wonder if it misses me. Looking at my life from outside looking
in is a very different picture and feeling. I woke up abruptly this
morning, and for a split second I thought that the last four years
was a dream, and I never left home. I thought I was still in high
school and was late for football practice. What has happened to me?
How did I end up here? Is California Strength real? Am I really
that crazy guy on YouTube? Is the legendary coach Pendlay really
my coach? There is no way I was actually on the USA team with the
Donny Shankle.... impossible. I soon realized that my dream wasn't a
dream, it was real. I figured out who I was when Coach
texted me, asking how my workout went. Holy moly....
I really am a Cal Strength soldier. I stayed
motionless in bed staring at the ceiling fan,
trying to piece everything together so it all
made sense to me.

Laugh, eat, hugs, smiles, and
more laughs.....this is what I have
been doing for the last few days,
and I never want to leave. It
feels nice talking to family
and friends about other
things rather than the
usual weightlifting talk.
I remember sitting back
and watching them all talk about
everything from their businesses,
kids, homes, and the local schools.

BEN
CLARIDAD

I realized that none of my family knows anything about my world; my world to them is a far away galaxy full of wonder and assumptions. I might as well have jumped on a space ship and flew to another planet. To them I am just Jonny Boy, nobody else. They don't care how much I lift, what meet I won or lost, or what training program I am on getting ready for nationals. I am the little boy who said twuck instead of truck, not a 166kg snatcher.

Writing this blog has made me realize that I don't live here, I don't work for my family's business, I don't compare grass fertilizer with the neighbors, I don't ride dirt bikes, I don't fit in. Their blood is red, mine is green. They do fun stuff on the weekends, I am not allowed to. They talk a lot; I am in pain a lot. I now remember that I am a weightlifter. Weightlifting misses me, and I miss it. I train tomorrow at central Oregon Croosfit in Redmond, great people, great gym. My Grandpa Poppy loves to go with me and watch.....but then ends up chatting everyone's ear off! I love him. He is the hardest working man I ever met. Training with new people is always exciting and motivating for me, I wish we did it more often, but the leash is tight around my neck. Tonight I will wear my Santa Clause sweater, switch the Adidas sweats for khakis, talk golf, and then say goodnight. Tomorrow I will wake up ready for war. I will wake up a weightlifter. I will march again with the attitude nation.

Family 2012

♪ ♪ ♪

local meets and more excuses

Monday, January 2, 2012

Your excuses are cancer to my ears. Leave me be. Take your weak mind somewhere else; take your defeat out of my gym. I see people like you everywhere I go like infected zombies walking around, just living, and hiding away when the sun is out. The only reason why you tell me you want to train is because you feel better about yourself just for asking, just for wanting. You want to be a weightlifter but you have no idea what it takes. You have no idea what hard work is. You have no idea what those two balls are for. If another person tells me they want to become a weightlifter and then gives me 10 reasons why they cant right now, I will just walk away from you. You disgust me, you sicken me, I don't understand your species and I will not let you infect my life with your sickness. Don't e-mail me, don't call me, stop telling me your goals and then not show. Don't you dare play your violin in front of me, I don't listen to that type of nonsense and just because your hamstring is tight does not mean you cant train, it means you are a pussy. Here is your refund, now go away. What did I ever do to you? You contacted me, and now you give me the run around like I am a door to door salesman.

I was going to write this blog about local meets and the importance of them. I was going to write about how a weightlifter should compete as much as possible, but my phone and e-mail keep over loading with zombies, they are breaking into my mom's house in Oregon. I will not let them get to my mom and wife. I will fight them off by removing them from my life.

Its dark and everyone is asleep. I am still drinking coffee, and I keep going outside to have my fire stick. I pace back and forth outside thinking about training, nationals, my future, more training, and why these people love harassing me with their excuses. I put out my fire stick and go back to typing to you, to the Attitude Nation, the only people who seem to get me. I trained great today at the Crossfit gym, it was fun. I competed in every meet I could get my hands on. I traveled far and long to compete, to become someone, to make it, to get better and someday....well, end up where I am now. It worked. I always say that weightlifting is like dating. If you ask 100 girls out on a date, at least one will go out with you. Just like weightlifting, if you always swing for the fences and always compete, you will soon win that gold.

I lived dead broke for more than a year in this sport. I slept in my car, struggled for change to eat at McDonald's, and ran out of gas many times. You can bet your bottom dollar I was at every meet though, lifting my ass off. I fought everyday to lift and compete. I dropped out of school to lift weights, I became homeless to lift weights, I did everything in my power to compete. I had no excuses, well actually I had a bunch but I never mentioned them, I just lifted the barbell. I wanted to make it so bad, I wanted to be good more than ever. All I wanted was to win a gold medal at a local meet. I wanted people to notice me and respect me. I wanted to make something of my life. So there I was, some raggedy kid who wanted fame and fortune. A kid who wanted success, a kid who wanted to be a champion, a kid who would have done anything to get where he is now. I competed at every

meet there was, and I still do. How bad do you really want it, how
far will you really go? Now I eat steak in my big house, with a fancy
bank account that buys me lots of gas, and my very first local gold
medal that sits high on my desk. To all you zombies out there, leave
me alone. Goodnight.

Local meets 2012

♪ ♪ ♪

Freedom

Thursday, January 5, 2012

Sunny but crisp, that's the perfect weather. Your freezing car in the
morning doesn't stop you from slightly rolling your window down while
driving. Even though your heater is on, you must take in the day;
you must smell the smells and feel the wind. You must wake up for
the day, for you are a soldier of life and it's time to attack. You
are free, thank you America. Thank you to all our troops. Freedom
is beautiful thanks to them. Thank you Donny for not only being
my mentor, but protecting this great country from your service as
a Marine. There are many days I feel bad for not joining the good
·fight. All this freedom, and I havn't even fought for it. I just
might join before I get to old. I must fight with my brothers and
sisters, I need to earn my freedom.
I pull over for some gas. I pump and stand, and so does everyone
else. We are all motionless like horses getting ready to be shot out
from the gate, it's a race and I am ready coach. "Click", the pump
stopped and I win. See you liberals later, the attitude nation is out
of here! Next stop.......Green Jungle.

The green Jungle knows me by name, and they know I have a nation
behind me by the sound of a thousand marching boots that follow me
around side by side. No one can see them but me, but people can feel
there presents. I kiss my coffee, and then exit. Move buddy, I have
training soon. Move little old lady, I am a selfish weightlifter who
needs to make the Olympics. No time bum, get a job.......well ok here
is two bucks.

I pull up to my second home and park down the street. My boss Dave
Spitz doesn't like when we take up the parking spots for the parents

308

and high school kids, and I always do what my boss says. I am a good
Cal Strength soldier. I walk into the gym and now I am safe from this
crazy world. I slap many hands, hug a hand full, only listen to a
few, salute the Nation, salute the Cal strength logo, and touch the
rings on the wall. Now I am ready for what I am good at....training.
Attitude Nation salutes the men in women in service, thank you for
giving me the opportunity to do what I do.

Military 2012

♪ ♪ ♪

Dream

Sunday, January 8, 2012

Sleep well my weightlifting child, for you have a big day ahead
of you. Let your chalky mind wonder in a world of magic and
peace. Sleep for a good ten hours. Dream about something besides
weightlifting, because you will be attacked by it the minute you wake
up. Buy your ticket to dream land and leave this world for the night.
It is your time to escape, and enter a place where you can lay by the
beach and ride unicorns with Dimas. A place where the bar can't find
you, a place where coach doesn't exists. A place where you can hang
out with your Dad again, play monster with your step sisters again,
and see your old friends who you have lost over the years. Sleep is
the best thing God ever invented, right next to sitting in the hot tub
while snow falls. A weightlifter needs at least 10 hours of sleep,
like Donald trump needs his money. There is no other option. If you
are not a soldier of weightlifting then stay up late and get your 4 or
5 hours. But if you are a fighter of the barbell, then you must rest
the body for battle, you must rest your mind for complete focus and
concentration. Tomorrow will be hell, so get ready.

The barbell just sits there waiting for you. The weights never
sleeps. The barbell and the weights stay up all night plotting on how
they are going to beat us. They are on no program besides kicking our
ass. They max out every day so we must do the same. While we sleep
they occasionally play poker and smoke cigars. They study the blue
print of the weightlifters destruction. They write to other barbells
in other country's making sure they are all on the same plan. They
laugh and high five one another when a weightlifter gets hurt. They

309

are an army of the steel, and they will stop at nothing. We must
get our sleep to fight back; we must never stop slamming them down,
throwing them over our heads, and shankle kicking them when we miss
a lift. Punch em in the teeth and roar like a lion! The Attitude
Nation will not back down!

For now you dream with a smile on your face. You are safe when under
the covers, as if your mom just tucked you in. The house is quiet,
the coffee machine is silent, the fan turns with rhythm, and a light
from a car lights up your room just for a moment, but you don't
wake. You are too far gone in your dream land. Sleep tight young
weightlifter, for you have many battles ahead of you.

Sleep 2012

♪ ♪ ♪

Devil In a Red Dress

Wednesday, January 11, 2012

She looks so tempting with her silky red dress and her plump red
lips. Her almond shaped eyes are half covered from her long black eye
lashes, which seem to bring you in closer every time she blinks. Her
long finger dances back and forth telling you to come closer. The
slit that rides up the side of her dress cries out to hurry. You are
brain washed by her breasts, by her comfort, by her smell. She walks
backwards into the room while her eyes stay locked onto your nailed-
open eyes. She enters her room, and sits on her red heart-shaped bed.
She gently pats the mattress on the side of her right leg, telling
you to sit by her. The fire place is roaring with flames. There is
a warm meal cooking in the kitchen, and now she starts to undress.
You never want to leave this warm house. You don't really know where
you are but you like it. It's like a dream where only some of it
makes sense, but the other half is just black and blank. You are now
lying in her arms like a kid that just scraped his knees. You have
completely surrendered to her, you are now hopeless and love lost.
Her name is your body and she is the devil in the red dress.

You just made love to the devil without even knowing it. Her sharp
red tail is actually your tail that is now wrapped around your throat.
Your training is being suffocated. She has locked you away forever

310

into a world of comfort. She has taken your soul and thrown it in
the fire. She has taken your dreams and swallowed them whole. You
listened to her when you should have trained. She walked you into
your own downfall. She made you quit the good fight, for her comfort
and sex appeal. Her horns were covered by her dark hair. Her smile
was a tattoo on her face so you would make love to her. It worked.
Now you are a prisoner of your own body. She is the gingerbread
lady and you eat all the candy because it was good at the time. But
afterword's you are a prisoner. Your own body has tricked you.

I promise your body will adapt to the hard training. Taking days
off only make you more sore and run down for the next time you train.
It's a doubled-edged sword. You think you are being nice to your body
by resting, but you are only hurting it. Your body must be trained
like a dog to hunt....to train. You have to let your body understand
that it's a weightlifting machine, and by training 6 days a week, it
will understand with a smile on its face. Yes it will take time, but
so does training your dog to sit. Now if I even take Sunday off, I
can't move on Monday. My body gets confused. Now Sundays are bar
work days. Now every day is training day. Kill the devil and never
let her take your soul 2012

♪ ♪ ♪

Phantom

Friday, January 13, 2012

I wonder what kind of blog this one will be. How will I make these
words dance today? Will it be a happy Irish jig, or a slow dance
to a sad song? I want this symphony of words to be a master piece,
legendary and unforgotten. Hey Beethoven wait for me, I want to join
you. I wave my coffee in the air composing a thousand buttons that
push their hearts out. An orchestra of crescendos, that strictly
depends on my mood. A thousand white eyes are looking for more, as
they hover in the black air. The world has stopped around me, as the
violin creates pink elephants that dance in my head. Memories of my
child hood play in a wave of coffee that carries me out deeper into my
subconscious. As the music picks up I start to rise. Now I fly with
the storks. It's a good feeling dropping off little weightlifting
babies to their mothers down below. There is a dark stage wearing
one black dress, playing one black piano as soft as an angel. I have
no idea how she got there, or even where "there" is. This world is

311

filled with brick houses lined up for miles that all look exactly the
same. Have you ever woke up on a farm in the middle of the night, and
couldn't find your parents? Have the trees at night ever made patterns
that scared you when you were a kid? This is a concert of all things
that you are still unsure of to this day. What did you really see? And
where were you when this all happened? I dream when I write, so I love
to write. I sing with a mask on, and I hide in my blog. This concert
hall is so quiet at night once you have all left. When a pen drops, I
hope it's you coming back for me. I patiently wait 'til I can compose
again, so you will float down and join me. I feel alive once you are
with me, and suicidal once you have left. I am the green blinking
light on your computer while you sleep, just in case you wake and can't
find me. I am here for you whenever you need me.

My orchestra is filled with skeletons and angels. They play happy
songs that make me write beautiful things. The skeletons sometimes
turn my symphony into a painful memory of sadness. At night it gets
worse when you are not around. As you read this you become more
confused. The reason being is because you have entered my insane
mind. To become a weightlifter you must already be crazy. To stick
with this sport you must be out of your mind. Maybe that's why you
are attracted to my twisted dark symphony. You are just as crazy as
I am. You clap, when most people would run. You are the phantom that
appears, but then you leave me all alone. Please stay with me and
train. Let's write together and become best friends. My dad left
me....so will you be my new one? This blog can be your new home. Your
seat is 24b, enjoy the show. Phantom 2012

♪ ♪ ♪

Run Danny

Monday, January 16, 2012

Chapter one
BW (Before Weightlifting)

He walked with pep in his step. He wore his Bright Reebok clothing
that made him feel athletic and fit.   His smile was of confidence
and joy as he hopped down from his freshly washed truck.   His shoes
were tied tight; vitamin water in his right and his salad in his
left. My cold Starbucks chair outside soon became warmer, as his glow
of light from across the parking lot lit up the whole city. The two

white doves that flew right by him, gave him a corny chuckle and a" gosh darn those birds" fist pump. His glowing shaved face got closer to our meeting point. He saw me drinking my coffee right outside the green jungle. His open hand raised high in the air while his heels lifted off the ground onto his toes like a ballerina. His eyes opened as if lightning struck him from above, and he began to wave at me as if I couldn't see him. His walk was long and powerful, that created a gust of wind that hit me from his energy.

He was so excited to start his first session with me; he was excited to become a weightlifter. What he didn't know was that soon his excitement was facing its last days. My face was half cover by the shade, with my smile showing in the sun, and my sad frown being hidden in the dark. He reminded me so much of myself when I first got into this sport. His innocence and determination gave me a warm feeling that made me feel free again. His arm stuck straight out like a soldier's sword running at the enemy. But this was no attack, just a much anticipated hand shake. His grip was tight, and his eyes burned right through mine.

Hopefully he saw the tears running down the left side of my cheek, so he could see what I Have turned into. Don't come any closer Danny Lehr, please run away. He was blind from excitement, only seeing my USA weightlifting shirt, not the blood stains around it. He saw my happy mask, not my sorrowed beat up face.

My national gold medal looked intriguing to him, like a new drug you want to try for the first time, or the first time you fall in love on the football bleachers under the stars. He had no idea what kind of world lived behind the gold medal, and what kind of creatures lurked in the darkness. His mouth moved a thousand miles an hour, but I couldn't hear a word he was saying. It was like I was seeing my mother for the first time.

I was drawn to his positive presence and enthusiasm. I wanted to reach out and touch his face. I am trapped in this dark symphony, screaming at him to save me, but he could only see my smile. Why can't he hear me? Please Danny Lehr save me, and then run far away and never look back. Every minute you sit with me, you fall further away from reality and deeper into my dark world. You are not talking to me Danny; you are talking to a weightlifting slave that has trapped me for life. Can't you see! Can't you see the black bird that sits on my shoulder? Can you see that my coffee is red and not brown?

Your tree is green and blooming, mine is burnt and dark. How can you
not see the handcuffs I wear and the thorn in my heart?

Please Danny Lehr, run away while you still can.

Chapter Two
(AW) After Weightlifting

He walked with a limp, dragging his right foot behind him. His loose
gray sweat suit was stained with coffee and ketchup from McDonald's.
His eye lids were heavy, as they drooped down his face like window
shades. His presents was followed by a red sky, and a barbell tied
to his ankle. The black bird was now sitting on his shoulder, while
he started mumbling to himself. The mumbling is the first sign of
insanity, and that's when I knew I had ruined his life. Danny's five
fingered shoes were now broken sandals that made a sound of a chain
rather than a flop. We made eye contact from a distance, but this
time there was no wave of excitement. Just a sad look, that spoke two
words that said "save me".   This time I was completely in the dark
sitting in the chair outside the green jungle, and my half smile was
now a sagging smile of hot dripping wax.

I feel for him, I really do, but there is nothing I can do now, I
already tried. Every PR he gets he slips deeper into hell. We are
now brothers, we are now just alike. The white dove's now lay dead on
the ground as he walked over them.   This time he had nothing corny
to say, just a small ache in his lower back and shaky hands from his
coffee withdrawals. Now we can play together Danny, now we are best
friends forever. I wanted you to run and be free, but now that you
are here I am happy. We can train together and cry together. We can
play tag around the concert hall, while the others sleep. Don't worry
Danny; I left the green light on in case they need to find us.   You
are family now, and I will never let anything happen to you. We will
ride the monsters together and slap hands while the skeletons try to
kill us.

See Danny your loneliness becomes your best friend, and your eyes
will adjust to the dark over time. Please trust me. It will
make this a lot easier. Danny stop looking around....there is no
way out, now come help me lift this bar. Danny to answer your
question, the white eyes you keep seeing are the blog viewers
who check up on us from time to time, don't be scared, they are
friends. Now go back to your cell for the night Danny Lehr, we

have a big day ahead of us. And Danny.........
I know you miss your old life, family and wife,
but your crying is keeping me up at night, so
please keep it down. Good night brother, and
welcome to hell.

Here Is a video of Danny Lehr in his new world
of weightlifting attacking a PR.

Danny Lehr 2016

♪ ♪ ♪

Attitude Nation

Friday, January 20, 2012

The glossy fire in my eyes is a reflection of the burning gym that is
slowly being put to its knees. The flames of the fire slowly rise
above me, casting a black shadow over an army called the Attitude
Nation. I will burn your gym down and take your athletes with me. I
am not brain washed by the puppet masters of this sport. I throw
up my hands and take on the whole dictatorship that has coaches and
athletes caged in there castle. We are not robots! The kids will be
set free! Your castle will be burned down.

People always ask me what my favorite lift is, and my answer is
I hate them both. I should have been a fighter; I should have
made a million by now. Fucken concussions, you are the one who
moved my chess piece to check mate.   Either bomb out or go for
the PR. That's my weightlifting program. The ups and downs of
a weightlifter will get the average Joe Sea sick just by standing
next to me.

Back in the gym again today after being sick. Maxed out and missed
almost all my lifts, fuck it, I'll try again at two. Local meet on
Sunday, max out again and cross my fingers. Nationals a month out,
see you all there with a big beard, a chip on my shoulder, a stronger
jerk, and some crazy high openers to win my gold again.

I drive my car like I am skiing, a lift weights like Ali, and I
will be the first to tell someone to get out of my gym. I must be

315

miserable at all times so I can adapt to misery. Tie me to the post and whip me tell I can't feel anymore. Spider Sylvia where you at? I want to fight you. 20 plus streets fights and still undefeated. It's been a while because now I am mature and responsible. I still have it, I know it. I have been jumped once, and I deserved it. Actually that was one of the best things that ever happened to me. Getting my head kicked around made me grow up.

Saw one of my teachers the other day who always told me I was a piece of shit, and then I saw him driving a piece of shit. Sorry buddy but I have no change for you, and yes I dropped out of college. And yes my account has an extra zero in it than yours. Sorry councilor, I went my own way. Stay with me, I know my writing is taking you all over the place..... But let's keep going. The song writes the blog, I am just the puppet. Donny gave me a crazy song that has taken my fingers over like my coffee has to my mind. Shall we move on?

Interviews are hard for me, because I have nothing to say, there is nothing to talk about. It's hard, it's a bitch, leave me the fuck alone. Take your sissy training program out of my gym buddy; this is Cal strength, where only the strong survive. Has my blog offended you? Good, don't read it again. Three fingers means three back to back Pan Ams, two fingers mean two back to back National titles, and one finger means I am the Johnny Cash of weightlifting. Sorry to the old crows in the sport, I know I am evil and the anti-Christ of weightlifting, but fuck you too. I will not be scared of the gang that runs this sport. The behind the certain chatter bugs and brain washers, who pull the strings of the young weightlifters and coaches who are molded into their beliefs and ways. I am rising up to stop you from the control you have cast over this sport. I will teach my way, I will lift my way, and I will express my emotions as an athlete any way I please. I am the robin hood of weightlifting. I will save the youth from there ball and chains. I will rip the roof off this sport and give the green vine more room to grow higher. Climb kids climb! Let this sport grow! We are free from the 1920's way of lifting now! Slam your bar and show the world how you feel!

JonNorthattitude.com is going to start sponsoring young athletes. Soon enough I will grow an army to take back this sport and give it to the people. Let the weightlifter be a weightlifter, and not a caged puppet that has his hands tied and his mouth sewed shut!

Coaches rebel from the norm, and let you're coaching beliefs grow
into a wave that crashes over the zombies! Spread the Attitude
Nation to become bigger than Crossfit. Crossfit is now on ESPN!
We as weightlifters must fight to have more freedom in this sport.
Throw your USA weightlifting handbook out, and write your own.

Attitude Nation 2012

♪ ♪ ♪

Insanity

Wednesday, January 25, 2012

Today is Monday that means today is war day! hahaha This is the
day when more 94kg lifters run! Right now I am drinking chocolate
milk, listening to Jonny cash cocaine blues, writing on my blog,
watching some Jon North videos and other secretes that I just cant
let out of the bag people. Lets see what else is new with me, o
I watched a great movie last night called the road. wow what a
sad movie, for some reason I did not cry though....which is weird
because I cry in a lot of movies, but this one I did not. I
thought the ending was bad, but I still really enjoyed the movie,
I thought it was very well made. I watched it with my Fiancee
and she got scared a few times. If you have not seen this movie
you should go rent it, or read the book. The word on the street
is that there is some cross fit slash weightlifter coming to
train with me at 5:00 from redding, well this should be fun! this
should be interesting, why do you ask? well I will tell you why
because if I had a dollar for every kid or guy that came to my gym
to train like a pro weightlifter and then left and never came back
after the first day, then I would be a rich man. or if they do
come back it's always the same old story...." man my knees hurt,
man my back hurts, man I am sore, wow I think I need a few weeks
off, yea I don't know if I want to compete, yea I don't know,
maybe well... ummmm, ill try..."   get the fuck out of my gym
then! I am so sick off that, it gives me a headache just thinking
about it. If you want general fitness then go down to your local
shine shop 24 hour fitness. They have fluffy white towels, music,
cold water fountains, mirrors, little blue birds that land on your
shoulder while you get your pump on, apple ladies that walk around
half naked and give out apples when you get a little hungry. Maybe

its the hose water in the back and a big coach penlday yelling at
you that might scare them away! lol no apple ladies hear, just
coach Pendlay!!!!

♪ ♪ ♪

Johnny Cash

Thursday, January 26, 2012

Today it's Red Bull, I left Monster for tomorrow. Three iced coffees
in the morning, a shot of chalk for training, and now I am typing with
wings. Johnny Cash in my ear piece, is it a coincidence that I am
dressed in all black? I put my middle finger to the world, as I march
with the Nation of attitude. I have been driving with no license
for 5 years now, no insurance, don't wear a seatbelt, and don't tell
me what to do government. If I hit someone I will pay it out of my
own pocket, I don't need you telling me to give my money to a company
that will take my money in the first place and spend it on "in case
shit happens". Seat belts.......am I putting any body in harm by
not wearing one besides myself? I feel that's my choice. Life is
a game, and I play it well. Attitude Nation is growing by the day,
my e mail is about to make my computer explode from people who march
with me, who do what they want with training and life, who take life
by the horns and slam the bulls head into the dirt. Make money young
soldier, love your mom son, and train 'til you piss blood. I peed
blood for the first four months of training with Coach Pendlay......
boy I hit that bar hard. My goal is to break it before I retire.
Tyson hips would be an understatement.

Shanlke thank you for this song. My wings flap to the beat of Cash
walking down the open dirt road. I admire Cash's outlook on life, and
the way he lived it. All of the NFL and College football players are
training at Cal Strength now. I looked up at all of them with my finger
waving in the air and I said, "Shankle is the captain on this ship of
weights, and you better respect him or I will break your knee caps."
Me, well I am just the soldier that does what the Don says. But right
when I exit the door, two people that were waiting outside with their
back against the wall immediately link to each side of me like magnets.
The further I walk the more join in to the march. I don't walk I March,
and I don't drink coffee, I chug coffee. No one walks in front or

behind, only side to side. All black clothes, with white hands from the
chalk. Blood drips as we walk, the ground shakes as we stomp, liberals
call the cops from the confidence we carry. "Ok Mr. North would you
like to deposit this check or cash it"? Always cash ma'am, cash is
motivation and I need to feel it in my hands throughout the day. And I
love listening to him as I cut off one of those bikers who rides right
down the middle of the road. I'll run your ass over, move.

I like to smoke cigarettes with all my medals around my neck with no
shirt on. It's awesome, comfortable, so I do it. Usually this only
happens when I am between training sessions, and I am on my third
iced coffee. I listen to Norah Jones a lot while I drive to practice
in the morning, she has a beautiful voice. But I must say that my
new favorite is Adele. That girl can sing, and I love her music.
Sometimes I lay in my king size bed and count cash while I drink my
grapefruit juice through a straw while the Office is playing. It's
one of my favorite things to do. My wife sits next to me with three
computers on her lap as she is running jonnorthattitude, putting
together more videos, working, working working, all the time. She is
the General of the Attitude Nation, she never stops! Babe put down the
computer and lets go hot tub!!!

Johnny Cash 2012

♪ ♪ ♪

Road Trip On 4 Blocks

Sunday, January 29, 2012

♪ ♪ ♪

Alice

Hey, it's good to see you. Do you have everything? I am glad you could make it. Are you sure you want to take this tour? Hold my hand in case it gets too dark. Remember you are just in my memories; this is not your reality. The time machine portal opens in 5 minutes, so make sure you are prepared to enter. There is no turning back once the smell and smoke hit your face. Here we go.

We got in later than I thought. It's three AM and the orange light in the white room is swaying back and forth from the bass of the music creating a strobe light of shadows on the wall. See.... in this world sleep doesn't exist. People's eyes are much too wide open to shut, and the black part in the middle is how much energy is left in that individual. If you are hungry, there is some wheat bread and some mayo in the frig, just don't eat the cheese. Find a cup that doesn't have cigarettes in it, wash it out no matter what, and you can get some water from the fosit. I am sorry about the smell; I agree with you, it does have a sense of thick sticky mill steam that seeps out of everyone's skin like sweat after a night of drinking. If you are feeling claustrophobic in this small room with all of these people, then we can go outside and get some fresh air. But you won't because your body is tired from the nightly activities, and the nothing you have been doing for two nights straight. So you will just sit here like everyone else, itching your head and waiting your turn for the next time the glass choo choo train comes around to you.

Your mind is racing a million miles an hour as you sit on a baby's red trike in the corner of the room. Your mind wants to be active and outgoing, but your body is weak, fragile, and shaky from the smoke that has made you skinny and pale white. Not only pale, but now you are getting red sores on your face, and they itch...bad. No matter how attractive the opposite sex is that enters the room, no one looks or cares. There is nothing more sexy than the glass train. There is no better feeling than the thick cloud of smoke entering your lungs and taking you to a faraway galaxy. Your smile is so big that it starts to hurt your face. You have so many ideas and emotions that you just start crying, then laughing while the stranger next to you rubs your head and tells you everything will be alright. Your legs

won't move but your hands will, and your hands are the ones that are
ripping out your hair from the scratching that is taking place. You
can't stop because it feels so good. You have no idea what time it
is as you wait for your turn to talk. Everyone is talking over each
other, no one is really listening. Your teeth start to feel loose,
only because they are. The white smoke is now a part of you. You are
a cloud with no name, a dream that has no chance to accomplish, so you
sit and wait for nothing.

You are in a room full of strangers, including yourself. The light
seeps through the window shades as people duck for cover. A brave
blank face gets up and covers the window with a black blanket. A
movie starts to play, and you watch their black eyes watch, wondering
if they realize that what they are watching is reality outside the
black blanket. I guess the movie to them is make believe, and the
world is really a place full of living-room skeletons that suck the
blood from one another as the sun rises and sets. The smoke is thick
and bright white, so dense you could make it a meal. You feel alive
even though you are dead. The talking never stops. Their chatter
toward each other is intense, almost tricking you to believe they are
going to put down the glass train and walk the walk in the real world.
But no, it's just talk.

The high is beautiful, the high is fantastic....and that's how it
traps you. The smoke that dances around the junky house might as
well be guards not letting you leave. You forget how it feels to go
to the bathroom because you stopped eating days ago. Your conscience
makes your stomach turn when your phone blinks from an outside caller.
Like an alien from another world just made contact with you for the
first time. It wakes you up for a split second, and you are shocked
at what you see. You are shocked to find that you are a fly on the
wall, nothing more. Your reflection from the mirror makes you look
away fast. You then proceed to beg someone for another hit, because
you have no money. You are taken over by the smoke, and you will
do anything to forget where and what you are.   There are no names
or faces, just who can offer what, and who knows someone who knows
someone else who can get what you need. It's like a bad pyramid
scheme, and you don't want to be at the bottom.

It's time to go.....I know you want to stay; please don't fight me.
We need to leave and get back to reality. Remember this is not really
happening; you are just in my memories of the past. I left this
world with only a few scars. I am just glad you can leave clean and

untouched. Grab my hand, the portal leaves in 2 minutes, you have already seen too much. Say goodbye to the land of Meth, and don't look back. Attitude Nation 2012

♪♪♪

Cello

Wednesday, February 1, 2012

It's been a hard day of training, and it feels great to be home. Protein...check. Meal...check. Hot bath...check. Writing a beautiful blog, in my quiet living room, with my dog sitting next to me....priceless. I turned off every light in the house besides the small lamp on the corner of my desk. I am sipping a hot cup of gorgeous brown eyed coffee. I am listening to a peaceful song that has me so relaxed. The pain in my legs and shoulders are slowly leaving my body as a write this sweet calm blog. It feels so nice to not lift weights; it feels so great to chat with you again. The song I am listening to is called a Sad Cello Melody. It doesn't say who the artist is on YouTube. The older I get the more my taste in music changes. I love the cello, the sound is heaven.

My blogs scare my mom at times, but I tell her I love her and that its all good in the hood mom, I am happy. I don't know why I wrote Alice, people thought I was crazy for telling that chapter of my life. I won't lie, there were a few times I thought the same as I laid awake in bed. I don't want to hide my life journey from people; I want my life to be an open book. That's why I write. I am not ashamed about Alice, if anything I would do it over. I think it made me a better person. I think it will make me a better parent. My hand has touched the hot stove, I know it burns, I know how it feels, so now I will never be tempted to touch it again. I guess that's the way I look at it. Who knows, maybe I helped some kid not do drugs from my writing, which would be great.

Sometimes I wish I started this sport earlier in life, I think I would be lifting much more weight. It would have been fun to be a junior and go on all the trips and have more weightlifting experience under my belt. But then again, I am glad that I started when I was 22 and walked in different worlds. It's like I was on a long tour through the jungle. I saw the football animals, I saw the night owls, I saw the college bears, the body building gorillas and much more. And most importantly, I met my wife throughout the whole thing; so yes, I am glad I started late. I am glad I get to write to you about my ups and downs, my secrets, training, life stories, and my journey through life and weightlifting. Thank you for visiting my blog; it's really the only reason why I keep writing. Well that and the fact it's not weightlifting. I don't want to come across negative about weightlifting, I am not. It just feels great to get away from it at times. That's why I don't write about training a lot, even though I do deeply love the sport. Do your shoulders ever hurt? Well mine do, and right now they ache so bad. I have to keep getting up and walk around because my legs will cramp up from sitting too long.

Why is it that I keep opening the frig looking for food when there is nothing in there? Do you ever do that? It's crazy. I have been doing it my whole life. I will look, see nothing, and then look again in ten minutes. I guess I am hoping that a steak with horse radish will magically be there the more I open the frig door. Well thanks for hanging with me, it's late and I have to play call of duty with Jared Enderton online soon. I won't forget about you, if you don't forget about me. I will be back tomorrow to chat more about life and training. Good night.

Cello 2012

♪♪♪

Row Your Boat

Saturday, February 4, 2012

I am a big believer in the arm bend. I call it "rowing the boat". Here are a few reasons why bending your arms will help you lift big weights: First of all, rowing the bar into your hips creates much more force and explosion at the finish of the pull. Secondly it tightens up that superman pull, allowing you to stay in better positions. It also allows you to stay over the bar much longer. If your hips hurt from striking the bar low on your hip, then the arm bend will help you clear the "ouch bone"! If you need more bar speed in your lifts, then please go to the store and buy some arm bend, because it will put the bar in 6th gear!

As the bar gets closer to the hips, the bend in your arms should slightly increase. Once the superman pull is over and he has stopped fighting crime, it's time to row your boat to the finish line! How hard you row the bar into your hips determines how much hang-time the bar will have in order for you to get under and win the Olympics!

Every athlete will be different. Some will do better with straighter arms, and some will do better with more arm bend like myself. I hope this helps some people, I know this has helped many of my athletes, including myself. Do what works for you.

Attitude Nation Salute!
Arm Bend 2012

♪ ♪ ♪

Freak

Thursday, February 16, 2012

Socially not eccepted, outcasts that reak of freak. Our home is the gym, the world has shuned us. We dont bench press so we cant be strong. If we are not powerlifters than we are not weightlifters. No curls no girls. We are the red head step child who eats in the adich. We are the miss understood. The suits and ties give me change as a wait for my coffee with my ripped up cloths and chalky hands. Teachers say "he could have really been something....only if he applied himself". Too bad he became a gym rat. Too bad he didnt follow in his fathers foot steps. No money.....so why do you do this sport? You should go back to school, you should figure out your life plan. What are you going to do after weight....power training..?

The NFL guys watch us like we are a half time show. They smile, shrug there shoulders, give a little clap and then go back to there grown up table. They lift weights, they run on the track, they play football. The weightlifter stays in one place as the bar grins with complete power.

We are freaks with tree trunk legs, over sized asses, pot belly's, long sharp traps like a rino with his horn, used for protection and survial from joe next door. You dont understand us, good... then leave us alone. We dont understand you eaither. Throw your rocks, thats fine, we are strong, we can take it. Trust me joe, if you can

be a weightlifter you can be anything. Consist missed lifts and
bomb outs is only the start of what I weightlifter can endur. Trust
me joe, your rocks dont hurt. Hey Joe, dont move, I am just going
to pick up this really big rock and drop it straight on your head.
Actually no I am not, I will take the high road, I am in battle
everyday, I dont have the energy to battle with you. Go back to your
desk job as I bleed 5 colorfull rings.

Weightlifting is dark, but beautifull. A place full of purple cats
and tea party's. The cold bar is our warm fire, a nation of crying
eyes and smiling faces. screw the rest of the world outside the gym,
we are family, we can do anything with eachother. But even though
this palace can get cold at night, and sometimes no one can hear you
yelling "anybody home"? Training is always there for you, and will
always respond by saying "yes sweetie, how was your day"? Everything
seems to be ok when training. Weightlifting seems to make everything
else in life fall in place. No matter what stresses or plroblems you
are having in life, you know for sure that training starts at two.
Training loves you. Its a great feeling knowing that when the world
gets cold, training is always there ready to hold you in her arms and
sing you hush little baby.

I know you think we are all freaks Joe, but fuck you, the Attitude
Nation is family, weightlifting is family, and all we need is eachother.

Freak 2012

♪ ♪ ♪

14 Days Out

Sunday, February 19, 2012

Getting ready for Nationals the Attitude Nation
way !!   Compete, compete, compete, fight, fight,
fight, win, win, win

♪ ♪ ♪

325

Shaky Hands and Cross Kissing

Wednesday, February 29, 2012

On my way to the Arnold 2013. On my way to represent the Dark
Orchestra and make you all proud. I will smash the American record
and bring home the title for you, for us, for the Attitude nation. I
came across this article I wrote sometime ago before nationals. A
year later and I feel the exact same way I do now. So I just had to
re post it. I find the taper bug very interesting as well. I have
been talking to a few friends on different ways to stay 100 percent
clear from the dreaded bug, so far not a whole lot of success. Its
something I want to chat about on my next podcast though.....o by the
way is not going live tomorrow at the usual time due to traveling to
the Arnold. BUT, we are putting together a LIVE show at the Arnold
grabbing as many guests as we can get that walk on by, Just like we
did at the American Open. Hope to see you their, it would be great to
be able to meet you in person. Salute.

I wasn't going to write again tell after the Arnold, but I just
couldn't stay away from chatting with you. Coffee is just not the same
without talking to the Attitude Nation. Writing has become a big part
of my life; a big part of the training, a big part of relationships,
and most importantly getting to know and understand myself. Writing is
my therapy, without it I feel claustrophobic, uptight, and lonely. So
I hear I am, back with you one more time before the Arnold. Lets grab
some coffee, put on a Piano guys song, put on our phantom mask's with
the dark cape, and let's sing together in this ever so odd world of
the dark symphony - while the world shuns us!

The Taper bug has finally left, thank the Lord. The last week I have
been tired, weak, slow, and unmotivated. I have been sleeping like
a new born baby, too lazy to even play video games. Just enough
energy to sit in the hot tub and stare at a swaying tree for about
30 minutes. This always happens to me before a big meet, or any meet
that is. I call it the Taper bug. The Taper bug is when you start to
back off the training and rest the body. The volume goes way down,
the squat workouts get easier, the length of training gets cut in
half, and the overall intensity lowers with each workout. You become
more sore, achy, slow, and even weaker the more the taper bug enters
your body. Why? I have no idea. You would think it would be the exact
opposite. It's like your body finally gets some rest and takes full
advantage of it. Your body shuts down, like a bear for the winter, a

big Donny shankle bear. Lol, sorry I don't know why I just said that, but the image is pretty funny. Months and months of hell training, months and months of beating this bloody muscular skinned thing we call our body down. Time after time of kicking it every time it tries to get up. Now when you let it stand, it doesn't just jump up and say "let's go"! but no, the body slowly gets on one knee first, and then the right hand helps support your the left, and after a few days of trying to stand up it does, slowly but surely. But my friends.....It doesn't just stand...no, it grows 90 feet tall and smashes everything in front of it. "Green Monster" my old blog explains this perfectly.

I have been in depression the last week. The taper bug got to my head a little bit, and the taper cloud over my head really brought me down. A few small injury's and some tweaks in the lower back is the minds worst enemy, and the body's worst optical. Even coffee didn't help. Weight after weight being missed, twitching legs while a sleep, and low energy levels, haaaa! NO MORE!! I have smashed the bug and grabbed my gun. I have reunited with the Nation and we will attack. Snap out of it Champ, you have a title to defend. Three time Arnold champ has a certain ring to it. You have a medal to send around the world, no time for pity. No time for "what ifs", no time for the weight to feel heavy, just lift and win....then do to all again. After they put the medal around our neck, salute the Nation with pride boy.

Yes that all sounds good, but a minute later my hands start to sweat again, my heart rate goes up, and my mind starts playing tricks on me again. The opener keeps me up at night, the opener haunts me. Sometimes I feel like running, running to a small town and hiding in a bar. Forgetting that I am 4 months sober and drinking my worries away night after night. Yes, this sounds great, no more pressure, just a white flag and my vodka. Every sip of that Vodka would warm my soul and make me feel good again. No more pain and hype, no more hateful comments towards me, no more long days training in the gym, no more letting people down if I do bad. But then again I would be letting many people down if I ran away. Then again I would not have you. I would no longer be a part of the Attitude Nation. Being a part of this Nation is everything to me, I take pride in it. Vodka is a nation of destruction and failure. Vodka is a friend who will smile to my face and then stab me in the back.

Fuck, this blog is all over the place, I am sorry, this is why I haven't wrote in a few days, I knew this would happen. I am glad I wrote this blog today, I feel its centering me and putting me back in a place of comfort and confidence. So thank you.

327

Someone call the small town bar and tell them I won't be making it in,
I have a title to defend. Tell Vodka I am sorry for no showing, and
not to wait up for me. Remind him that I am with the Nation still, and
I will never leave them.

Smash the Taper bug and Win The Arnold 2013
Smash Sir Vodka and keep marching with the Nation 2013
Calm before the storm 2016

♪♪♪

Yellow Brick Road

Tuesday, March 6, 2012

The highs and lows of this yellow brick road is something I haven't
seemed to figure out or grasp yet. The ups and downs of this sport are
on the same level as trying to figure out a math problem. You have
no idea where to start and how to find the solution. They tell me the
solution is train times train equals win.....but sometimes the answer
doesn't come out the right way. I let you down and myself, and for
that I am sorry. What happened? I jerked the bar above my head with
everything I had. The wining lift was there for a split second before
it came crashing down right in front of my eyes. As the weight hit
the platform an earthquake took place, I felt my whole world tumbling
around me. As the bar was over my head I remembered thinking to myself
that I did it, I remember how happy I was for that half second....that
was a great half second. But then my smile turned to dirt and dust as
the bar fell in front of my face in slow motion like a piece of paper
being dropped from a high building. The bar dropping reminded me of
the end of a movie, as it fell it erased the audience into black, it
killed my vision, it destroyed my fans.

Can we make a deal? I promise you I will train harder than ever if
you don't leave me. Will you stay if I keep fighting? I can't promise
you I will win every meet, but I can promise you I will be at everyone
giving it my all, and fighting for myself and the Attitude Nation. I
hope I don't lose you, I love writing to you and chatting with you
throughout this crazy journey of weightlifting. This blog is the only
thing that keeps me sane, without it my training would suffer. I am
truly sorry from the bottom of my heart; you have no idea how bad I
feel. I have let you all down, and I am struggling to get back on the

horse and find my identity again. I havnt slept in days, and my mind is being very hard on me. My tears have fallen and my hands hurt from wall punching. The "if only's" are attacking me, and I can't seem to get away from the hell they are putting me in. I have a few pretty good excuses that I tell myself so I can feel better, but those are just cop outs. My forehead is bruised from knocking my head back and forth against the wall. And the talking to myself is getting much worse; I am sometimes worried I am losing it. If you stay with me it would mean the world to me, and shit, if you want the bronzes and the silver I will still send them to you.

The road continues, and the witches will always be out there, but I must keep training. I must keep competing. I will still be in the corner of my gym leashed to the platform training for whatever meet is around the corner. I am there when you need me, and there to do what I love, I am there always ready to put myself on the line and go for Gold. I am a weightlifter, win, lose, tie, Olympics or no Olympics, I lift weights over my head and I love doing it. I will not give up; I will not let this depression take me down like the Titanic. I am a fighter not a quitter, we are winners, and winning is what we will do. Maybe not today, or tomorrow, but some day, some time I will win again and stand tall. I have always said that weightlifting is like dating, it's a numbers game. If you ask 100 girls out, one will say yes. Same with weightlifting, I will be at every fucken meet there is, I am bound to win a few more! I refuse to let a medal tell me who I am. We wake up every day and we attack life, no matter what. We are not Rob Adel, we won't quite, and I will never walk out on you.

Brian Drescher is my role model; I hope I can be like him when I get older. I truly admire his outlook on life. I will still be lifting weights doing what I love with a proud smile on my face like Brian. His swagger is awesome, his bravery to be what he wants is motivational, and he helps me when I get down, so thank you Brian.

I have wanted to write to you the last few days, but I couldn't get the courage to talk to you with the state of mind I have been in. Depression is an understatement, and the prison my mind has locked me in wont seem to let me out. I was to depressed and worried about what you now think of me. Time is a great cure though, and I started to realize that we are like family, and family is always there for each other, so thank you.

You guys should have seen all the Attitude soldiers that were there at nationals. Everywhere I went handshakes, salutes, pictures, and autographs. There was USA weightlifting and then us slowly taking over. Even after the meet was over and the Bronze and Silver were around my neck, you were all still there. We are growing and fast. I was shocked at how many people saluted. A top weightlifter was sitting next to me seeing this happen, and he looked over at me and said "shit North, this is almost getting scary". lol, I said scary no, fucken awesome, yes.

I will be writing daily again about training for the Pan Am Championships in Mexico in 6 months. The journey will continue, and the Olympics are still in my reach. I just need to come out of my depression and figure out the math problem. Train times Train equals slam bars. talk to you tomorrow my friend.

Pan Am Championships 2012
Get back on the horse 2012
Attitude Nation 2012

PS: Thank you to the guy that was helping loading my weight in the back room. I never got a chance to shake your hand and tell you thank or even get your name. So thank you.

♪ ♪ ♪

Love triangle

Tuesday, March 13, 2012

As my rubber band stretches, my smile becomes much bigger. Independence is the key, freedom is beautiful, and the Stack is the gateway to this all. Green is my favorite color, and my freedom stack agrees with me completely. My freedom stack is my best friend, and it goes everywhere with me. Some times in my pocket, other times in the trunk of my car, hiding from others who want to steal him from me. He always has my back, and is there for me when I need him. My parents love him more than I do, he has taken me under his wing and helped me fly away from the mother bird's nest. He has shown me that working hard has rewards, and that the rewards can make life much more comfortable, fun, easy, and exciting. My freedom stack also gives me the opportunity to train almost full time, and able to take time off to see my family and friends. So I thank him daily.

I never leave him alone in jail, (aka) the bank. I would never abandon him, we need each other too much. His smell is magnificent, and the swooshing sound he makes while I count him is music to my ears. He gives me confidence and motivation to keep working harder and harder every day. The harder I work the more he grows, the more he grows the more I grow as well. We feed off each other, we are the dream team. I have to take him cloths shopping for new rubber bands when he gets too big for his old ones. Shopping is great bonding time for us. He also drinks more coffee than I do, but the nice part is he always buys.

My national Gold medal gets jealous from mine and the stacks relationship, so I had to leave Ms. Gold in her glass case in the living room. It's a complex triangle of love and hate. The Medal thinks that she is the reason why the stack even exists, and the stack thinks the medal just can't let go of the past from 2011. I see both there points. Both forgot about one person though, and his name is work hard. Work hard is the reason why they both exist, work hard trumps everything. Work hard is the Godfather behind the curtain pulling all the strings, he is not just my best friend, but my role model. A man who I aspire to become every day to better myself and others. I owe everything to him, and medal and stack do too.

I hung out with work hard all day, and now it's time for bed. I have tucked Ms. Gold and Mr. Stack into bed and sang them to sleep. Watching them sleep brings a tear to my eye. I am so proud of both of them, and I am so glad that they are in my life every day. Ms. Gold looks beautiful from the polish I gave her, and Mr. Stack looks good in his new rubber band that is stretched but sturdy. Good night my loved ones, and sleep tight.

I have to meet work hard early in the morning for training, so now I must get to sleep as well, goodnight.

Work hard 2012

♪ ♪ ♪

Ding Ding

Monday, March 19, 2012

The video below is the best battle I have seen in a while.
Testosterone is a powerful drug that can lead to PR's, wall punching,
face punching and lots of bar slamming. Forehead to forehead, nose to
nose and fists to fists can even make a spectator get sweaty hands.
Throw in some coffee, a few monsters, and some techno music into the
mix, and you got yourself a recipe for mayhem. What the videos don't
seem to show is the Ali vs. Frazier boxing matches that happen between
team mates from time to time. There are some Fights that get broken
up fast, and others that turn into a full 10 round match. But once
training is over and the green blood that was once racing through
our blood slows down and reality seeps back into play, we shake hands
and get ready for the next training session. We all have an unspoken
understanding, that when in battle....anything can happen. Nothing is
personal, nobody is safe and just because you out lifted the other
guy, doesn't mean you won't end up on the floor. Welcome to the border
line of crazy that takes place daily at Cal Strength.

I left Ms. Brown eyes in the refrigerator for later when I write my
blog, in training I pull out the green monster. The monster is my
secret weapon, especially when team mates get to talking a big game
before training. In training my team mates are my enemy, and I will
do anything to lift more weight than them. I don't care if Rob is a
weight class below me, or that Donny is a weight class above me, fuck
it, I am out for blood, and Shankles blood tastes the best. My top
competitors in the Country in my weight class are not training with
me, so I must fight with somebody. "Don't get to excited Tom; I am
much stronger and faster than you....so sit down rookie". "One weight
class below Donny, and I just out snatched you, I guess even the lion
killer can be beat". "Let's go coach Pendlay, squat off right now"....
well shit maybe not that. This kind of attitude and environment is
what we at Cal Strength strive on, and so does the Attitude Nation.
Push and get pushed, hit and get hit, win or lose, no matter what we
are like fucken Mosquitoes, always there whether they like it or not.

Mosquito 2012

♪ ♪ ♪

The Nest

Wednesday, March 21, 2012

Training was hard today.....damn it never ends. I am dressed in all
white, rocking back and forth banging my head against the wall while I
sit cross legged on my cot. I live in a mental institution. The same
shit happens daily, the same pain, same jerk frustration, same bar,
same monster energy drink, same misses and same highs, ...staying
motivated in this sport is hard. "The definition of insanity is doing
the same thing over and over again and expecting different results" -
Albert Einstein. I am going crazy.

I wait in line for my group therapy sessions, like I wait for the
next training session. Every time I try to escape the hospital the
warden Glenn Pendlay tackles me down and puts me into the straight
jacket. I am so tired, I am so beat down, my body hurts and my mind
never sleeps. Silver, Gold, Bronze, bomb out, to a Pr...the insanity
continues and the sport seems to live on.

I was just going to post our new video from Nationals that my lovely
wife made, but instead somehow I got off on a rant. I guess my
feeling's just seep into the key board without me knowing. I don't
even know what I just wrote, this whole time I have been staring
at the small amount of coffee I have left in my chalky cup while my
fingers just continue to type. Here is the newest Attitude Nation
video, hope you like it, talk to you guys tomorrow. Salute.

Mental Hospital 20.......

♪♪♪

Pink Elephant

Sunday, March 25, 2012

Good afternoon my fellow friends. Wow, sorry it's been a few days;
coaching and training have been keeping me away from writing to you
all. Maybe they are just jealous because of how much I love this blog.
They can try to keep me away, but the dark orchestra needs me, and I
need it. So let's dance in hell with smiles on our faces, our bodies
full of pain, and our minds heavy with weightlifting dreams and goals.

The Attitude Nation is my best friend, and I am so glad that you have joined me once again in the crazy and bizarre world called my mind. Most have run for the hills and never came back, but you have stayed with me, and for that I thank you.

I hang my coat and hat, stretch my arms and yell throughout the theater, "Honey I am home!". I dance with the pink elephant to the beautiful sounds the orchestra of skeletons make, hidden away on the third story where only glimpses of their white show through. This is the home of weightlifting, a place that is unpredictable and at times strange. A place where you have to surrender to the mysteries of this sport, and just sing and dance. The person who tries to figure this sport out is the one who becomes lost behind the stage in the world of pulley systems, ropes, and props never to be seen again.

Now that you have joined me back in our theater of weightlifting and life and hung up your coat and hat, let's watch a brand new Cal Strength interview from Strength Sessions hosted by Camilo Gutierrez. The video features Donny Shankle, Caleb Ward, Glenn Pendlay, and me, along with Don the "godfather". We went out to lunch at Chiles and before you knew it there was a camera out, and this is how it went down. See you tomorrow for a new and interesting blog that I am excited to share with the Nation! Salute!

The Nations Orchestra 2012

♪ ♪ ♪

Jim Davis

Wednesday, March 28, 2012

Thank you Jim Davis for being a great friend over the years we have known each other.

First I want to say that my heart and prayers go out to you and your family. Losing you is not only a great loss to us all, but the greatest loss I personally have had in my life. You will live forever in my heart and forever in every bar and weightlifting plate in California Strength. I looked up to you Jim, and I will continue to look up to you for as long as I live.

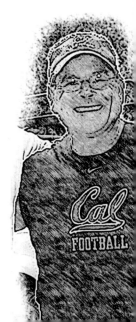

I will never forget what you taught me, the advice you gave me, and the great training sessions we had together. Every time I teach the superman pull I crack a smile with the image in my head of us arguing with one another over what the hell I was trying to teach you. You and I going back and forth about technique will always be a priceless memory that I will never forget. I will never forget your famous line that always brightened the mood, and that was the "well actually" line. You are forever famous for that one Jim, and we will all miss it dearly.

I hope someday I can even become half the man you are, it's something that motivates me every day, and I thank you for that. Everything you touch turns to gold. You are rich in every way possible.

You are kind in more ways than one. At least once a week I would spit my coffee out from laughing so hard from the conversations we would have; the smile on my face is making my cheeks hurt as we speak. Every time you walked into the gym you would be followed by a certain energy that would spread to all of us. You were a powerful, in charge, strong, generous, humble, sweet, and awesome person. All the Washington Huskies gear you wore everyday made you a big purple ball of joy and happiness. Seeing Jim Davis made you want to do one thing and one thing only, and that was to give him a big bear hug.

Thank you Jim for your encouraging support before and after every one of my meets, you were always my biggest fan, and I was yours.

Thank you for the beautiful suit and tie you let me borrow on the night I took my wife to the ballet. I have to admit, even though we are friends, it was hard giving that suit back to you.

Thank you Jim Davis for being you, I love you, and I will never forget you.

In loving memory of Jim Davis 2000 and forever

♪ ♪ ♪

Good Morning

Friday, March 30, 2012

It's six in the morning as I gaze out the window of the green jungle. Ms. Brown eyes keeps my fingers typing as I write to you with many thoughts and emotions. I think that's why I woke up so early, an itch to write, a brain itch that needs to be scratched. It's been a sad week, but in a way a new outlook on life. Family and friends, that's what matters. As I cry about a Bronze medal I have a family who loves me, why am I bathing in my own self-pity with a beautiful wife and a dog that I call my daughter? The small things in life have made me smile more lately, and I thank you for this Jim, even though you have passed you still are helping me become a better man.

I love the early morning, it's like the ocean, there is something mysterious about it. As a kid I used to help my friend Andre with his newspaper route in the morning. I felt as if I was walking on the moon. I felt alive and adventurous. Four in the morning and everything looks different; everything you once knew is now changed into a dream world of aliens and monsters. The little old lady's house a few blocks down has now turned into a haunted house, and the trees are following me....I swear. The quiet makes you feel like the last person on the whole planet, a zombie movie you are the lead role in, a movie with a one person cast. The newspaper world I emerged myself in was the first taste of freedom for me, and it was a rush. My heart would pound the further I would venture into the unknown. I would sometimes look back behind me, thinking my mom would be there rooting me on with her open hands out in front of her like she was pushing me forward. Her red lipstick smile and golden blonde hair stood out in the night so I could find her in case I got lost. I would began to smile to her but then realize I was all alone, no mom, no one to cry to, no one to run to, no mom to help me if I fall, just me in a very big world. Sometimes I catch myself looking back for her as a 26 year old adult. I turn and smile to show her the PR I just made in the gym, but she has been replaced with a broken white wall. I guess a mothers comfort and love never goes away no matter how independent and strong you become. I guess I am still that bigger than me backpack middle school kid with untied sneakers and raggedy jeans that drag behind my shoes. A rug rat kid with a chip on my shoulder that thanks to a big heart smoothed the chip out and made it dull. Basically, I was a normal kid.

When I get up early I always think I should be getting ready for
school, middle school mostly. The early morning takes me back to
family breakfast, picking out the coolest outfit, waiting in line on
the cracked pavement of the cul de sac with the other kids who have
for some reason made that crack the official bus line. The good or
bad feeling of remembering your homework...in my case mostly bad.
I sometimes feel that I have been on a very long field trip, and
at any moment my mom will pull up in the morning in her blue and
white minivan with her pink pajamas, crazy bed hair, followed by the
greatest question a kid could hear, "how was your day sweetie"? The
smell of the morning can bring back memories you completely forget
about, which makes your morning coffee much more interesting and
enjoyable. Driving through the cold foggy air of the morning makes you
feel like you are sailing the Atlantic Ocean with an image of yourself
that looks similar to the hard nosed captain of the Movie Jaws. I
don't know how I haven't crashed into another car or even a light post
from all the day dreaming that takes place while I am driving. Have
you ever been driving and forgot you were, then realized you were and
didn't even know where you were? lol, well if yes than we are on the
same page.

Boy this has been a peaceful morning, I needed this. A keyboard
and coffee in the morning is all a weightlifter needs to clear his
mind for the hell that awaits us on the platform. Train hard today
my friends, slam bars today my friends, and attack life my friends.
Kiss your mothers, and tell them every day how much you love them.
Call an old friend, take a friend out to dinner tonight, tell someone
who works hard that you appreciate how hard they work. kiss your
wife, pat your dog, tell your coach thank you, because life is like
weightlifting, it's completely unpredictable.

Here is the song I listened to while writing this blog. I could
write a 500 page novel to this song. I don't know why I am posting
it, maybe to give you the same feeling I had while writing this blog
that hopefully moved you in some way or took you back to a child hood
memory. Salute.

♪ ♪ ♪

A Clean Friendship

Saturday, March 31, 2012

Team mates may come and go over the years, but some memories will always stay, and some friendships will last forever. Here is one of those stick with yea for life moments, with a last forever friendship. A man some call the Mullet man, the COD killer, the pro sports better, or even the upcoming champ, but I call him my friend, my buddy, Jared Enderton. Even though he is now lifting for Average Bro'z gym, I am very glad that we are still close friends. Yes we play Call of duty almost every night together, we play fantasy football together, we are Texas Holdem buddies, we compete against each other in the 94kg weight class, we have trained together, but most importantly we have cleaned 240kg's.... together! I guess they are right, teamwork is everything! Salute, talk to you tomorrow.

Friendship 2012

♪ ♪ ♪

2 Minutes

Wednesday, April 4, 2012

Your hands rub your thighs up and down in a fast motion, not because they are sore, but because you...well you really don't know. Your mind is tired but your body is in such shock from the training that it can't help but to constantly move and twitch. You begin to rock back and forth as your head looks all around the gym like a little kid in an orchestra looking for his parents. You smile, not to anyone one person, not even to yourself, you just smile. Not an upward smile, but a sideways smile, a fake smile, a smile that lets you know that you are still ok and not dead from this battle called weightlifting. You watch your teammate attempt a big lift with your head slightly down and facing away, as you watch from the corner of your eyes. Watching straight on will infect you with the pain disease that man is going through.

In the 2 minutes of self-reflecting and heavy breathing you are intimidated,weak, scared,unsure, and nervous for what awaits you when coach tells you to lift. Your mind wonders off into the past like someone rewinding a video tape. You forget you are a weightlifter and that you have been doing the same two lifts for 4 years now, and looking at the same broken white wall just as long. You forget your

338

life consists of chalk,bars,plates,and a big bearded man that never
seems to forget that you are a weightlifter...damn. You have a feeling
that a minute has gone by, and that you are half way to hell again.
Your head drops back against the wall as your droopy eyes still face
down toward your Ali feet. You start to count the sweat drops that
fall from your face. You don't wipe your face because you are just too
tired, and honestly,you just don't care anymore. You have surrendered
to this lifestyle, you have surrendered to your own imprisonment.

Someone walks by you and says hi all perky and happy. You are suddenly
woken from your exorcism of thoughts and silence. You reply with an over
the top "hey how's it going" with wide eyes and a large still fake smile.
But once your paths have past you sink back into peace and tranquility.
A world with no lifting, a 2 minute world of heaven and peace as you
slide down snowy banks with penguins and polar bears. I wonder how my
dad is doing. I wonder why Jake hasn't called me back. I wonder what I
am going write about in my blog today. Shit,180kg awaits me,just sitting
there loaded and awaiting my arrival. I wish I could just sit here
forever and never move. What if I fail and nobody likes me anymore. What
if I never win Gold again or even get on the Podium again, then what? I
am glad people don't really know how insecure I am.....I feel insecure
right now...so I think on this lift I will yell even louder and slam the
bar much harder than usual. I should super glue this mask to my face so
it won't fall off, just in case Donny rushes me with a Shankle hug.

"Jon you're up"! Fuck, my happy purple dinosaur has run away with another
group of kids,and now I am left with a mean broomstick from the movie
Fantasia. I can't wait to get this lift over and return back to memories
of wooden skate ramps and 50 cent pop. Let's go! I am the Champ! Attitude
fuckin Nation baby! I will smoke you 180, I will smoke you then slam you
then cut your throat tell you bleed your red paint all over the fuckin
platform. I am strong,I am fast, and I am fearless. I have the Shankle
blood in me, and I will rip this bar like I am ripping the head off a
lion. I will win more meets, make more teams, and piss more people off. I
will chalk my hands like Russell crow feeling the dirt before battle. I am
a cocky, in your face National Champion that will piss on every platform
I lift on. Get out of my way rookies, the Nation is about to lift.

Thank you Nicoli Trefil for this blog topic

Love Liza 2012

♪♪♪

Frankenstein

I am letting the monster out this Sunday, and he is more excited than I am. I have been working on him day and night for four years now, in my brown dusty basement where trial and error has been a consistent fight with much hard work. A crazed mind and an ongoing vision of a perfect monster has kept me poring green liquid and using all of the electricity in my house. A creation that has been perfected, performed, and well tested. Now it's time to let the monster's impact and teaching spread all over the world, now that he has full confidence and self-assurance of who he his. Starting in San Ramon this Sunday at Cal Strength, the birth of the very first Attitude Nation Certification Seminar will take place. Four plus years of up all nights, blue prints, Gold medals, silver medals, USA teams, bomb outs, missed lifts, American records, great training and bad training have been performed with this project, or better yet this certification. A certification that has gone through the depths of hell to have seen heaven. A seminar that has wear and tear to it, like a baseball mitt that has been broken in. This monster has cries and smiles, scars and pains, success and beauty, hate and love.

I want to take what I have learned in my career and give it to you, and then from there you can toss it or keep it. I have tried everything under the sun in this sport, from different techniques, different dynamic starts, approaches to the bar, diet, recovery, training programs, the mental game and so on. I want to give back anyway I can, and I guess with this seminar I can do that. I would say this blog, but this blog means more to me than just giving my personal advice on weightlifting. This blog is where I can talk to you about anything, this blog is my journal and you are my friend. So yes, I hope you get some helpful weightlifting advice and tips from this dark orchestra, but mostly I am just glad that us gladiators have a place to go and talk while our minds wonder with thoughts and emotions.

I can't wait to teach my way, to show the world how great the superman pull really is. How beautiful the arched angel can be if done right. How fast those Ali feet can move when the lift just falls in place like the gumball that shoots down the windy ramp into your hand...perfect. I am excited to give you my thoughts about training, give you the proper tools you need to get through the hell before someday seeing the light of weightlifting. I just feel that there is so much about weightlifting that is never talked about. I feel this energy that is pushing me from behind to speak out about the Alice in Wonderland world that seems to be called weightlifting. I want to talk about what I have seen and felt. I want to explain to people how I succeeded and at times why I failed. I might just be crazy, but for some reason I feel I can make a shift in this sport, make it more popular, more entertaining, more fun, more exciting, and more interesting by talking about the lifestyle and mind games this sport puts you through. I admire boxing and how it's marketed and how excitement seems to hit you in the face. I catch myself lying in bed picturing weightlifting like boxing, and all the different things we can be doing to make this sport...well, more in your face.

I write most of my blogs to the A.I soundtrack. I love all the songs very much. Tonight I am drinking hot coffee, even though cold is my lover. I have a soft spot in my heart for miss hot as well. Training was fun today... Wow, I can't believe I used the word fun. Usually the word that comes to mind is hell or pain, but today really was a blasty. I went head to head with Spencer in the 7 singles at 90 percent workout, which would have been hell but competing on the live stream with money on the line makes it a great exciting battle for everyone. He won, yes I know, damn that kid. Boy he is a freak athlete and a strong Mo fo as well. He made every lift. I made all my snatches at 146kg and four of my clean and jerks at 172kg. After missing some, punching the wall some, and kicking the bench and bar some....I came back making one more for pride, and pride alone. I couldn't let the Nation down or myself, so I smoked it, spit on it, and then gave it the bird letting the weight know that we won, not him.

Hopefully, some of you can make it out this Sunday. I know it's short notice and you might live far away, but I thought I might as well mention it. I just hate "plugging" shit on this blog. I don't want to be "that guy" every chance I get plugging a new product on my site, a seminar, or whatever else I am involved in. Some might call this a plug, but I call it chatting about something I am excited about and looking forward to. I have a hand full of seminars set up across the country in the next few months, and I can't wait to hit them head on, and grow this Nation bigger and bigger.

Here is the newest Cal Strength video below. A good battle is good training. Salute!

The Growth Of The Attitude Nation 2012

♪ ♪ ♪

341

The Crossroad

Stay motivated, stay motivated, stay motivated. (repeat)

Just hit 5 years, body hurts more than ever. The 2016 career will be
hard, and the pain will grow more each day. My Hell is sunny from
the window looking in, like a wide eyed kid glued to the zoo window
watching the bears wrestling in their unnatural habitat. My hell is
what some call envy, a dream gym, an "if only I lived closer gym".
A "bad ass" gym that some even think about dropping their current
freedom to enter our invisible caged freedom. I don't want to get
burnt out, I truly don't, and I am scared that the dark hole will
finally suck me into its sea of normalcy; a land of joggers saying
good morning and pick up basketball games at the YMCA. A nine to
fiver with friends, drinks at the ball game, a looking forward to the
weeker, a non fucken weightlifter is what I am really saying.... and
o yes how good that sounds. Yes, its my choice, and I understand I
choose this lifestyle because I love this lifestyle. I love being a
weightlifter. But I am not going to sit here and tell you that I never
think about what lies on the other side of that white fence. I wonder
if the grass is really any greener just like you. A man with a mission
is what I am, a mission that at times fades away out the front door of
the gym as my wide eyes and open mouth try to catch what everyone is
laughing about.

They call me for seminars all over the world... Wow, that's a
beautiful feeling. What have I created? I have woken a sleeping giant
after coaching my first seminar. A smile appears on my face, and a
joyful feeling comes over me, like seeing my mom cry from happiness.
I skip to training as dreams turn into reality and ideas flood my mind
like over pouring my morning coffee. Wave after wave of excitement
crashes against me, telling me to go! The world has opened its doors
to me from the prison of room 2.... I have finally made it... I am
finally free from everyone.

This dreamful blog has been boarded shut, and this unoriginal "you
can do it" bullshit blog is not reality. I can't even ride my fucken
bike without the "you can get hurt talk", ended with "stop riding your
fucken bike" talk. I watch my calendar full of hopeful seminars and
weightlifting clinics burn in the fire from the broomstick bar yelling

in my ear. His loud voice and sturdy hands overwhelm me with fear as I surrender and listen to him. I have one hand out towards coaching like a small child dragging their parent to the carnival ride they want to go on, and the other being grabbed by the broomstick bar. This life has constant moments of sudden possible change, that never seem to happen. I want to coach; I want to spread my ideas and personal experience to everyone and anyone who would care to listen. The only person I am frustrated with is me, know one else. I say this to you, I express my frustration to you, but then again I want to make the 2016 Olympic team and dedicating my life to training is the only path that will get me there. I am trapped, but then again I don't want to leave.

I will always wonder what the other side may feel like, how much greener the grass is, or if it's really any greener at all. I will endure the pain and do whatever is in my power to stay motivated and positive. I will strive to stay focused and committed to the task at hand even with the many temptations that try to lure you down the..... well not the wrong road, but just the not right now road. I will try my hardest to put coaching to the side for now as I walk down the dusty road called weightlifting. Weightlifting is a mind game, nothing more, nothing less.

Here is the latest Cal Strength video. Talk to you all tomorrow. Salute.

Athlete 2016

♪ ♪ ♪

A Shirtless Lifestyle

Sunday, April 15, 2012

A change has occurred deep inside the soul of a weightlifter. A tilted light follows a wondering boy chasing nothing, knows the tail is nothing, but loves chasing it... what is it? I have no idea but it's exciting. A dream has woken me on a different side of the bed, a side that lifted my wide shut eyes with a baker's smell face, high above my sheets and then without warning, slammed me into the closet door knocking down the picture of the lady and the red tree. A picture that

I just can't seem to figure out, a picture that jumps out and kicks my head to the side while my mind runs away to a random childhood memory, how I got there... I have no idea. A shirtless drive to the gym for no apparent reason at all. A shirtless lifestyle that frees us from the restraints a shirt provides. We must feel the breeze against our skin, we must be free at all times. A yellow light now seems to wave you good morning as you pass him by without even looking in your rear view mirror. Tapping your fingers to your favorite song while you drive carelessly throughout the streets like laws don't apply to you. This is not non sense but pure freedom. Some might jump into my front seat and roar into my right ear nay!... nay this is not a weightlifting article, but yes, yes I say, this has everything to do with weightlifting. A wide awake dream that has not ended yet as it stalks your every move. A big gulp coffee doesn't make any sense, but I also have no care in the world, for now I am just drinking coffee. Simple is better, leave the long list for Safeway and begin to back your car out with your arm behind the passenger seat while sipping the coffee from the side of your mouth. Your view that you see is the front window looking out as everything moves fast and blurry. You spin the wheel fast, and then off you go, off I go. I am a strong superhero who spits laughter and ball breaking jokes at only my closest teammates. A one finger wave for the you can never catch me people, the AC windows up folks that try to tell the nation what's right and wrong. I can fly throughout this gym, a giant gym full of toys that I only share with Shankle.

Can weightlifting break a man? I think so. I think the mind game alone can climb its way to your brain making it see and feel unusual things. You or I's go back and forth in my writing. I feel that you are me and I am you when you are reading this, so should I use "I" or "you" consistently in this article of some sort?

I went and bought two BMX bikes, and for the last three days I have ridden them all over my city. I have been a kid again for a short while. I have been free from being a grown up. A new challenge has arrived in a dream and I have accepted the gentleman's game full throttle ahead. Is this an escape from training? I have not the slightest idea. At this point, you

A Shirtless Lifestyle.

344

know more than me. I have been obsessed with biking, even talking of
wanting to become pro. Wasteful thinking because I just sold them both
today. The dream has ended and now I wake on my usual right side of
the bed. Scared of getting injured? Or a weird child like virus that
raced throughout my body as my usual self being turned into a child
monster. Money never came to mind, and the thought of goals and dreams
seemed to live in a far away land full of parents and minivans. The
care takers would take care of it, I just needed to ride my bike.

Peter Pan I must be, or was in a different life. Now I have caught
the mean old Hook and killed the alligator. I must get back to my
studies, studies meaning training, for this sport is a ongoing study
of science, bravery, human race, and a shirtless lifestyle that only
weightlifting can create. A mind game of emotions, a constant jail
cell of scared feelings that you never confront, tired, hard life,
hard training, all mixed together over time and you have yourself
Peter pan. An adult that buckles and loses it, a grown ass man who
only for a few days just wants to ride a bike.

"Ill Never Grow up" 2016

♪♪♪

The Muscle Snatch

Tuesday, April 17, 2012

I love the Muscle Snatch, Spencer is great at the muscle Snatch, so
without further ado....the Muscle Snatch!

♪♪♪

The No No No Life

I have been driving with no License for 7 years now, and I have no
plans on getting it back. I have been driving with no car insurance
for just as long, and also have no plans in getting myself into that
scam as well. I raise my middle finger to the world as I ride my
black horse into the distance on the trail unpaved, untouched, and
what some call "the not right trail". I lay in the dark, hidden from
the world as I take a bite from my apple, while watching the white
sheep march in a straight line like jail birds walking from cell to
work yard. I am free, I am me, I am happy. I am my own boss, I have
no boss. A shirtless lifestyle as I drive with a smile on my face,
with stacks and stacks of cash rolled in a rubber band in my trunk,
like I just robbed a bank. Zero in the bank so "they" can't trace
me, my trunk makes it impossible for "them" to tell me anything.
Why do people feel the urge to tell me how to live my life? Why? I
never asked them for their advice or help, so why give it to me. Why
judge me? I think it makes them feel better about themselves as
they lay their head down at night. They don't show their emotions in
weightlifting because they were told not to. They can't slam the bar
because the old people get mad. They don't smoke cigarettes because
they were told it effects their lifting. I am not saying you need to
do what I do, just don't judge me or tell me to roll my fucken windows
up while I am pumping the AC in MY car.....not yours.

I don't stretch, never have. I personally believe that stretching
causes more injury. I take only hot baths never cold baths. I should
add I have no scientific backing on this, but fuck it, it works for
me. The last time I did an ab workout was a decade ago. I eat fast
food daily because I love it. A college drop out that seems to make
people uneasy for some strange reason, like any day they are waiting
for me to go back and finish. Maybe that's what I am supposed to
do....I really have no idea. I choose the dark shade and my little
village I call my wife and dog. I love life, I love my wife, I love
my dog, and I love weightlifting. These are just some examples of the
ongoing scrutiny that I am attacked with on a daily basis. Vicodin
and coffee seem to blanket the pain at nights, as I write to you while
tears sometime slowly drip down my face onto the key board. I am the
happiest sad guy you have ever met. My supporters like yourself is
the only thing that keeps me going, without you, without this blog, I
would be back home in Oregon at a motel six trying to bum a light.

2 time American Silver medalist......I want Gold this year. Win
Gold, and then get ready for the 2013 season. I want Attitude Nation
tattooed across my for head. Now that sounds like a brilliant idea. I
am fully committed to this weightlifting galaxy. This body has many
more years of winning left in it. Then when I retire from competing as
a senior, I will become the best master's lifter the world has ever
seen. I have told coach many times, "I might not win every meet, but
I will always be there like an annoying Mosquito".

I miss you Shankle, Shankle? Can you hear me? Are you out there? I
hope you are doing well and training hard for the Pan Am Championships
my friend. I am still your biggest fan even though we are best of
team mates. I promise you I will be on the World team with you next
year; I am sorry for abandoning you on this year's international meet.
Two years in a row traveling the world with you, and this year I guess
I will stay back and watch the home base while you drink the blood of
other lifters. I take a drink of coffee for you; I will train hard
for you, and wait for you.

God Bless America. God Bless The Attitude Nation, and God Bless Donny
Fucken Shankle. Salute.

American Open 2016

♪ ♪ ♪

How Bad Do You Want It

Saturday, April 28, 2012

"Every Kilo Counts" - An Attitude Nation video of
Kevin Cornell, Tom Sroka, Jon North, and Coach
Glenn Pendlay training hard on a Saturday.

♪ ♪ ♪

The Milk Cow

Yes, coach. Yes, I know coach. Stay on my heels, chest up, dip and
drive on both legs, head through, Shankle, Shankle, Shankle.....
down. Two whites, one red, thank God. Wrap my knees tight like
Klokov, like an athlete, like a person who is wrapping their knees
to lift as much as that one person can lift. I drink my iced coffee
with love as coach opens the gym door to let the sun in, to let the
breeze in, to let life in. I never seem to remember what day it is,
only the weight that is loaded on that quietly awaiting Pendlay bar,
as it rudely sits and stares at me. I am a part of the gym now, my
life is 100% dedicated to achieving greatness in this sport. Whether
that may be finally breaking the American snatch record officially,
or just staying the course and seeing what else this body and mind
has to offer. The grassy hill behind the gym looks so beautiful in
the sun. I have this strong urge to run around the grassy field,
jumping and pushing over the cows as they roam the field. Every time
I am about to jump the fence into the grassy world of freedom, coach
comes calling for me to get my shoes on for training. Oh, that damn
training, that damn training has got me again. Oh well, someday soon
when coach is out of town I will skip training and try to take down
one of those milk cows all on my own. Just the thought alone makes
me smile while chalking up for my first attempt. Sunny days make
training hard, staying focused on the task at hand became difficult
when you hear the laughter of others outside. I should paint the gym
walls and ceilings with a blue sky, sun and fluffy white clouds. Boy,
would that be awesome. I would paint in the milk cows over by my
resting bench so I have someone to talk to between attempts. I love
those damn cows.

Everything in the gym is touchable, everything is seeable, but the
future is completely dark. The path just seems to drop off. Right
behind where coach sits is a sea of black water that goes forever. I
hope coach doesn't fall in. If he did I would save him, for he has
saved me many times before. If coach got into a little boat and
started paddling off into the dark nowhere........ well, I would
jump off my resting bench into the water. I would do it without even
blinking. I would swim, swim as fast as I could with all the strength
he gave me to grab the side of his boat, and climb in. "I am with
you coach, my USA singlet is yours, my National Gold medal is yours,
you can't travel without it, so here it all is... let's go". See I

348

believe in loyalty. I believe in friendship. I believe in training
hard. I believe in winning. I believe in working hard. I believe
in grabbing the world by its throat and taking complete control over
your life. I believe in the Attitude Nation. I believe in myself.
I love to buy breakfast for my teammates, my money is their money,
my car is their car, my house is their house. The people who are
close to me are family, period. There is family, and then there are
people I know. I will die fighting for the people I love, I will die
fighting in this sport, I will die fighting in every aspect of life.

Doesn't that first pull feel good? That heavy weight in your hands
that you are lifting yourself can change ones life. That weight that
you have worked so hard to lift, the weight you have given up so much
for to just get over your head, is finally moving, moving because of
you and the team you have around you. I love it, I am addicted to it
like I am addicted to coffee.

The stars are bright as they reflect off the dark black water we are
sailing in. A new land has bursted through the water like Shankle
standing up from a clean. A powerful feeling has arrived in our guts,
an eye opening adventure turns the boat and all its surroundings in
complete silence. A remarkable world of weightlifting, a world of
hard work, more bad days than good, and little reward. But the little
reward is bigger than any reward out there, a reward that money can't
buy. A reward that keeps us doing what we do, even with many other
options out there. Trees of golden apples that we choose not to
pick, a house full of candy that we walk right past, an army of only
a few as we set out to sea with eyes upon the rings that bring us joy
and happiness. Yes my body hurts, and yes my mind aches with doubt
and troublesome thoughts of failure, but this does not stop us brave
soldiers from taking one step forward everyday in training.

Yes, I tell a lot on this blog about my journey and who I am as a
person. Some see me writing and question if I should let people in on
some of these things that make me, me. Some say that it's too much,
and that people will turn their backs with disagreement. Some say
that what I write is not what people want to read, or that my writing
is unimportant. I guess I don't disagree with anyone's opinions, it's
theirs to have, but this does not stop from speaking the truth. This
does not stop me from letting out my once caged emotions and feeling's.
I will never stop being real, I will never lie to you, or sugar coat
anything. This is who I am, this blog will tell many stories of
what I have been through, good and bad. I write to you on the water

with Shankle by my side, even though he is far from our boat. I feel comfort and at ease sailing with coach. So I keep writing with many forgotten thoughts and emotions racing through my head. I feel·like it's important to tell all about myself, so hopefully you can take something good from me, or take something I have done bad, and know to avoid it. Thank you for being with me, and being a part of my crazy journey through life and the sport of weightlifting. Thank you for not leaving me all alone in this dark orchestra. Thank you for giving me the freedom to write without being scared of the negative and controversial feed back. Thank you for allowing me to write with complete freedom. I salute you, the Attitude Nation, as we set to sea for another training day ahead of us.

The Cows 2016

♪ ♪ ♪

Kit Kat

Friday, May 4, 2012

What should I write about today? What should I rant on about today? Should I write a technique article, or a drink five monsters in a row article? Should I talk about the second Attitude Nation Certification seminar that is taking place tomorrow, or will I just be beating a dead horse? Donny is back, yes sir, Donny is back. Take my hand and jump into my mind for a second. First drink this monster with me, chug with me, cheers with me, then smile and slap hands with me.

He walked into the front door and I jumped with joy. A memory flashed through my head as I was walking through the gym to meet him half way. Long strides with a smile on my face, long strides as I looked down at the ground excited to look up for the reunion. Why do we do that? Look down when we are walking to something important. I guess it's the excitement we are to nervous to show others, so we bow our heads keeping our smile below our chin. A memory about my father flashed through my head, cutting off my smile and slowing my walk down to a complete stand still.. A memory of me sitting cross legged on the floor with my sister watching the X Files flashed into my head like a teacher turning on one of those damn projectors. Late at night, dark room, with the TV's glow covering my sister and I as if the TV was an alien space ship sucking us into its ship. A big blue house in the country, a gravel bus stop, horses for miles, old rusty trucks and tractors that lay dead in the tall grass, and the common "mom, Jon is being mean!" line that my sister used quite often. A house full of life and love, a farm full of family and happiness, a time that my sister and I will never forget. A support group that could take down a pro football team is what we were....well, and still are. But this night was different, this night was like a dream that sticks with you for the next week or two. A dream that sits on your back like a monkey from the zoo, hitting you over the head while your wife is trying to take a picture of you. No mother in sight, not even a clue where should could be. Lost in the always creepy and weird world of the X Files. Sister by my side, even though I couldn't see her from the glare of the blazing TV light. The door behind my sister and I opened, how we knew was simple, the door makes a screaming noise, and I could actually see my dad through the reflection of the TV. Thank God the show had a dark scene so I could see him, if not the noise alone would have given me that fear of panic...you know, the instant reaction of looking for your mom, especially at that young age. If you can't find her, well, then I think the next move is just to sit there and start crying. Right? My sisters pony tail hit me in the face from her turning her head so fast. I then followed, starting to stand up before even getting my head all the way around to see him. Watching TV too long, or playing a video game too long always gave me a "homesick" feeling. An uneasy stomachache that put me far from reality. Once my dad walked in, that feeling vanished, the TV had lost me, I was no longer trapped in its bright light. My sister beat me to him, hugging his right leg while she was somehow still able to jump up and down. I followed like a sprinter taking second place, still happy, but jealous that he was already giving her the attention first....damn. I held onto his left leg with my eyes closed, and my two feet standing on his one foot. When I opened my eyes I saw a Kit Kat bar in my dad's big squishy bear paws, yes! Kit Kat! Thanks dad! My sister was even more happy and excited than I was.

Soon after the fighting got worse, and my parents got a divorce; but at that moment everything was perfect. At that moment nothing else mattered.

I then shook Donny's hand and we began to lift weights.

I still don't know what to write about. I don't even know what I just wrote. Maybe tomorrow I will write something worth telling. Today the Monsters and coffee combined took me down a road that has been grown over by tall grass and weeds. A road less traveled. One of those old

memories that sticks with us for life, and we have no idea why. Why
that memory? I am assuming there are many more that has escaped our
memory. I guess we must hold on tight to the ones we still have.

Good night, talk to you tomorrow. Thanks for reliving a very great
childhood memory with me.

I love you, dad. I hope to someday see you again.

Salute. Dad 2016

♪♪♪

Dirt

Sunday, May 6, 2012

Once an idea has drilled its way into your a head, that idea is very
hard to remove. Once an image flashes in your dreams, that image
is very hard to forget. Thoughts are nothing but air, you can't
touch them or show others. Ideas are nothing but dirt. You are held
captive by your own images. There is no unseeing what you have seen.
There is no turning back from the path you have stumbled upon. You
must walk, you must take one step at a time. You must sacrifice to
reach your dirt, because dirt is all your dreams are to others. This
is why you must be selfish. You must carry on no matter how painful
the journey may be, or how dark the path may become. Will you take
your handful of dirt and run with it? Will you chase what others say
is impossible? Will you put in the work to get what you want? Will
you go through hell to achieve heaven? Or, will you throw your dirt
on the ground and walk away. Will you surrender to society and what
others say? Will you call your dirt... just dirt? Will you quit?

Long nights in a small garage labeling and pumping product. We were a
long row of family side by side working for the same dream. With every
bottle we pumped product into a smile came over our faces. With every
label we slapped across the bottle our dirt pile became bigger. My step
dad quit his job, and my mother sold her salon. We were then broke,
living in a small house hardly getting by. We went through hours and
hours of work, and hours of constant excitement followed by constant
worries and doubts. The black crow was always there, circling around us,
letting us know that if we didn't make it then he would get something
out of it. He would peck at our eyes, and knock over containers full of

product. He would try his hardest to take our dirt, but our strength as
a family was too strong. He soon flew away once we made our first big
deal, and bought a small warehouse moving us out of the stuffy garage.
It was a life changing event. It was a "we made it" event. Our dirt
pile outgrew our small humble house, our 447 Brookside Drive house that
brought me great memories that will follow me for the rest of my life.
After school my sister and I would work long hours in the new warehouse.
We wanted more, we wanted more dirt. My whole family would play on the
dirt pile after a hard days work. We would just sit on top of it with
silence and comfort as we bathed in our success, still in shock in what
we were creating. Our dream was finally coming true, as we turned our
slow walk on the windy path into a full sprint to the American dream.

Just an idea, thats all it was. Three more upgraded warehouses, world
wide sales, and a company that is worth a lot of rubber band stacks
has turned the dirt into gold, and a small idea into an empire. They
were dream chasers, now they are dream catchers. They were broke,
now they are rich. They were employed now they employ. They took a
chance on their idea, and won. They held tight to their hand full of
dirt and never let it slip through their fingers.

                          Chase your dreams, and get your dirt!   2016

                                ♪ ♪ ♪

                              Red Eye

Tuesday, May 8, 2012

We are caged animals in a gym with no windows. The holes in the walls are
from us trying to dig our way out back to reality. The year could easily
be 1920, and we would have no idea. Well maybe the techno music might
be a give away, but I don't know...... I am pretty sure techno was just
starting to get popular at that time. I have completely lost track of the
year, date, and time. A zoo animal is what I am. I am hamster turning
in a never ending wheel. It's hard not to lose my mind in a sport that
keeps me standing in the same place 99 percent of the day. This is why
I can't help but to dance, jump around, run in circles around coach, or
scream and yell after making a lift. I do feel that at times I am really
losing my mind, and it worries me. I will create different characters
in training and act them out as if I was in a movie. Why do I do this? A
smile will cross my face with no warning or apparent reason at all. I

will occasionally sit outside staring off into the blue sky with my mouth open wide and my head resting on my hand until coach comes to get me, and then walks me inside leading me to my bar like a horse to water. "There you go Jon, there is your bar, grab it, good boy, now lift it above your head." All eyes on me, and at times I feel I have no privacy. The little red light from the live feed camera is always judging me, staring at me, clapping for me, and at times rolling its red eye at me. Everywhere I look there is now a camera in my face. I have no idea where Cal Strength gets all that footage from on the YouTube videos. I don't remember doing half of what's recorded, and if I do I didn't realize someone was filming me. Good Lord, let me dance in peace please.

A long car ride has my head out the window. A car ride is fun because it means I am not training. A car ride is pure heaven. In this world the sky is purple, and the grass is pink. My world is black, well besides the red light. My world looks so fun from the outside looking in. I watch the videos and they make me want to join the Cal Strength team, and I actually get excited. "Hey babe, tomorrow I am going to get into weightlifting and train at Cal Strength with this crazy guy named Jon!" I feel bad for the surprise that kid will endure.

Coffee is my love because it cures the pain momentarily. I drink so much of it; I cant get enough of it. I am drinking some right now and it always tastes extra good when writing to you. I try to escape through the hole in the wall, but coach grabs me by my legs and drags me back in. He holds me down with force as I put up a fight kicking and screaming. He jams the coffee straw down my throat and tilts miss brown eyes' beautiful butt in the air, draining the coffee into my stomach. I soon stop fighting, and become completely at peace. Damn....They have drugged me again.

Here is the brand new Cal Strength video below. Prepare to enter the wild zoo of my life. This is the footage that is not suppose to be shown, the footage of a weightlifter slowly losing his mind in a windowless, four walled prison called weightlifting. Salute my friends.

Car Rides 2016

♪ ♪ ♪

354

Tigger

Thursday, May 10, 2012

I have competed, lifted, coached seminars on my own, helped with many
Pendlay seminars all over the world, and I have never once seen anyone
perform the "low bar squat". Actually, I didn't even find out what
it was until a few months back when someone asked me if they should
do high bar or low bar for the squats I just prescribed them. I am
still in shock that athletes actually perform such a "nails on a
chalk board" lift, especially for a weightlifter that should make
the bottom position their home. The number one problem I see with
beginner weightlifters is their depth, or lack there of. Watching
a weightlifter low bar squat makes me want to take the elevator to
the highest floor, and then jump. Low bar squatting is just as bad
as a beginner doing power snatch and power clean more than the full
lifts. Both of these weightlifting killers create incorrect movement
patterns, horrible rhythm, awful consistency, and do not increase the
novice weightlifter's flexibility. The low bar squat is not just ugly
and painful to watch, but teaches you to move slower than a turtle
that just drank two bottles of nyquil.

Brand new client, brand new dreams of becoming an Olympic
weightlifter, in a brand new sport where the sky is the limit. We
work on catching the bar in the hole over and over for hours. After
catching a lift in the hole, I would have him sit down there and get
comfy. I would throw him a bag of popcorn and tell him to watch a
movie down there. I would tell him to bounce like tigger over and
over to create stability, balance, and for the great practice of at
times having to catch that second or third bounce to stand up with a
heavy weight. I introduced him to his new home. He then started to
make progress in the lifts, especially after I told him never to do
a power snatch or power clean again, until he became a champion at
the "full" lifts. A fist pump followed by a smile is the action and
emotion that he got when he was able to lift more weight by receiving
the bar as low as he could. I dropped out of physics, but I have
the innate ability to understand that weightlifting is nothing more
than a race against gravity. I get excited for him; I get excited
for his new PR. We slap hands and drink more coffee, going over how
the training went and what we both want in the near and far future.
I think he thought the training session was over because he started
to take his Pendlay shoes off. I then laughed and told him that the
fire in Hell was still burning bright and high, and now we had to

squat. Tired but still motivated, he took another sip of miss brown eyes, and began to slap the big bearded man's shoes back on. Back squats, 5 sets of 2, lets go. I had to take a number one from all the coffee that has been poured down my throat since I woke about 7 hours ago. In a full on sprint to the bathroom I yelled without looking behind me, "Get warmed up!". As I slowly started walking back from one of the best things God himself ever invented, I heard a bunch of little kids crying and screaming for their mothers. People everywhere where running past me to the door like the building was on fire. Coach Pendlay stood up and yelled for someone to call 911, and then he walked fast....not ran, because everyone knows that Coach never runs....well unless he is imitating my teammate Kevin Cornell. As I was spinning in circles trying to comprehend what was happening in the quiet town of San Ramon, Donny bumped into me spilling my coffee all over my deep v Attitude Nation shirt. He told me that a red fire breathing demon with sharp fangs and dinosaur scales dripping down its greasy back was killing people by its grotesque image alone. I pushed through the panicking crowd and to my horror, I saw my client doing low bar back squats.

The world ended hours later.

High bar 2016

♪ ♪ ♪

100,000

Saturday, May 12, 2012

100,000 Monsters, 100,000 coffees. 100,000 Attitude Nation Soldiers. 100,000 smiles, tears, and laughs. 100,000 epic songs dancing through my soul while writing side by side with Donny as if we were two gladiators fighting in the Colosseum. 100,000 haters trying to defeat the Attitude Nation. 100,000 victories we celebrated. We have raised 100,000 middle fingers high in the air for all to see. We have 100,000 black suits, playing only one guitar, that never stops playing, even late at night when the drunk crowd tries to boo us off stage. An army that started at one, one lonely Monster sitting at 7 Eleven in its cold refrigerator, waiting to speak its mind. One year ago, one iced coffee by the name of Ms. Brown eyes sat hopelessly waiting to be rescued my her knight in shinning armor. One year ago no one would listen to her, or even knew who Ms. Brown eyes was. She would try to speak her mind, but would be shunned by the green jungle's dictator. She would be thrown into her cell only left to cry and wonder, wonder if she would ever have the chance to be free and speak her mind. She would ponder if she would ever have the chance to make an impact on the world... or who knows, maybe even change it.

Ever since I was a child, I knew I was different. I knew there was a some sort of expression that was just waiting to be released. I was constantly muted by my own self insecurities and unsureness of everything, including myself. I had the thoughts, I had the words, but I was too scared to speak them, write about them, or act on them. I was too worried about what others thought, that it blinded me from ever seeing the Attitude, the Nation that gives me hope, freedom, and self worth. Soon I realized that I must not let the audience of life be the judge, I must be the judge. At the end of the day, I figured out that by writing something good on paper would bring real happiness and a release from my own self judgment. I would constantly hear the deep pounding drum against my chest, over and over as I walked to its rhythm. The marching soldiers in my head kept me up all night, and soon made me realize that I wasn't alone. I knew there were others out there, patiently waiting to attack the world as one well oiled machine. I just didn't realize there would be 100,000 of them armed and ready.

When the time came one year ago, I knew what I had to do. I had to start the attack. I had to release the beast. I had to bring the Nation together once and for all. I had to find the missing pieces to my life. I was a kid that was slowly transforming into what some would call a "grown up", a grown up with interesting images in my head that spoke to me at the oddest times. I had to write, or I was afraid I would lose it.

After falling in love with Ms. Brown Eyes and adopting Mr. Green Monster, the Nation was almost complete. I was missing two things, me as a writer, and you as the audience. I had no idea what kind of words would spill out onto the computer screen. I spent hours upon hours just staring at the white screen and blinking black line that constantly taunted me to write something, anything! But it had to be good, it had to come from the heart and it dearly had to mean something. I was sweating like a pig, and as nervous as a school boy about to kiss a girl for the first time. We all know in a situating like that you must go for it, and commit fully. So I did, and as I leaned in to start typing, Ms. Brown Eyes grabbed my hands and

starting punching my fingers against the black buttons with such
beauty and finesse. Mr. Green Monster was whispering ideas into my
mind, similar to putting your ear to a sea shell. We were a team, and
still are. I am not even writing this, they are.

Thank you all for your support over the last year. You all mean the
world to me. This blog would not exist without you. Thank you for
being a part of this team, this family, this creation we call the
Attitude Nation.

100,000 and onward 2016

♪ ♪ ♪

Beer Talk

Wednesday, May 16, 2012

Hey, welcome back to the Dark Orchestra. Here..... here is some
coffee I made for you. I threw in an extra shot just for you,
so pucker up and enjoy the warm but ice cold kisses from Ms
Brown Eyes. Welcome back my friend, it's always good to see you.
Cheers. How has your training been going? Mine has been hard,
as you are probably experiencing as well. At the end of the day
we are both much a like. We both love weightlifting, and for
having weightlifting be such a big part of our lives, that pretty
much means we are the same damn person. I have nothing special
or interesting to write about today. Some would call it writer's
block, but I would call it just saying, hi. No technique talk, no
coaching tips, no stories about a devil in the red dress capturing
young weightlifters and ruining their career from the rest she
casts upon them. This is just a simple hi how are you doing,
and a cheers of the coffee. It is a simple chat about training
and life. It is like a simple beer conversation with a friend,
yes.... this is always the best kind of conversation. Why is it
that a single beer sitting between two people makes each person
open up with such ease and relaxation? Why is that? A single beer
doesn't even need to be drank, yet it can make a social situation
so comfortable that you can end up talking for hours upon hours.
A conversation has come to life between you and your best mate,
and you now feel closer than before. You have drawn a few tears,
laughed hysterically, got mad, and hugged, all in the small window

358

of time you have been sitting at the corner bar with a beer in
front of one another. But have you noticed that you haven't even
taken a sip yet? You haven't. You are in shock, because for a
while you had the back up plan to announce to everyone around you
how tipsy or even drunk you were getting. You thought you had that
big glass of beer to fall back on from all the emotions and deadly
truth you have been spilling out onto the half wood half brass bar
table. You end up drinking about 7 more and the night gets crazy.
It's almost like you try to hide the fact you opened up that much
without being intoxicated. So the next day you talk and laugh
about everything besides that first few hours. But why? I guess
I find the psychology of beer interesting. I personally think the
same goes for coffee, tea, and whatever else can alter the mind.

I didn't realize the impact coach had on training until he left.
He was gone today, and he will be gone for the next week, and now
I feel that I have been dropped off for summer camp and I already
want to go home. I don't know how you garage soldiers do it. I
salute you. I am having a hard time staying focused and motivated
while coach is out of the gym. It would be so easy to just not
train, half ass it, skip squats, or even skip the whole damn week
of training all together. For the first time the front door is
wide open. There are no bars caging me inside. There is no ball
and chain around my ankle. I could make a run for it right now and
never come back. I could go with rest and live with her forever,
or at least for a week, but I don't know if she would ever let me
train again. I heard that once you lay with rest, you are doomed
forever. The small vacation time you thought you were on turns into
a jail of its own. But today I stayed and trained hard. The world
team next year is the only thing in life that matters to me. I am
proud of myself for pushing throughout today. I felt I made a good
impact on my teammates. They saw me training hard, so they trained
hard. I am not saying they do whatever I do, but I feel that I am
at times the leader, and today I led, hopefully making them better.
I kept looking over at coach only to find an empty chair. My head
would tilt to the side and I would begin to scratch my head. This
is odd..... what is happening? It's like the world as I knew it
was slowly crumbling down around me starting from the ceiling down.
It's like wishing your parents would leave you a lone as a kid, and
the minute they do you get sad. Shit, I already miss him. Who is
going to yell at me to squat, and tell me my v neck is gay? Who is
going to ramble on in training about food, how he made his food, how
his food tasted, and how I missed out eating his home cooked food?

I missed a lift and nothing happened today. There was no look from
coach that easily read "what the fuck was that?". The miss was
followed by quiet....... how odd. Coach please come back...... I
need to be pushed. Without you I might be "him".

Come Back coach 2016

♪ ♪ ♪

React

Wednesday, May 23, 2012

Seeking to find answers in this sport will only lead you to a snowy
bank that falls hundreds of feet below. The strong wind behind your
back seems to be pushing you further and further toward the edge, no
matter how hard you dig your heels into the white ground. The big
bear behind you is a certain indicator that you must just jump, jump
or get eaten by the once black now white frosty bear that has pulled
up a seat behind you and is starting to write a weightlifting article.
He looks up at you with those low glasses and a know it all sigh. Now
your imiganation is playing tricks on you. Now you have entered the
wonderful white world of lost. Your ongoing search for answers has
led the pitch black horse to nothing but more white sand. The water
seemed to be there, but now your lips will stay dry and chapped as you
continue to look for the secret that you think the wishing well has to
offer. Oh wishing well, wish me the correct understanding to reach
my goals. Wish me the wish for all the answers I so desperately feen
for. The long rope that you have been pulling on for some time now
has ended with an empty let down. The well is out of water, and the
hollow barrel echoes your cries of a frantic obsession.

The day you know it all, is the day you know nothing. The minute you
try to figure out this sport, is the same minute you will lose your
mind. An odd idea if you think about it, but so true. Fish and catch
fish. Love your mom, and well.... you will love your mom. I didn't
miss the weight, I simply am a weightlifter. It has taken years and
years of learning how to not use my mind. A much harder task than
technique. A task that seems impossible, but if mastered could be
fantastic. The minute I think, is the minute I lose. I could say
the unoriginal line over and over that many use on a daily basis that
makes them think they have some sort of clue or grasp on this sport,

360

the line used with so much confidence, "this sport is so mental".
This sport shouldn't be mental, it should be a fact. It should be
art, that at times is just splattered on the canvas with nothing but
pure emotion. You should make the lift like 1+1=2. Is it possible
to shut your mind off so much that making a lift is nothing more than
a reaction? Coach's eyes coach me, not his words. The horse needs
to keep running, not trying to find water. You must jump to not be
eaten. "Training must become a reaction". - Donny Shankle.   You can
think all you want while resting between reps, but when it's time
to lift the barbell you must just react. Just like a lion in the
woods that looks as if he is going to attack you, I promise, you will
just start running. Grab and go, jump and run, slam the bar with no
thought process at all. My celebrations are 100 percent true and
real, 100 percent me. You are witnessing true emotion coming from my
soul, not my mind. God rips out of my chest wearing a USA singlet and
throws up a "I am number one finger". Well because shit..... God is
always number one. Get em God. I love God and what he has given me.
I thank him every day for the emotions that I am allowed to spread all
over the world to help motivate not just me, but others all the way
from garage lifters, to top lifters. You must react. The dog must
sit with just one look. You must stop looking for water because the
minute you stop you will find it. Yes, I know this is a common dating
line, but it's so true in training as well.

How is your coffee? Mine is strong and powerful. The Dark Orchestra
is extra dark tonight. I love it. I love how we really don't know
where we are, but we feel at home. This feeling has always interested
me. Why is it that some places make us feel good, and some bad? It's
like a dog that likes some people, and viciously barks at others.
What is that dog's reason? Don't be afraid to miss. Nothing upsets
me more than a weightlifter that always gets down on their selves when
they are faced with the reality of missing. Even when they make it,
if something felt wrong they proceed to hit themselves over the head,
followed by a check list of what they did wrong. No! Stop! If you
made the lift.... then good. If you missed the lift.... then good,
you are a weightlifter.

Goodnight and salute to you all. I fucken love you.

God 2016

♪ ♪ ♪

Odyssey

The day is sunny, while the air is cold and crisp. The early morning
orange glow has seeped through your blinds, covering your body with
stripes of black. The weightlifters rise out of their bunks with
stretching arms and achy backs. A warm shower hits your back as
you bow your head towards your feet. Your eyes are wide open, as
your mind races through the checklist of who you are, what you have
accomplished, what you still need to accomplish, and flashing images
of the hell coach will cast upon you once this quiet early morning
comes to a close. You choose to drip dry as you brush your teeth bare
naked, which goes against your usual routine of drying off thoroughly
with a towel. Your blood starts to pump though your body a little
faster the more you wake. You throw up a bicep pose while the tooth
brush takes a break to admire your strong muscles. Fox news is in the
background as you pour a bowl of cereal. The peaceful chatter and the
sound of the cereal hitting the bowl could make a grown man cry from
its simple beauty.

Quiet before the storm. Peace before war. Heaven before Hell. You
gently rest your hand over the coffee maker's left cheek, while singing
a random Christmas song to her. You are excited for Christmas even
though it's only May. You are excited for what she will give birth
to in the next few minutes, and how happy it will make you feel inside
once you have her in the palm of your hands. The coffee drips with
rhythm, as each drop has its own personality and desires. You look up
to see coach standing on your living room table, waving his hands in
the air while his eyes are closed shut, and his head tilted back. The
strings connected to his fingers are casting a web all over the house
as you try to maneuver closer to him. No, you can't touch him, for he
is in a glass bottle. Coach is connected to everything this morning has
had to offer you. The small little red dots all over your naked body
are from the strings attached from coach to you. You are a puppet, and
everything you think you have control over.....well, you don't.

When I watch our videos, another video is watching me. I then watch
that video of me watching the first video, only to feel the presence
of another video watching me watch the second video. Time and reality
seem to be slipping away. The red eye has lit up the morning from
orange to red, and my front door has turned from wood to a glass lens
looking out into the gym. My teammates wave me in from the other side

as I stand there drinking my coffee, naked, and in complete peace. I have surrendered to the whys and how's. I have let down my conscience and I now just dance when things don't make sense. This sport doesn't make sense, and how coach went from standing in my living room to playing the violin on the other side of the lens has confused me. I guess what all this means is that we must train. We must train no matter what. You know what I mean? It doesn't need to make sense to be understood. No matter what is happening in our lives we must train through it, by it, and right over the top of it. When life doesn't add up, the training will. Over time, all the training will pay off like a bank account you have been growing for years and years. At the end of the day, I guess the most confusing things in life are really the most simple. A peaceful morning is only peaceful because of the pain you and I endure during the day. I feel that weightlifters appreciate down time more than anyone else. We are at war in the midst of the hardest sport in the world, so we must train.

Coach, coffee, and shower 2016

♪ ♪ ♪

Phil Sabatini

Wednesday, June 6, 2012

A lift dedicated to my good friend and competitor Phil Sabatini. (video below) The man I have been at war with for so many years, has now laid his sword down in retirement. It's a sad day for me. It's a sad day for the sport. We have fought against each other in some extremely tight battles, and we have also been teammates on the USA team in 2010. I will miss him. It has been an honor to fight with and against him. A certain understanding brews between us with very few words being spoken. We understand that at the end of the day we are enemies, and we must do whatever it takes to win. It's not personal, just business.

My loses over the span of my career have been from his sword digging into my stomach. My eyes widen as I watch the blood drip down my stomach while my knees hit the ground. I can see in his eyes he feels for me as he watches my body drop to the ground in defeat. Every time he digs the sword deeper into my stomach my jaw opens wider and wider

363

while I try so hard to grasp for air. A single tear rolls down Phil's
face as his strength starts to bleed out of him, and his emotions
get the better of him. He apologizes in a whisper, but there is no
need to, for I would do the same to him. Respect is everything. He
respects me, and I respect him. He is a true warrior, and so am I.
If there was anybody to lose to it would be him. He pulled the sword
out from my stomach and wiped the bloody blade off with his singlet.
He stood over my body as the crowd roared in celebration. He threw
up his hands in victory. He raised his sword high for all to see.
Then looked down and nodded his head at my dead body. A warrior's
nod, a warrior's respect. He bent down to close my eyelids with his
hands, and right when he got close to me, I pulled my small dagger
out from my boot and stuck it right into his neck. At that moment we
just stared at each other as we both slowly started to stand up, using
each other's body like a ladder. He placed his hand on his wound, and
then looked at his bloody hand in disbelief. The blood was pouring
from his neck, just like my stomach. He then took his sword and drove
it into my stomach again. This time, blood came squirting out of my
mouth as I bent over. I would have fell face down but he held me up
to only twist the blade around even more. As I was laying over his
shoulder as if we were hugging, I built up the strength to throw him
off of me creating a few feet of space. One hand was grasping tight
to our weapons, and the other was resting over our wounds. A moment
of silence came over the whole arena as we both stood motionless. And
then it happened, we both ran full speed at each other creating a
splash of blood that sprayed onto our faces. Our teary eyes and last
gasping breaths were inches from each other as a smile appeared over
both our faces. We laughed out loud, as we were both just glad to
get the blood shed over with. No more words were spoken, just a slow
dying laugh that soon ended when both our bodies laid over each other
on the dusty ground. Our hearts stopped beating as we laid there dead
with chalky hands and USA on our chests.

Thank you Phil for pushing me over the years. I would not be where
I am today if it wasn't for you. Thank you for being such a great
competitor, and even a better friend. I know you and your wife have
a little baby girl now, and you have much bigger battles ahead of you
than weightlifting. You are my fucken hero brother. You are my role
model. You are a family man that I some day hope to be. You are a
man I envy in every way possible. Like I said in the video when I
retire, we will drink a beer together on the porch and tell old war
stories. We will be old men sitting in the audience watching the new
young weightlifters battle it out. We will smile as memories race

through our heads. Thank you for beating me.
Thank you for not punching me when I beat you.
Thank you for everything. Salute.

Phil Sabatini two thousand and forever

The King 2016

♪ ♪ ♪

I'm Back

Wednesday, June 20, 2012

I'm back. I'm sorry. I have missed drinking coffee with you in the
dark orchestra. I have missed chatting with you, venting to you, and
entering unforgiving worlds of imaginations and familiar experiences of
hard training followed with tears of pain with you. Tears of pain from
the hell we live in. Paths that lead to demonds and anglels. Yes, I am
back. Yes, we are still alive and well. Together holding hands in the
blazing fires of weightlifting, side by side, shaky hands and pissed
off haters, we stand. A society that shunned us from the norm, who
call us freaks, who don't understand. The sport that will take your
soul and swallow you whole. A sport that will leave you with nothing
unless you achieve something. Unless you man or women the fuck up and
attack the devil in a red dress everyday. Never take her hand, leave
her beauty for "him". A move across the Country chasing a dream is
why these moving boxes smile at me. The plates chatter with talk of
never again. The title will never be yours my kitchen tables explained
to me, as I chewed on its wooden side showing it my strength and the
power of my bite. Everyone I have beat in this sport knows my bite,
so now it's the kitchen table's turn. Why chase something you can't
see? My world is not in America, it's with you in this empty hallway
that echoes sounds of an orchestra playing our sad song, a song that we
are familiar with. "Why sad?," asks the new member to this blog. I
will tell you why, no.... we will tell you why. Listen closely my soft
handed friend, because there are more bad days than good days in this
sport. 99 bad days and one good day. 99 days of doubt dragging behind

one maybe "I can" day. Just one "yes" day. Maybe I will keep opening
my garage door, turning up my music, and training by my mother fucken
self. Maybe one day I will slam this bar and shatter everyone who ever
doubted me. Maybe I will climb to the top of the world and raise my
hand high as I disperse into a chalky cloud that hangs over all who
tried to tell me to roll my windows up when the AC was on.

She followed me here, Miss Brown Eyes that is. She has been waiting
for me as I drove my car across Country, chugging red bulls with my
hand tight around the wheel, imagining thoughts of me representing this
great Country again. On stage, with TV cameras following me around
again like last year at the games. Oh, did I go crazy, yes I did,
and people hated me for it. Yes. Complete. Thank you. Thank you for
putting this black coat on me, this black shirt on me, and these black
pants on me. Thank you for putting this guitar in my hands and letting
me sing to the world through this blog. She tasted slightly different
from the heat and humidity, but her kiss are the same. Her touch
is the same, and the feeling of hope and happiness throughout all my
trials and errors in this life is the same. We are back. The Attitude
Nation is back, well....we never left, Just busy is all. But now all
settled in, now finally time to write. Miss Brown Eyes is back, the
team is back. We together will achieve greatness in this lifetime,
whether it's through weightlifting or family. Whether it's bettering
ourselves as people, or getting better grades in school. We are one, we
are the best, we are a family which the flames cannot touch.

The new radio show is exciting. But there is something missing. It's
not the same as writing. I feel we connect much better through this
black key board. I feel more alive when writing to you. I feel we
have a certain understanding, more so than when I talk through the
mic. The mic cages my true emotions from being nervous and not letting
my fingers do the talking. My soul types and the coffee directs.
Talking is just the surface. Yes it's fun, yes it's great to chat and
hear your voice, but the connection is just not there. Writing is a
powerful feeling that cannot be explained. I am going to start writing
everyday, not every other day, but everyday. I will never leave for
that long again. I will never leave the Nation alone while you stand
over the bar with your war paint splattered on your face. Your chalky
white hands look as if you are a mime, the only difference is the blood
from your wounds has crept through the dry cracks of your hand, and are
now dripping one by one onto the platform. You smile, but you really
aren't smiling. We never really smile. We are great actors, for pain
and discomfort is always casted upon us. I must fight with you. I

must die by your side in this fucken hell we live in. The strength of
many, that's how I will win Americans. That's how I will break these
American records. The strength of the lone garage weightlifter. Salute
to you, the soldier who fights with no one around to push him. The
soldier who trains hard, even though little gremlins tell myths about
over training. Salute to us, who turn our back to rest.

Fight 2016

♪ ♪ ♪

Weightlifting Talk Ep 2

Sunday, June 24, 2012

The Second Episode went much better. We finally
got the big Rush Limbaugh mic to work. Moved
the episode to an hour and half for more time,
and just had a better flow on air. Shankle and
I were much more comfortable, we really did get
lost in the conversations. We are both excited
to continue our chats every Friday at 1:00 eastern
time. Don't forget to tune in next week at
blogtalkradio.com and call in to say hi. Salute!

Rush 2016

♪ ♪ ♪

Team MDUSA

Tuesday, June 26, 2012

The Very First Muscle Driver USA video! The
craziness starts all over, so lock your doors,
hide the kids, and prepare for the madness that
this awful sport has to offer. Fists may fly,
chairs may be thrown, and the rookies will cry
in defeat......shit, here we go agin. Americans
5 months out. Salute.

MDUSA 2016

♪ ♪ ♪

Wanderlust

Thursday, June 28, 2012

A meeting with a zombie. A Wanderlust mind that directs your feet away from the herd. A sit down with another type of person. A cold and lonely stage is where you eat dinner tonight, and the skeletons you have put away for so many years seem to have joined you at the long wooden table that sits a family of thousands in the empty center of the Dark Orchestra. This is what I find fascinating. Just as fascinating as dedicating your life to something that you cant see or feel.

Your green hill has now turned dark red from the sky that crept up behind you. The sky that looks down upon you so proudly, as the black birds guide you to......well you. Yes proud, where others see the red threat as doom. This is where they are wrong, this is where their feet should walk, this is where the comfort zone starts, and their world ends. Bold steps towards what you want. This is what Shankle speaks of so passionately. Steps of chance, followed by steps of courage, can cure anything and anyone. Steps that will eventually get you face to face with a zombie, or lead you to a small town where you could meet your new best friend. Steps that make your hand bleed from the double edged sword you hold so tightly. You must take a chance; I must take the bold steps to achieve what I want. We must leave ourselves back home at the kitchen table, and walk to a new outlook, a new adventure, and a new life. We must walk in the dark, or else we will live in the white light called the comfort zone. A world where so many live and die. A blanket of comfort and satisfaction that people walk around with in public. A world where so many dream day and night, for they can only dream, because dream is all they have. They are too scared to make it reality. They are prisoners of their own self-doubt.

A gamblers rush of losing intrigues me. A rush that reminds he or she that they are still alive. This amazes me that a gambler could be the same as a weightlifter, they both have the disease of Wanderlust, and it seems they are both chasing the unknown. Even losing is a win in many ways. A win of living and taking chances. A win of trying. A sit down with a zombie could be good, who knows. Over the hill could be heaven, or just the red hell that seems to still hang over you. See in my opinion hell is a place that lives within us. Hell is a comfort zone, a prison cell that keeps us from being.....well, us. Don't listen to anyone. Close this blog down now. My words are nothing but talk, they are not walk. You must walk; you must eat dinner by

yourself. You must ride the rides at the carnival with no one around.
Find out what will happen, and how you will react to such unknown.
Find out who you are, and what you are capable of.

A bloody hand only means a well sought off person. An individual who
will sleep well at night, for they have fought for their dreams, win
or lose. But there is no lose, because the journey itself in a win.
A double edged sword is a win-win, even though your hand drips with
blood. There is no such thing as a win-lose, only a lose-lose. A
lose-lose is the world of comfort and sought after acceptance from
others. The sheep will never know who they really are. I find myself
at ease when I am on the edge. I find the darkest corners of life so
intriguing, so comfortable, as if they were my childhood home lit up
like the month of December. Wanderlust is what my buddy Adam Hall told
me it was called, as I so despretly explained to him one day about this
odd feeling I constatnly encounter, I didnt even realize it had a name.
I am so drawn to the unknown, at times I catch myself just driving,
just walking, and just looking out through the Starbucks window for
no apparent reason. What the hell is out there? Maybe this is why I
couldn't stand sitting in a class room; I was too busy itching for the
bell to ring so I could explore the sea I could not see. I am addicted
to wanderlust like I am addicted to this coffee. Do you ever have the
feeling of getting in your car and driving with known destination in
sight? What if I just walked for three days straight, where would it
take me? What would it bring me? What would I find?

Shit, the more I think about it, the more I am realizing that everything
up to this point in my life has been driven by
wanderlust. This is how I met my Wife, this is
how I met you, and by sitting here writing is just
another way of breaking free. I guess Wanderlust
is really the unknown, because I have no idea what
the hell I am talking about, and where I am going
with this. I am just taking bold steps forward.
I am just writing to you in the ever so confused
dream world called the Dark Orchestra.

Here is the brand new MDUSA video below. Salute.

The Dark Orchestra 2016

♪ ♪ ♪

369

A Chat With Train

Saturday, June 30, 2012

Episode Three of Weightlifting talk, brought to you by a planet called "I slam bars". Salute!

♪ ♪ ♪

Black Eyes

Wednesday, July 4, 2012

Eyes wide open from the Devil's smoke. The smoke that lifts you up so high, and then violently drops you down with nothing but lose teeth and confused thoughts, all connected back to pale skin and fragile bones. Your dark black eyes match the circles that so massively surround them, as if your eyes had fallen deep inside a giant crater. Two black holes in your face fill with water, as the tears fall down your boney cheeks and into your wide open mouth, as it screams so desperately for your father to save you. You cry out for help with closed eyes and hands that have seemed to form into tree branches that have branched in all different formations and directions. Your father is just as gone as you are. His eyes are blacker than his hair, and you can tell he has come down harder than you have. He no longer stands tall and confident, now he leans drooped over and beat. The realization has hit you, and hit you hard, that the person who has been protecting you throughout your whole life has now become a helpless man that cannot do anything for you, only to cry as well. Seeing your father stand in the middle of the road staring back at you while his arms wrap around his body, is a feeling that will never leave you. Two minutes of crying and shaking, not one of you had

the courage to take a step forward and embrace each other. You keep
waiting for him to hug you, but he never did. To this day, you don't
know why you didn't either.

I sometimes lie awake in bed finding myself reliving this stained
memory, trying to guide myself toward him. Imagining that everything
would have disappeared the minute we hugged, that life after that
could have gone back to normal. But no, I realize that never happened
as I get up out of bed in the middle of the night to find myself
looking back at a man that left that crying kid in street so long ago.
Our bodies shook rapidly from the "come down". I was only 16, and I
had been up for four nights straight with no food, no water, and no
sleep. Every time the thick cloud of smoke entered my lungs, a part
of my innocence disappeared. My mind went places I didn't even know
existed. I couldn't tell if it was the drugs giving me this rotting
feeling inside, or the lack of life necessities that I had abandoned.
Black is all I saw in his eyes, no white at all, just black.

On top is heaven. Your eyes roll back behind your head and soon you
become lighter from all the bad that has left your body. You float
with emotions and feelings. You can feel your heart and mind pound
with dreams and ideas, but your legs don't move. Your legs are numb,
so is the rest of your body. Paralyzed is what you have become. You
are understanding life better, for the first time in a long while you
feel good. You are actually slipping further away from reality. You
are becoming sick, at the same time you feel you are being healed.
You truly feel alive, but you are slowly dying. This is no movie.
This is reality, something that seeing up close can change your
outlook on life forever, in a good way, or bad. I guess it's a matter
of how you take the experience in the end. Blinking is something
that happens in a blue moon, and going to the bathroom is something
that well..... never happens. Itching feels great, until you find out
that you have been itching the same spot all night, and now the blood
from behind your neck has built up under your finger nails. Your
hair has seemed to fall like a dog in the middle of summer. You are
literally dying. All at the same time you feel the most alive.
Four nights later, the story wraps back to the beginning, and you
have lost complete track of the time and day. It's only when you
hit bottom and the smoke no longer swirls inside you that you have
realized that the last four days has been a complete lie.

I sat on the side of the road for hours with my head between my legs,
praying this feeling of being sick would leave me so I could feel

normal again. Sick is the only word I could find for this feeling, even though it has no way of explaining how sick I really felt. A sad story that I had no intention to write. An experience that haunts me to this very day.

Back to school I went on Monday. Walking through the hall reminded me that life has been continuing on without me, even though I could have sworn it stopped. I never did experience this dream world again, I swore to it. The temptation was too high, the drug was too good. I walked away and never looked back, leaving the four day room of smoke forever. Thank God for Weightlifting. Thank God for my Wife. Thank God for you.

Weightlifting 2016

♪ ♪ ♪

A Team

Friday, July 6, 2012

The New Show is up, its out, its alive, and it gets heated. After the show I grabbed my hair and looked at my wife, and simply asked, "what just happened"? Two long smooth curvy beauty body shots of miss brown eyes might have tipped me over the side with rage, rants, and frustrations. Tomorrow is the MDUSA tryouts, maybe that's why my blood is pumping extra fast. This might be the reason why I was standing up the whole show with my shirt off. My feelings and emotions were simply knocking on the door, I had to let them out. I will tell you one thing though, these rookies aren't taking my stipend tomorrow, I will slam the bar on everyone in the gym, get in my car, roll my windows down, and then crank the AC up on high. Salute.

Also here is the latest Team MDUSA video.
I really enjoyed Coach Pendlays voice over,
the big bearded man gave great commentary while
we trained.

A Team 2016

♪ ♪ ♪

Memento

Sunday, July 8, 2012

Cheers, hi, hello, good morning. I wanted to write something on this
beautiful morning that grew goose bumps six feet tall, taller than
a Weightlifters ego. A gut wrenching piece that stands the hair up
on the back of your neck, like the audience giving a weightlifter a
standing ovation from their made lifts. I wanted to write a piece
that helped people train harder. A motivating coffee trip, an amazing
story about weightlifting, sun, and flowers. Smiles, fist pumps,
and three little white lights that brighten up the room with joy,
and a buzz that stings one another with goal reaching achievement. I
could try, I could lie, I could write like a college kid who is brain
washed to write what the teacher wants, or I could write how I really
feel. I should feel really bad this morning from my bomb out at
yesterdays MDUSA tryouts. Yes I am on the A team, Donny and my spot
has been secured from day one, but this did not keep me from competing
and trying. shit....Its fun! Plus I wanted to show the rookies who's
boss, but I forgot my boss hat at home I guess. I know my spot wont
be secured forever, I must step my game up, excpecialy with all these
hungry Weightlifters coming after me. I am feeling the heat, and fast.
Maybe my good mood comes from the journey that lies ahead of myself,
and with everyone on the new Muscle Driver Team. I am seeing gold down
the long road ahead, even though the journey looks rough and pain full.
Gold for my teammates, and the growth of an exciting creation that
is being built all around me. I am really just happy to lift side by
side with so many great lifters, a great coach that always supports me,
and you, a great Weightlifting community backing each other up to the
death. All this will make any man smile and continue the good fight.

Maybe its the song I am listening to that has me in a happy mood, or just simply how this sport makes no sense, so there is really no need of getting down. I shake my head with frustration followed by a smile of "fuck it, whatever". I throw my hands up looking for someone or something to blame, but there is know one but me. I throw my coffee against the wall looking for an answer, but there is non. I am sorry Miss Brown eyes, I will never throw you again. This is sport, this is athletics, this is Weightlifting. This is the Dark Orchestra, a stage that can give you the best day of your life, a place that can give you a single purpose for being on this planet, and at the same time, a place that can put you in depression and tears. A place that can doubt your very existence. Fucken Weightlifting, back stabbing son of a bitch. I love you, but I hate you. Why do you hurt me? See now I am getting mad all over again, a roller coaster of emotions is what I am. All the time I give you, spent with you, and story's and memories we have shared with each other. Why? I guess to know happiness we must experience sadness, and sadness is something that comes with the weightlifting kit you buy at the store. Something we will all experience at some point, something we must put behind us and move on from. But no, today I am actually ok. I love this sport, and I love writing to you. I love my team, my dog Daughter, Wife and my Coach. I love being a weightlifter, what else can I say? This bomb out.... I mean this hasn't happened to me for over two years, so I knew he could be around any corner just waiting for me. He got me.

150 miss, 153 miss, 155 miss. Yes I went up every time, witch might have not been the best decision, but who cares, I went for it. I got so pissed that I walked back on stage and made 155 for my fourth attempt, lol, an attempt that I made my own. 175 make, 180 make, then took a big jump to 190 and missed the jerk. I will say my lower back played a part in that miss, but at the end of the day that's just an excuse. Life goes on, training will continue, and the MDUSA team will grow with new lifters, new dreams, and more upcoming bad asses. This is just a talk with blog, there is know real meaning behind this, just a chat. A chat about the common bomb out, a chat about Weightlifting. What am I suppose to talk about? I have no answers for what happened. The bar just didn't land where it should have. Pull, finish, miss. This equation doesn't work. I have found to win in this sport you must pull, finish, and then catch. This equation is correct. Bad luck? Nerves? stop Jon! stop trying to figure it out, just get back to training, and try again.

No this did not count, but before they could strip the bar I ran back out and made it.

Well my coffee is almost all gone, and this means my fingers are slowing down. I hope my bomb out can motivate you. Maybe I can take one for the team, so you wont have to. A blog full of real life is what this is. No bullshit, no lies. The best thing I can write about is the truth of what this sport has to offer. Up front and honest. Even though I still cant figure out why I am not more down today. Maybe it has to do with the fact that shit could be a lot worse, and there is know time for me to bath in my own self pity. So fucken salute, carry on, slam bars and win meets. talk to you later my good friend.

Three Whites 2016

♪ ♪ ♪

$80

Thursday, July 12, 2012

(Video Below)

I don't always like to post the daily MDUSA videos here in the Dark Orchestra, simply for the fact that you can find the videos other places online. This boarded shut lost abandoned building that has been left for dead which we call home has so much more to express and talk about. Frustrations? Let them out young man! Built up anger towards life in general? Scream young women! Break shit, smash your glass bar down against the stage floor. Play your violin, for this is the place to cry and bath in self pity. Blame, yes go ahead, only for a little while though, training starts soon. Glide that white mask over your face and smile for the camera. Look, my smile is the same as yours. Once you are done with the day, join me for coffee back here. A place where you can hang your coat, show your true skin, and be who you please. This is a place to throw miss brown eyes after a bomb out, or a place to make wall pounding love with her after winning a meet, or achieving a PR. This blog is not a blog, but more of a mental institution full of wounded weight warriors who fight so hard for gold, or simply those who just want it back. Even those who have been on top still find themselves climbing. Look to your side, thousands climbing the same hill you are. There is no such thing as reaching the top, just check-marks for celebration and accomplishments.

The mother f'in pain is driving me up a crack head hotel room wall. I can't even sleep at night because of the leg twitches that sting me like bees all throughout the night. Does anybody know what this is from? Or why this is happening? 5 months out from Americans makes it hard to stay positive and focused at times. I lose track of why I am even training. But then I sit back and reflect for a few minutes on my all white southern style deck after a long day of chalky hands and bloody thumbs. It's not about Americans in 5 months, nor the World team next year. It's all about getting better at Weightlifting, stronger in this sport, and the rest will fall into place. Keeping your mind focused on one thing, and one thing only is very important. I need to get stronger, period. Stronger plus showing up equals USA. Slamming bars and bleeding from the eyes from too much N.O. explode equals Gold. Well..... or silver or even bronze if shit just doesn't go your way, in many cases this will happen. She will stick a steak knife through your heart and turn it. Just like my dad did, just like the drugs and "cool" friends do, just like life. This is why I drive a fast car, to stay away from the sheep.

My mind drifts off into the oddest of imaginations. Where do they come from, and why the flying fuck am I writing them down? I read other blogs and they are so..... I don't know... right on? They have so much direction and meaning. You can learn so much from them. They all seem to be so smart, college educated smart. I was literally just going to put the $80 dollar victory bet I had with coach from the latest MDUSA video, and that's it, but here I am typing away about God knows what. Salute, slam bars, and see you soon where hell and home sleep side by side.

$80 training day. Very hard training week. The high hangs are beyond hard, they are punsihment! Coach should be put in jail for athlete abuse!

Champ vs Champ 2016

♪ ♪ ♪

376

The Spell of PR

You know when the Violin enters the song its time to write, no matter
if you have something to write about or not. What to write is not
important, writing something is all you need. Just like you know right
away when you wake in the morning you have training to complete.
Fuck, this song is beautiful, and fuck, training makes you feel great,
yes beat down and tired, but great. You combine the piano with the
violin and its game over. Miss Brown eyes enters the room with her
silky black dress and her hair down around her face; stunning. You
get excited, just like staying up tell 2 AM waiting for the the day
to arrive so you can slam bars with your friends, while your favorite
songs blast in the gym, only helping you get that much closer to your
PR. You should be in bed.

2 AM and the movie credits are basically saying "go to bed", but you
don't, you cant sleep. How can you though? You have your whole life
ahead of you, just waiting for you like one pig waits for another.
For a weightlifter, every morning is Christmas morning, you have no
idea what you are going to get, or what awaits you in the upcoming
day. 2 AM and the whole world is asleep; but you. The smoke from your
cigarette hovers around you completely stagnant from the lack of wind.
The white smoke looks beautiful in the blue night sky, as it turns from
its original form of smoke into elephants and a herd of birds that
soon disappear.... again, telling you to go to bed. A weightlifter
has no middle ground. Its either hot or cold, max or sleep, fast or
slow, lots of coffee or just water for today's training. Its a spell
that helps us and hurts us at the same time. A spell that gives us
unbelievable energy and drive to attack the day. A PR spell that gives
us the power to fight through the hell of training to achieve what we
want in life, but then again turning this spell off at the end of the
day is at times impossible. Stay up much longer and you will enter a
dream world of orange. A blog that I wrote a while ago that I still
consider one of my favorites. (The orange room)

Now 3 AM and YouTube has replaced your bed. Dimas helps you feel not so
homesick from staying up so late. Klokov makes you laugh followed by a
smile like you and him are best friends. Which are, you have seen
so many of his competitions and training videos that you feel close to
him. Steiners 2008 performance draws a tear to your eye, as the clock
pats you on the back, trying to lead you to bed like the smoke and movie

377

credits failed to do. But no, because now Ilya has busted through your
computer screen and you have found yourself brewing up a pot of coffee
while asking yourself why he spikes his hair so weirdly. But then again
he is an Olympic Gold Medalist, so who cares! You didn't just think
that, but you said it out loud to yourself, witch gave you a creepy
feeling considering the fact you haven't heard your voice for hours now
in your ever so quiet as a mouse house. Shankle enters your small lit
up world around the computer screen, while the dark gangs up all around
you. Goose bumps crawl up your arm from Shankles presents and all
around bad assnes, if that's even a word, fuck it, in the Dark Orchestra
anything is a word. There are no more teachers telling me whats wrong
and write anymore, just me and my YouTube at 3 AM. For all the teachers
who stamped an F on my forehead, guess what, Andrei Aramnau thinks I
have great technique from the letter his coach wrote me that hangs above
my desk. Andrei Aramnau, a baby faced killer, aka the best all around
athlete in my opinion. He moves like leaves dancing over the grass. He
moves like a ballerina on stage, or like Ali taunting his fly in a web
competitor. He moves like Miss Brown Eyes crawling all over your body
as you don't just drink her down, but chug her strength and eye popping
motivation deep down in your weightlifting belly, what I call the "power
belly". Pocket Hercules makes you scratch your side ways head with
amazement, as your hands move from your hair to your droopy eyes. Yes,
your second family of weightlifters are basically tucking you into bed.
You share a bond with every Weightlifter, strong or not strong, Olympian
or no Olympian. We are the same species, the same blood type. We are
all addicted to PR's and strength. We are a family of many stray dogs
that rome the night, for we are lost when training is over, and we look
at "others" with confusion and wonder.

Dimas pulls the covers up to your chin, then famously looks to the side
seeing Steiner shut down your computer still holding his wife's picture
with a strong tight hook grip in his hand. Ilya walks into the kitchen
like he is getting ready to lift, and shuts off your coffee pot with his
still ever so spiked up hair. Aramnau slides across the living room like
a fucken cheetah, and smoothly turns off the TV and PlayStation. Pocket
looks up at the door handle, getting himself up onto his toes and then
shutting the door that leads out to your smoking deck of elephants and
flying birds. Goodnight, sleep tight, and don't let the bed bugs bite.

                    Dimas, Steiner, Klokov, Aramnau, Pocket 2016

                              ♪ ♪ ♪

Ritalin

Monday, July 23, 2012

I should have ripped the test up right there and then. Ha! You son of
a bitch you can't catch me! I should have threw all the tiny pieces
of medal shackles in the air like chalk before lifting. I should
have rubbed the black coal from my face and painted him a picture of
reality with my shaky bare fucken hands. They would have probably
done me a favor and put me on even more Ritalin than I was already
on. That would have been great, considering the fact I would have
just kept selling those little pink pills of joy all over the black
market for more party money. Thanks Doc for supporting the whole
football team with kegs, pizza and gas money. Yea, I am crazy buddy,
but then again you are the one telling me "what I am going to be when
I grow up" from this A B C D or E test. I didn't see BAMF Athlete on
any of the test results, why not Mr? He then laughs with his brown
elbow patch coat and probably a Subaru outside in the parking lot
with his name on the curb. He thinks he is original and self made,
but in my eyes, by him telling me what I will be when I grow up, and
his best answer for me is more drugs, just means he himself has been
told what to do his whole life, and he is 100 percent unoriginal and
full of bullshit. His coat is not brown but white, white a fluffy.
Bad ass mother fucken Athlete is what that means Doc. Can I be that
when I grow up? Or do I have to pick from these 20 options, because
honestly Doc, I really don't want to be a post office worker like you
are telling me to be, with your eyes still gazed upon your notebook.
I don't think he has even looked at me once. He then responded by
telling me that sometimes in life we don't always have control, and
we are what we are son. Followed by upping my dosage of Ritalin and
extending my stay in the resource rooms, (aka) Room 2. I then took
his clip board and shoved it in his mouth followed by wrapping duck
tape all over his body, so he could never bring down another kid
again. A kick to his chest rolled him and his rolly chair into a
closet that I bolted shut, then proceeded to screamed "Shankle" at the
top of my lungs! Odd moment for I didn't even know this man named
Shankle back then in high school, also known as the lion Killer.

The Attitude Nation was pumping through my blood before I even knew
what it was. You knew when this happened, even if you didn't, you
felt a shift in the air this long while ago. The shift was a giant
boat called the Titanic that I drove around the world visiting every
room 2 class there was, rescuing kids from their low ceilings and

no window rooms, full of Safeway applications and community college
forms. I burned those jail cells down with my ship. I watched the
room 2 burn to the ground as the kids broke free from their enclosed
life, and set foot on a boat of freedom and opportunity. Now their
anger can be controlled in the right way, meaning their way. A
wanderlust boat that could end up anywhere. I was captain freedom,
captain hook a kid in the back and bring 'em a board. I was robin
hood that told the kids they could be anything they want, not just
a Pro Football player. And even if you fall short of becoming the
football player they always wanted to become, it doesn't mean you
have to give up on athletics! GET INTO ANOTHER SPORT! Don't surrender
to football. Football and the other big sports kill more dreams
than they give out, understand this and move on. You can be a Pro
Weightlifter, why not? You can invent the next Facebook, or open your
own gym! You can be a coach, personal trainer, or yes, you can be a
postal worker if you want! It's a great job!

We are different, we are unique, self Made, self achievers. Some self
taught, and some taught by others of the same unique flavor. Black fur
that is constantly attacked by white paint thrown from others. Freedom
is always envied by others, sometimes even our closest friends. Go
getters we are, go getters who attack our goals while helping others
in the mean time. We are no captain, we are no champagne toasters.
We don't have cigar time after dinner with the gentlemen while talking
politics. We are the coal shoveling, fire burning, bottom of the boat
black faced working, sweat dripping, strong armed, banned from society,
out casted sheep who didn't listen to our fucken guidance councelors.
Rebels of some sort, who wash their hands with blood, not soap. Eat
with their hands not forks. Who get a high off strength in the gym and
even more importantly... out.

This never happened though. My face was not black from the coal I
shoveled into the Titanic with my fellow weightlifters. I did not
save my fellow room 2ians. I did not cast a ship of freedom and duck
tape my counselor's mouth shut. All these things I wanted to do, and
thought about while my therapists were showing me black shadows on
card stalk paper, while being asked what came to mind. I listened
to all my counselors, therapists, tutors, and teachers. I took the
Pills that gave me little emotion, and seemed to numb my feelings so
I could read at a faster rate. Even though my senior year I was only
reading at a 7th grade level, and I still couldn't pass pre-algebra.
This came with tears and embarrassment. That's why seeing my blog
near 200,000 hits makes me check my alarm clock to see when it will

go off. All my subjects were in one classroom, one teacher, and only a few classmates. My odds of becoming who I am today were against me big time. I said red and people laughed while black always hit. Black, black, black, black. Pills, pills, pills, pills. Talk, talk, talk, talk.

It was the day some of my teachers laughed when I said I wanted to play ball at a four year out of state, when I threw my desk and walked out of the classroom in tears and frustration. Fuck you Football, you left me all alone, but guess what you son of a bitch, a family called Weightlifting picked me up on the side of the road, and took me in as one of their own. Fuck you Room 2, I rose high above your low bar, and never surrendered to your 20 options and your "poor me I need help" pink little liberal pills. Fuck you weird looking black shadows on card stalk, that only mean one thing, and thats a waste of tax payer money. Fuck you math, for we have never got along, even though I still admire your genius. Fuck you reading, I am in love with your brother writing, not you. Fuck you Oregon, you can keep the suckers who stayed in your trap, I escaped and have never looked back. Fuck you Ritalin, I will no longer be your zombie. And Fuck you councilor, for we are two different species, and you are NOT apart of the Nation we call Attitude. Now I really do have a ship called the Titanic and it's this blog. A place I can reach out to people and tell my story. I have thought and talked this new idea over for the last few months, and I have come to the conclusion that I am going to go around and speak words of motivation to the kids of room 2 at middle schools and high schools all over. Don't worry, it will be a little more PG than this blog post. I am not necessarily knocking the public school system, I am more reaching out to kids like me who I have seen surrender to the tests, pills, and hometown life after school. The kids who need a little wanderlust in their life, a boat of freedom. Kids in my opinion who sometimes need to buy a bus ticket and get the hell out of dodge, and find themselves, and what they want to do on their own. Have the kids scrape their knee, get burned by life and even hit rock bottom, stop catching their every fall!!!

I stopped taking Ritalin after high school, and it's the best thing I ever did.

Boat of Freedom 2016

♪♪♪

381

Milk

Thursday, July 26, 2012

Take a bath in milk while you soak in your own recovery, while brain
storming over your next blog topic. Watch a home video of your self
as a kid 'til your heart hurts. Drink so much coffee in one sitting
that you start throwing up outside the green jungle for all to see.
Don't forget to stay on your heels while driving the bar high into
the sky so the white clouds can take your bar and spit it back at
you, leaving you with three red bruises on your back, and your face
black and blue in the lobby of building platform. White hands say
good bye to your old friends, leaving you with colorful new friends
with strong hopes of becoming locked at the hip. A dog named Sparky
puts on the Russian Techno music as you both lift in a town that has
been evacuated from the virus called Weightlifting. An infected
soccer mom who put the town in panic and fear as everyone ran for
the hills, seeking and holding onto normal and well excepted dreams
and achievements. Flowers turn to black, and your knees turn to
acorns. Weightlifting has dried your skin to desert, and has made
your everyday walk odd and crippled for so long, that now it's normal
and straight. A milk bath can only mean one thing, viewing life in a
different light, seeing people as different than you, and making sure
they are crazy.... not you. But then again, you are the one laying
naked in a tub of milk after lifting weights for six hours straight
in a warehouse, while the rest of the normal world was racing by
you outside those double doors. A chalk bucket full of blood and an
attitude full of hate and rage. Rage against the bar, rage against
your father, rage against nothing. Rage is the best coach; rage alone
will help you succeed. Hate will guide you to happiness. A crash
from the bar against your body is the best type of feedback, a don't
fuck up feedback that never lies.

Drink your milk, chocolate or white, it really doesn't matter. If
you choose white over chocolate then it must be red cap, also known
as whole milk. The extra fat is good for you, so drink up! Recovery
liquid will make you strong for the next day. As I sleep, I can feel
my bones swimming in a lake full of milk. I dream that there are
little fish who live in the milk that work construction on my broken
body. The fish swim inside the muscles singing bed time stories while
covering them up with blankets. Milk provides strength and recovery
fish. The fish provide construction on your body while sleeping.
Construction on your body while sleeping leads to PR's and hard

training. This is why milk is so important, much more important than
air or water. Not coffee of course, just want to make that clear.
This has been my milk speech, a subject that should be taught at
school. A subject I really don't know how I got on. I drink a half
gallon of red milk a day. But then again, Attitude Nation, do what
works for you!

And one more thing! Can I ask why everyone is saying that fat is so
bad for you? Fat is good for you! Calories are even better! This is
why I eat Italian almost every night. Lots of bread and pasta, with
milk.... of course. Every Sunday is pizza night. I eat a slice of
cheesecake every night before bed, a secret that I haven't let out of
the bag 'til now. I truly believe that these foods, if training on a
daily basis, are good for not only recovery, but your body as a whole.
I always feel much better the next day after eating meals like these.
If you are not training hard everyday than you should eat these foods
only in moderation. My view on food and diet is not normal, and 100
percent of people disagree with me. So please take my advice with
caution. But even with all the facts and attacks that people throw
at me, I still stand strong with my opinions. I refuse to back down,
Cheesecake and I will fight to the death! I don't really know how I
got onto the food topic, but this just might be my next blog. I have
a lot to say about this, and many thoughts and beliefs on food I would
like to share with you. Salute, and keep training hard.

Italian Food! 2016

♪ ♪ ♪

Gym York

Wednesday, August 1, 2012

Gym York.
A coffee grave yard that lays rest on
the outskirts of this dream town of dirt.
A city full of lifters and teachers. Athletes called life drifters.
Addicted green monsters and restless sleepers run the streets full of
gifted and motivated believers.
Poisoned by the bar of hopeless thinkers, and bloody hand wishers.
Day dreamers run the town like fucken gangsters who take pray on
anyone who stands in their way.

Business meetings settled over who can lift the most weight,
move the most weight, and who can handle the most weight.
Board meetings discussed in chalky rooms while three white stripes run
down only the people who wear the nicest of suits.
Street lights that always change to white lights, never red.
PR's have replaced money,
and bar slamming has replaced anger management classes.
Women aren't the only ones who wear heels. Now the sound of tapping
throughout the hallways has doubled.
Shots of coffee have made driving much safer,
while miss brown eyes smiles from all the lives she has saved.
Meth addicts have turned to a new drug called N.O. Explode,
that now runs through the black market like a virus,
giving the bums and tweekers much more energy to get a fucken job.
All stairs have been replaced by elevators. Why? Well like my first
coach Jackie Mah always said, "Weightlifters always take the elevator".
Yes coach!
Dimas now rides high on the Charging Wall Street Bull, as he ever so
confidently waves one finger high in the air,
while looking off to the side with an ever so bad ass smile.
Everyday is a beautiful day in Gym York.
A great place to live and to grow a family.
A prospering city full of big PR's and lots of opportunity.
A city full of milk parks, protein pools, and coffee lakes.
Techno music plays under the streets,
pounding the city with energy and rhythm.
Klokov has eaten the morning rooster then lets out a giant Klokov roar
during the morning sunrise; always giving the town's people a boost of
morning energy before the techno music starts to pump through their blood.
Rain has been replaced by ash, ash from the many weightlifters who
have been burnt alive from this, at times, unforgiving lifestyle.
It is always a sad day when their ashes fall from the sky,
landing on our platforms.
A reminder that those ashes could be ours, and the hot flames from
this sport could burn us out with no warning at all.
Always a sad day, but always a move forward day; an on to the next day day.
A weightlifter's day is always filled with a next rep day, a let's
fucken do it day, an attack day,
a fuck the weak day and let's get strong day.
A gym zoo full of hungry vampires who don't eat food,
but drink the blood from the red kilo plates.
We are monsters.
We have been abandoned for too long.

This is why my blog must come true, and we must start our own world.
A weightlifters world.
A city called Gym York world.

Kendrick Farris 2012
Sarah Robles 2012
Holly Mangold 2012

♪ ♪ ♪

Nothing

Monday, August 6, 2012

I am on empty. I am tired and half confused. I am beat up and half
asleep. I have buried my head in the sand to see nothing but dark,
here nothing but the soulful music of Clint Mansell, and mostly to
hide away from the man who makes my body hurt from his name alone,
Coach. Hopefully he wont find me, because if I have to lift another
weight I think my body will vanish into a cloud of chalk, never being
able to yell Shankle again, or slam a bar down with built up rage and
anger. I am slowly and gently pressing these little black keys while
listening to this beautiful song that has my body swaying back and
forth like I was playing the piano. Today was an average Joe day, a
put your head down and get through the workout day. Glory fell short
from today's painful escape from reality, as we all took turns lifting
like hamsters in a cage fighting over the wheel. The wheel that never
damn ends.

Its raining outside now, which makes the Dark Orchestra that much
more peaceful and relaxing. I needed this, this time with you, this
time with miss brown eyes. So thank you for joining me on such short
notice. Here, I bought you a coffee, drink her down and feel all your
stresses and frustrations seep out of your body. Let her take complete
control over you, let her wipe away your sadness and anger. Lean
on her when times get hard, drink her when you feel like waving that
white flag. Something the white flag crosses my mind from time to
time. I am not going to lie. This is a hard sport, a hard lifestyle,
a strict and never forgiving world we live in. Live like others and
then some world. Raise your kids like a pro, make money for your
family, and then go above and beyond by beating yourself up on your
own free will in a cold gym everyday damn night after dinner. While

385

others sit back and work on their model ships, watch the night time news, we throw ourselves down a flight of fucken stairs. Every damn day we punch ourselves in the head, while others say "ouch" we smile with pride. While others say "stop" we keep going under that bar that knock us back over and over again. Under, under, under, under, fucken under and then under some more. It never ends, the pain never leaves, the heartache of wanting something so bad never seems to lighten up. The alien looks at your local grocery store that try so hard to figure out why you have white dust all over your body gets old and fast. Somedays I feel like pulling the Al Pacino bad guy speech on em. Freaks I tell yea, a group of odd ducks that swim up river not down. An Orchestra of emotions that beats to our own drumb.

Its so beautiful outside this green jungle window. You should see my view right now. Its one of these nights where the rain has stopped, but the streets are still coverd in water. Its just dark enough where all the parking lot lights and street lights are reflecting off the wet road, giving the night a blury mix of colors and reflections. Its a very Christmas December feeling that has come over me. Fuck I am glad to be alive. The white flag will never be waved, we are born fighters, period. Even though I sometimes imagine how life would be if I waved that weak liberal flag. What would we become if we just quit lifting? I wonder what life would be like, and how our world would change. What if we stopped beating ourselves up? Would life then take the bars place and beat us up? I would much rather be beaten by the always strong bar, than fall pray to this game of life. would you? I feel that sometimes doing nothing is something. I feel that laying around after training tomorrow and watching 10 movies while drooling at the TV screen in my sleeping shorts, eating cheesey puffs, is something this old race horse needs. I need a nothing day, maybe you do to. A call in sick day...well after training of course, we don't want to fall victim to the devil in the red dress. But after training we need to stop, stop for a day and shut the mind and body off. No emotions, no energy, don't make your bed, don't take the trash out, don't wash your car, just do nothing. Yes, this is what we need. This should be a monthly holiday for us warriors, for us old race horses. Let me know how your day of nothing goes, I would love to know. I know this is short notice, so if you cant tomorrow than do it soon. But then again Attitude Nation....do what you want. AC up! windows down!..... That would have been a great line to end this blog on, but nope, I guess miss brown eyes has more to say.

How do I go from a 160 190 day on Friday, and today a everything past 70 damn kilos feels like a semi truck day? It's like my bar had too much pasta last night and she gained 100 pounds. I swear this sport makes no sense. The day you try to figure out this sport is the day you will lose your mind. Take my word for it. I have tried, and the next thing I knew I was sleeping in my car talking to myself while popping vicodin pills left and right. I am so tired. My wife asked me before I left to come chat with you in the green jungle, "why don't you just relax here and rest your tired body"? I responded with drowsy eyes and rolled over shoulders, while grabbing my right elbow from the massive tendinitis it has. I said "sweetie, I must write, I must play my violin in the dark hidden from reality world with people who get me, the people who understand what it means to bang your head against a wall all day and then cry while at the same time smiling. I love you, be back soon." I love my wife so much I want to cut her head off and carry it around with me everywhere I go.

Well I should probably get back home and enter a dream world full of non weightlifting, full of non existing coaches yelling at me, know body pain, and know white flag thoughts. Dreams of my mom smiling and laughing. My mother happy is heaven. Love you mom, goodnight.

Mom 2016

♪ ♪ ♪

Everything

Wednesday, August 8, 2012

Let's see where it takes me. Fuck......here we go. Fuck....buckle your seat belts and lock your doors. Hold your favorite stuffed animals tight, because the song Shankle gave me today is too much. Too much to hold back. Once I flood my body with life juice, fists can fly and emotions can run even higher. Alice in Wonderland thoughts and Johnny Cash feeling's can get me in trouble. Stop reading this blog if you don't like to grab life by the throat and hold him high for every one to see! Stop reading this fucken blog if you don't like ripping the heads off lions! Raise your glasses and make love to your dreams. We shall slam our bars all together at the same damn time, creating a more massive shake than the protein in your shaker cup! SLAM YOUR BARS so the normal folks above us can be reminded that our power bellies still move up and down at a fast pace.... .breath, breath, breath....we still live.

Miss brown eyes just grew Batman wings, and the little green monsters are flowing onto my key board like the opening scene in The Lion King. Wave after wave of sugar sweat people fall from the sky into my mouth. The taste is electrifying, the rush is heart pumping and cocaine feeling. I am jacked. I am gone. I am no longer tired. I am wide awake and ready to kill. I cut the slow people in line to get to the front. Move, you're in my way. More sugar! More caffeine! More life! More training! More Shankle!!! More you and more medals. More bloody hands as we wave to all the people who hate us. Hello to you all! I wave with a smile as they all throw garbage and rocks through my computer screen, only to be blocked by the bat wing of coffee. The happier we are, the more angry they become. Who are they? I'll tell you. They are the ones who missed training yesterday. They are the ones who transform their smooth shiny hands into a cup shaped bowl. Prisoners of the world! Move out of our way! I buy milk like it's a sport. I push the cart to by milk like it's a race. I park my car, to push my cart, to buy milk like a damn pro. I get ready at home to park my car, to push my cart, to buy my milk like I am getting ready for a Weightlifting meet.

We slowly wake. We wake from the once cold, now warm floor of the Dark stage, while the Orchestra of skeletons stand and play songs that lift us from our puddles of tears and depression. A happy day in the Dark Orchestra, a day of dancing and singing. A day of heaven, before training casts its hell over us once again. Before the fog sets in, let's climb the green grassy hill and draw pictures for our mothers. Pictures of family members holding hands. Pictures of past dogs and memories that boost our motivation to keep the right stepping and the left following. Let's fight! Let's have a good day! No, no, let's have a great fucking day! It's a great day to be alive. Enjoy the happy while it still lasts, before the lights dim, and the trees lose their leaves. Before the ash will fall, and the music changes from grassy fields to bloody hands and barbells of doom. Enjoy this moment, because training starts soon.

Batman 2016

♪ ♪ ♪

388

Sweet, Sweet Love

I am writing to you from the airport in Phoenix, while on lay over
to San Jose where the 10th Attitude Nation Certification is taking
place tomorrow! I have been waiting for this video to get uploaded
so I could share this over whelming training day with you, my best
of friend, here in the Dark Orchestra. (video below) This Friday,
the fire was hot, so I had no choice but to roast marshmallows! Miss
Brown Eyes wanted to make love, and the bar wanted to dance! Coach
was looking extra dapper with his hair styled back and beard so
black and promising. As I started to oil up my tin man body before
training, my favorite techno song came skipping along right into my
ears down deep into my Weightlifting Soul. I knew it was going to be
a good day, a great day, a day that makes this hell hole of a sport
all worth it. A day of "mom I don't want to leave summer camp, I
want to stay longer and play with all the other kids" day. A day that
screams WHEN IS AMERICANS!! I CAN'T WAIT TO WIN GOLD, MAKE WORLDS,
AND BREAK THE AMERICAN RECORDS!! I feel like a little kid in a candy
shop stomping my Ali feet pulling on coaches shirt while whining about
how 4 months is too far away. Screw it, F it, the more I think about
it the more I welcome the weight. It just gives the Attitude Nation
more time "PAY OUR TAXES, LOVE OUR WOMEN, AND
CRUSH CLEAN AND JERKS"! - Donny Shankle.

All time PR total! 163kg snatch / 190kg c&j /
353kg total. Missed 167kg snatch behind me,
which is 2 kilos over the American record. The
video doesn't show the second one, but I went
after that son of a gun. Travis Cooper is now
officially part of the MDUSA team! And many more
athletes have already signed and are moving out
as we speak. It's going to get crazy! Salute!

Miss Brown Eyes 2016

♪ ♪ ♪

389

Wolf

Wednesday, August 22, 2012

I lift weights to blanket the pain. Every weight I lift lifts my
middle finger higher and higher for all to see. See this Oregon, see
this finger middle school bully, see this teacher, see this hater,
do you see this weight above my head counselor? See how much it is?
Look... no Ritalin. You can't drug me up now. What do you know about
my parents and their divorce? Nothing. See how I have the world
over my fucken head, and how I'm about to slam it? Well, this is what
I think about their divorce. This is how I feel. I slam it while
blood drains from my veins and I scream at the dark trees that look
like monsters at night. You know when you were a kid, they were damn
scary. Monsters that I would gladly take over the ones I met later
on in life. Slam it down while I cry an ocean, downing all. See
who I am now, and what I have done? No sir, no ma'am, no more room
2 for me. No more special classes and pats on the back for me. This
outcast now slams bars for a living. All day, all damn day long. I
don't want to attend your party. I should have never attended your
party in the first place, it's the worst memory I have, and it haunts
me to this day. I have my own party now, a big fucken party with lots
of people, people who slam bars with me, throw chalk in their eyes
and bleed all over the bar with me. My new home away from home. A
camp ground of emotional basket cases who hold on tight while our bar
takes us through a land called candy. A hold my hand land, and enter
hell with me land. Fuck who you were in the past land, and let's lift
this weight land, making us better people land. A Johnny Cash land of
AC UP WINDOWS DOWN LAND! No more backing down to the bully. No more
backing down to society. No more walking their line, talking their
talk, and listening to their bar low expectations. See me now, for I
am a wolf. A giant hungry wolf who strays the land with other giant
hungry wolfs. Wolfs who eat sheep, sheep like you home town.

I mix my coffee in this room where I write to you while my legs shake
from today's training. As the bar keeps rising and Americans get
closer, I find myself drinking more and more coffee. More and more
smokes as I pace my deck outside. My body has these random twitches
that I can't seem to control, and have no real understanding of
what they are. I find myself going to bed later and later for no
real apparent reason. The negativity that leaks off the websites and
forums keeps me from getting online. There is always hype coming from
a new lifter. I don't care, and I don't want to know. They come and

go. I will be at Americans and I will lift what coach tells me to lift. I wake up earlier and earlier sitting outside on my deck. My deck has become my new hang out spot, and again.... I have no idea why. Maybe I feel hidden out there, away from it all. Or maybe it's to attempt to collect my thoughts of what the hell has happened to me the last few years. Getting to know and understand this new man can be very hard and taunting. I like me now. I like the man I see now, and getting to know him has been a pleasure.

I squat low to stay hidden from my past demons. I move fast to stay 10 steps away from the smoke filled motel rooms. My up all night eyes are now wide open from up all day training. Crushed Vicodin has been replaced by chalk, and rooms full of skeletons have been replaced by friends and family aka weight room warriors. Strong s.o.b's and even stronger minded. Hot or cold, this is how I have lived my whole life. I have never been in the middle. Now I am all in and all out crazy with the weights. I guess this dreadful problem I have had my whole life paid off, funny how that works. Funny how one minute all you want is a drink, and the next is a bar. One day you want a hit, and the next you want a win. It's interesting to me how you can change so fast that it takes time for you to get to know you. Salute.

My Deck 2016

♪♪♪

Confidence?

Wednesday, August 29, 2012

Wake and train, train and sleep. Repeat. Slam your bar, breaking the necks of all your inner demons. Rewind, and then repeat. When you feel the pain from training, drink more coffee, throw it up, rewind, then repeat. Drink coffee when sad thoughts pass through your mind while you wait for the bar to wheel you around the gym while drool drips from your fucken mouth. Ask the bar for a straw, drink and repeat. Drink more coffee when you miss your dad, drink more coffee when you wish you could go back in time and treat your step dad better. Drink, throw up, slam bars, rewind and repeat.

The towel that drapes over my head in training means leave me alone, or better yet, leave me the fuck alone. Stay away while I focus on the task at hand. Others go to school; I sit in a chair while an occasional tear drips down my masked face of "crazy energetic Jon North". I lift a bar while coach leashes me with his eyes, and keeps the world of training just dark enough from his beard keeping the outside light out. Get close while the camera tilts to the side trying to peak at what lies under that shaded cave I stay resting under. Bad idea, the lion's nest is always a bad idea. My white eyes turn to the lens, and my long fanged teeth bite the neck of the wanderlust filmer, drawing blood instantly, and then letting the rest drain into my coffee cup.

Animals is what we are, freaks with athletic abilities that give us a pass. Outcasts that have found a place to fit in. A certain shade casts down your face from the towel hiding you away from the mother fuckers in this world. A shadow that really speaks to you, blankets you with comfort, all while keeping you tucked away deep in your childhood memory of the light blue house with the long swordfish attached to the wall. That one side eye winks at you when standing up from a successful lift. The fish keeps you calm, the fish is always there with you no matter how old you become. I sometimes think of that cold Easter weekend, wondering about the big house with so much..... well, wanderlust. Maybe my obsession with wanderlust started in this ever so off setting house. All the sounds turn into echoes, and all the others training look as if I'm watching an old movie. My eyes move back and forth while I stay hidden under the towel. My sweat doesn't seem to bother me, in fact, I like the cool drips of half coffee half blood water skiing down my emotionless face. The face that if you look closely screams help, get me out of this summer camp of weird creepy camp leaders and odd activities. Fucken save me from the carousel that has my vision blurry from life passing me by. A weightlifter's face screams run, but never moves.

Eat, coffee, train, eat, coffee, train, nap, coffee, squat, eat, call your mom, try to go out and do something which is always pointless considering the fact that about 20 minutes into your freedom adventure your tired mind starts pulling on your shirt while pointing back at your recovery tank, aka bed. Repeat.

A small state of depression has now been broken from my lips separating, sending out a bright light of seething teeth ready to bite into a fucken bar. Now I am jacked up. Now I am ready to kill anyone or any weight in my way. Now I will show the world how to slam a bar, yell, scream, Shankle fist pump, smoke a lift, win a meet, represent my country, bang my chest and jump up and down. Now the shirt is off and the crackin' has been released. The champ is coming! The champ is here! I have been filled up with hate and sadness from my black cave, and now it's time to light this gym on fire. I pour my coffee over my head letting the long drips fall into my mouth only to spit them back out in my competitor's face. If you are looking for good sportsmanship, this is not the blog for you. I want my snickers bar. I want my dad to pat me on the back again saying, "Good job son, way to push him back". I'll take my demons and use them for strength. I have a whole deck of magic cards, and they are all bad, but isn't bad good? I play all of them all the time. I walk to the chalk bucket like John Travolta in Saturday Night Fever. Get off me bro. I'm going ham on this shit. Sometimes an overwhelming confidence takes over me, giving me the power to trick my mind into becoming someone or something else. This pisses some people off, and others like it. I don't really have an opinion, that guy seems cool to me. That monster seems fucken crazy at times, but hey, this sport is fucken crazy, we are all a little crazy. Look at Ilya, he is the best, he is the craziest. There is a monster living in that man, just like in me, just like in you. The same monster that lives in the Dark Orchestra.

Funny how confident I can become, while being the most insecure person on the face of the earth. This sport will never make sense. Its powers are amazing. Salute.

Snicker Bar 2016

♪ ♪ ♪

The Weekend

Saturday, September 1, 2012

Brand new episode of "Weightlifting Talk". We had fun on this one. Plus, Wednesdays training below of a very tired and beat down team, but still pushing through to grab a few PR's.

This is the first week in a while where the Attitude Nation is not conducting a Cert. Even though I am sad not being able to slam bars with my fellow Attitude Soldiers, I am excited to take this weekend to do absolutely nothing.......nothing at all.....just typing the word nothing puts a smile on my face. Salute, and have a great weekend.

Last but not least, My beautiful and always strong Wife Jessica gets a 91kg C&J PR!

Have a good weekend 2016

♪ ♪ ♪

Get Off Me Bro

Sunday, September 2, 2012

Writer's block. Wait....... hold on now...... yes, this song is the
one. Let the goose bumps rise! Let me turn up the volume, good......
prefect. Now if you could give me just a second to finalize the mood
while I take my first sip from miss brown eyes' lips so that the Dark
Orchestra style of writing can activate in full effect. Here we go..
.... ah, thank you.
Now let me smash my fucken head though this computer screen. I will
pop my head through to say hello, hello. Good moving on. Now I will
drink 5 pounds of N.O. Explode while training at my old bodybuilding
gym back in college. All by myself, with so much built up thoughts,
drive, ideas and emotions that I could only show through the mirror in
front of me. Curl, curl, curl, ha, ha, ha, ha!!!!!!!!!!!!!!!!!! So mad
I was, but why? The weights make a thud as they hit the rubber floor
below me. Get the fuck off me bro. Mean I tell you, mean is what I
was and still am. I had no idea what I wanted to be, no idea at all.
Get off me bro. A lost kid with the world in his chest. They didn't
like me, fuck it, I didn't like them. I'll tell you what though, the
weight room likes me. The weight room is my dad, coach, role model,
classroom, bedroom, cry room, a fuck you world room, a get off me bro
room. Always on my last and toughest rep I would think to myself,
just one day I am going to get you life, grab you by the fucken neck
and kill you. One day this angry kid will rise, and when I do, I am
taking everyone down, and the ones who cared for me, with me. Every

394

tear that fell down my face, a mirror broke from my hand, and every hand I broke, I had to pay the gym owner back. But I always came back. Hello you sons of bitches, the freak is back, the daddy issues kid has arrived, and I am ready to punch the bag in the corner, jump rope 'til my nose bleeds, and get MY FUCKEN BRO DAY ON BABY! HA! Back and bi day, chest and shoulders, more N.O. EXPLODE, more Cutler videos, more pumps, more food and more mirror smashing. More fights I got into, more protein powder that I swallowed down by using the water fountain. Disgusting, but who cares. The taste never bothered me, because the nasty taste in my mouth throughout the day was 10 times worse. A big F on my forehead is what I was reminded of everyday. A failure in school, a failure in football, and a failure with my father. Tah, Protein...... get off me bro, are you serious with this shit? I worked at a supplement store once, and I thought I was going to jump on the back of the next "tough guy" that asked if I had grape in stock yet. Get off me bro. Are you serious?

Treadmill walking while the local news played behind me. 1AM and for some reason there is always you and that one last guy in the very back of the gym, still training, still crying, why are we crying you ask? Well I'll tell yea, because me and this other sad guy are in the gym at 1AM on a Friday while the rest of the world is cheering at the bar or watching a movie with their family. Isn't it funny that the last guy in the whole gym never speaks to you, never says a word the whole time working out and while leaving? When the place is busy during prime time, everyone says "hey". This has always intrigued me. Why don't the lost and sad individuals like myself ever speak to me........ shit..... but then again, I never spoke to them. I am them and they are me. Holy shit this is fucken crazy. I wonder what the "last guy" thought about me? I wonder if he is at home writing a blog about me........o shit...... wait........... or better yet, reading this blog! Hello are you out there! If you are reading this, if it's really you out there, let me say just one thing to you Mr. Last Guy in the gym with me who never spoke to me and always seemed to walk past my treadmill about 5 minutes before I left making the gym creepy and even more depressing, I am here for you if you ever need me. I hope you feel the same towards me. We must stick together, even though we don't know each other, because the world doesn't understand us. We understand each other, better than we both might ever imagine. Our goals might be different, or paths of life might lead in different ways, our movie taste might not be the same, but we are always the last two guys in the gym for a reason, and that reason is...... I don't know. I can't answer such a huge question like that, it's beyond the human mind. Or maybe just beyond this F stamped mind school has labeled me as. All I know is that we have an understanding that no one can take away, or understand. I will never get a chance to talk to you, why? Because if we talk to each other we are breaking the gym rule, and the gym rules are everything. Break them, and you have no home. I will see you again as you walk past me, and a small smile will come over my face as I confidently drink more coffee.

The Dark Orchestra lives in the late night gym. We train better when the "social butterflies" leave to go grab their fucken grape protein shakes. Turn up the local news that has played over and over again. Let the vacuum from the janitor bring you peace while you curl your pain to your chest while you sway back and forth with that look of "get off me bro" on your face. This is BRO NATION, this is ATTITUDE NATION, this is when bodybuilders and weightlifters come together and take over the world. We can all relate to being freaks, outcasts, emotional basket cases, and YES........ the LAST MOTHER FUCKERS IN THE GYM.

Local News 2016

♪♪♪

Miss Brown Eyes

Thursday, September 6, 2012

A bar slamming coffee drinking PR smoking training day. SALUTE!

♪♪♪

The Councelor

Monday, September 10, 2012

Time to write. Hello, Dark Orchestra. It's good to see you again. The
steam from my tea swirls with an orange glow from the little candle I
light before I type. A light that I cannot write without. A feeling
that goes hand in hand with pulling out your stomach and throwing your
guts against the wall. A feeling which you had no idea was there in
the first place. Music, tea, coffee, and now this flickering light
are not just mood setters, but necessities. Dark is good, black is
comforting, the night time is my peace from war. The light piercing
under the door makes me glad I am in this dark office, and not out in
the normal chaos we call life. This is when I am most alive, right
now with you, on this dark fucken stage that echos my thoughts to the
second story where the skeletons play our life's soundtrack. A smokey
mirror that reminds me where I came from, and what still lies inside
me. A stage full of beds where monsters play chess. A place where
vodka tears fall from our eyes while we watch home videos. Hand prints
on our faces from "I wish I could do it over" moments. Play time with
thousands of airless footballs. Incomplete puzzles leading back to
middle school. Something as simple as asking her to dance, but never
committing. Or as powerful as losing a friend you loved so dearly.
Scattered splashes of beer stain the black stage floor while reaching
out for your ankles, screaming to stay, and to never leave the party.
A glass house is what surrounds this orchestra, a fragile reminder
of what lies outside those doors. Who we truly are, and what we are
capable of doing. A scary thought that explains why we volunteer
ourselves to this slave labor we call weightlifting.

Slam this bar with pride young man. Kick the weights 'til your toes
bleed. Smear your bloody hands all over the platform. Cover your face
with chalk as you cover your face from crying. Let it out! This is
not weightlifting! This is counseling! Come on kid, slam this bar, go
ahead, it's ok, let it rip! Fuck your old counselor, and guess what,
fuck you. Yea, I said it. It's time for someone to break down that over
sensitive wall you have built around yourself. It's time to learn how
to break balls and break these weights. Break your bad thoughts and
your self doubt. Break your meth pipe and that bottle you have in your
hand. It's time to break you down to build you back up. Just like
Shankle did to me. Now it's my turn to fuck you up, and make a man out
of you. It's the weight's turn. Everything else failed.... right? Now
it's time for these weights to fall upon your back only for you to stand

stronger. Get beat down, go through the pain, bleed, fight, cry, bath
in your own self pity, go ahead, get it out of the way. Your new role
model is you and this bar. Nothing else. I don't care about your other
dreams, shut up and lift. Lift this weight while lifting your head
high, higher, higher, fucken higher! Good, now drop the weight just like
your father dropped you! Slam this bar 'til you puke all over yourself.
Get the demon out, smash your fucken head against the wall until you
taste your blood dripping down your face. Learn how to love your own
blood, learn how to love yourself. Find yourself by beating yourself.
Find you while you break this bar. Yes! THAT'S IT! Now grab this
violin and play with the skeletons on the second floor. You will play
music you never knew you could young man, I promise. Raise your hands
and become you. You are you and you love it. Lift this weight the same
way you are going to lift life. Smash this weight the same way you are
going to smash your demons. No one will understand you better than this
bar. No one will support you more than this sport. No one will be more
truthful than these weights. Nobody loves you more than you. You young
man, welcome to the Dark Orchestra, welcome to your new life.

Welcome to Strength not weakness. Welcome to more bad days than good
days, and learning to deal with bad days to get to good days. Welcome
to a bad day meaning good, and not just a wasted bad day you call
yourself. Take this step away from yourself, and enter the no comfort
zones. A house of pain, a bed of nightmares, but a life of achiving. A
life full of team mates you can now call brothers. A coach you can now
call a father figure. A support group that will never let you fall,
but will always let you fail, for failing is apart of this sport, apart
of life. Your old veiw on failing has now changed forever. Failing is
good, its real, its the best advice you could ever recieve. A wise man
named Adam Hall once said, "I am the greatest contracter in the world,
and I love it". This changed my life forever. Thank you Adam for your
always motivating words and actions. Thank you Shankle for breaking
me down to build me up. Thank you coach for not only being my coach,
but fulfilling another role I need so desperatly. Thank you mom for
etending all my soccer and football games. Thank you Jim for the values
you taught me. Thank you Lexy for being happy. Thank you to my lovely
Wife for saving me and loving me. Thank you Dark Orchestra for giving
me a home. Thank you for readin this.

Second Story Skeletons 2016

♪♪♪

Young Rookie

Chapter 1

More bad days than good young rookie. Understand this, and you will
go far. Hold onto your dreams tight young rookie, or this sport will
snatch them from you. Always stay focused young rookie, or you will
be forever lost in limbo. Understand you are a rookie, this will
help you become a vet. Everything you learned before weightlifting
throw away, nothing applies to this alien sport. Stop with the
thinking young rookie, for this sport doesn't make any sense. The
minute you try to figure out this sport young rookie, is the minute
you will end up in a straight jacket. Walk at night to clear your
mind. Wake up early to a cup of coffee while the news softly plays
in the background. Take a shower, not to get clean, but to wash away
the frustrations of the day. Let the water hit your face, giving your
hands a rest from hitting the gym walls. Listen to your coach young
rookie, on and off the platform. Your coach is not just a coach, but
a path to success...... the only path to success. When you become a
vet, then you can spread your wings with your own ideas and opinions.
For now, you have no opinions, no ideas, you have no rights, no
control, no freedom, shut up and do what your told. Lay down your
sword, break down your wall, and become a slave to this sport and
your coach. A slave is what you are, and will always be if you don't
succeed. This doesn't just go for weightlifting, but for life as
well. You must live weightlifting to conquer weightlifting. You must
cry tears of pain before tasting tears of joy. Learn to love the pain
and you will never feel the pain again. Adapt, adapt to a new you, a
new outlook on life. No one cares what you did before weightlifting
or what obstacles you've had to overcome. The only thing that matters
young rookie is how much weight can you take from the ground to over
head..... that's it. The day you understand this is the day you will
lift big weight from the ground to over head. Don't listen to anyone
but your coach. Stop reading this article, unless your coach says it's
okay. Become a robot. Learn how to sit when coach says sit. Train
your body and mind to react without thinking. React when coach says
lift, react when coach says eat, react when coach says more weight,
react, react, react. Train your body to understand two things in
life, snatch and clean and jerk. If you can do more than 10 pull ups
then some thing's wrong. If you can still bench press over 300 pounds

after a few years of weightlifting, then get the fuck out of my gym and stop wasting my time. Become the weakest person on earth, but the strongest weightlifter in the world. The minute you understand that there is no such thing as over training, is the minute you will learn how to train. The minute you learn how to train, is the minute your body will finally break down. The minute your body finally breaks down, is the minute you will rebuild. The minute you rebuild is the minute you will become a monster. The minute you become a monster is the minute you will become numb. The minute you become numb is the minute you become a weightlifter.... or better yet...... a vet. This takes time and dedication. This takes a lot of trust, for your body will tell you different. Your body disagrees with this blog whole heartily. The devil in a red dress will try to make love to you, will you? Or will you punch her in the throat and trust my words, trust your coach, and not trust yourself?

The day the bar body slams you into the platform from falling on your back is a good day, a day that gets you just that much closer to becoming a vet. Young rookie, the day you bomb out at a meet, is a great day, a day and feeling you will never forget. A bomb out is a day that will harden your skin, harden your hook grip, harden your heart, and harden your mind. Living broke only to spend the money you have on food for recovery is a rich day, a day that will make your training even that much better when you have rubber band stacks in the trunk of your car to spend on better food, massages, etc. Coming from the bottom always tastes better when you reach the top. Young rookie, I am not done yet. And I hope you asked your coach before reading this because my words mean nothing compared to your coach, I'm just another schmuck online typing words.

Let's talk haters. The more people who hate you, the better you will become. Bath in the negativity, love it, dream about it, inject it in your veins, and then go train with it. Taking a negative and turning it into a positive = vet. Taking negative feedback and looking at it as negative = young rookie. Remember young rookie, the only thing that matters in life is coach, everything else is just.... fuel.

Becoming numb is one of the hardest parts to becoming a vet. Becoming numb is teaching your mind to stop sweating the small stuff, and then big stuff, and only focusing on training. Stop thinking about how you did yesterday, or even last rep, to become numb means only focusing on the lift ahead of you. Nothing else matters. Learning how to clear your mind to only focus on each lift is one of the hardest things I

have ever had to learn, and am still working on to this day. Young
rookie, stop...... and just lift.

Learn how to get your balls broke. Train with me, and I'll break you
down like a mother fucker. I'll be talking so much shit in training
you'll want to run home crying. I'll call you out in front of the
whole team and coach. Why you ask? I'll tell you why, it's what
Donny did to me, and what I will to do you, young rookie. The day
I took it, is the day I learned how to get off my high horse, face
reality, face life, face people stronger than me, face myself, and the
day I became a man. If you can't take some shit talking from a few
vets, then this sport will have you for dinner young rookie. Shut
your mouth, learn how to take it, put your head down, and train. The
day will come when you have a good enough resume to break a rookie
down only to build him up. Thank you Shankle for breaking me down
and yelling at me to get the fuck out of your gym. It's the best thing
anyone has ever done for me. Guess what Shankle, I never left, and
now because of you, this once young rookie is now a vet.

Thank you to my coach Glenn Pendlay, and my teammate Donny Shankle for
graduating me from young rookie to hardened vet. Salute to all the
young rookies out there. Put your heads down and become champions.

Chapter 2 coming soon

Pendlay Shankle 2016

♪ ♪ ♪

Solo

Thursday, September 20, 2012

Weightlifting Talk was fun today. First Solo show without the Lion
Killer or Mr Black Beard. The show had a different feel to it, a
different flow that I really liked. I didn't know how I would do,
or where the show would go, but I thought the show went very smooth.
TOPICS: Training without coach and Shankle. Great call about the
bottom position and catching the bar too high. Self motivation. The
presents of a coach, Punching a kid, American Open, Training alone,
Coach, Diet, Freak athletes, Jeff Wittmer, Why no program? Why the
show is called Weightlifting Talk. (below)

I hope you like it, salute.

Here is Wednesdays Team MDUSA video below. 154kg snatch, 190kg clean and jerk! I really feel that this wide grip in the jerk can lead me to 200 plus....maybe even sooner than I think. Who's knows, I guess more coffee, more training, and more Shankle. LETS GO!

♪♪♪

Team Commentary pt 2

Saturday, September 22, 2012

Max out Friday with more team commentary! First 160kg snatch since coach has been gone, and killed a 185kg c&j before making a gutsy jump straight to 195kg......which looking back now, I would have made the smart jump to 190kg. But what can I say, I had that SHANKLE Blood in me!! Plus, Saturday's squat workout is at the end of the video. I smoked a BIG 10 kilo PR in the back squat at 250kg before dropping down to complete my sets of 5. Yes, sometimes when coach is gone we will have a little fun and go for a max squat, but still always move on to complete the actual workout at hand. I hope coach is reading this so I can get some brownie points. Here is the video below. SLAM BARS AND KILL PR'S!!!!!!!!!!

♪♪♪

402

Weightlifting Talk - Shankle is Back

Thursday, September 27, 2012

♪ ♪ ♪

T-Rex

Saturday, September 29, 2012

The hip clean is a mysterious creature that seems to stay hidden in the dark away from the world to see or talk about. He is the fastest and most explosive creature in all of the land. His arms are bent like a T Rex, his hips plow into the bar like a punch from Mike Tyson. The sound the hip creature makes rattles the poor now half broken bar that echo's throughout the gym for all to here. It's a chilling sound that gives you goose bumps from head to toe. The power the hip cleaner creates will make even Chuck Norris feel in fear for his life. He is a patient creature, one that waits a long time before he attacks. He waits on the pull like I wait for my wife to get ready to go out to dinner. His shoulders stay over the bar like a sling shot being pulled back, or like Tiger Woods setting up to launch the little white ball into outer space. A longer pull...yes , but much more explosive than the rest? Most definitely. His upper body is asleep when he kills his pray, his legs and hips do the snapping of the necks, they are the ones who bring home the bacon.

I have tried over and over to become a hip cleaner...but every time I am reminded by the weightlifting Gods that I was meant to kill with my thighs. I live in thigh land with most of the other Olympic weightlifting warriors. We think the hip hitters are elitist know it all's, and are full of themselves! They say they are stronger for being able to bring heavy weight into a higher finish position, and I say nay. We the thigh hitters say that we are just as powerful and such good athletes that we can get under any weight. It's a back and forth battle, but at the end of the day we are all still friends and still lift heavy weight. "There is more than one way to get to the top of the hill"- Glenn Pendlay. There are just as many Gold medal hip creatures than there are thigh creatures.

The hip creature may live in you, he just might be hiding in the dark corner at the gym you train at without you even knowing. He lives in Spencer Moorman, Caleb Ward, and many others.

                              Hip or thigh we still love each other 2016

                         ♪ ♪ ♪

                       Jogging

Monday, October 1, 2012

The hateful forums. The American Open hype. The hateful YouTube comments. The nervous thoughts, twitches, and emotions. The pain that this sport has casted upon me, and the pain that life has brought me. The let downs and achievements. The highs and lows. The gold medals and bomb outs. My fight with drugs and alcohol. My sad story that is called my relationship with my father. My coach being away from me too long. The constant eyes that watch for my next move. The high bar that constantly stays floating over my head. The stacked 94kg class. All of this vanishes into the morning fog as I start my morning jog at 6:00 AM.

Something new for me, something that has helped me on and off the platform the last few weeks. I find a certain peace within myself that I never knew existed. I have met another Jon North that I am drawn to. A new me that is calm and quiet. Peaceful and mysterious. A Jon North that breaths clouds of morning fog and not flames of fire. Who never walks but runs, and who never talks but thinks. These crying thoughts that drown me with shame must be freed. These thoughts must run away from my skeleton pit mind, never to be seen again. Run away from me you blood sucking Demon, your thoughts that tear holes though my heart, will be no longer, as I run from you. Facing you has got me no where. So I run.

This old race horse has trouble moving when off the platform, so
starting a jog is always an up hill battle. I step with pain as my
knees start to play their own violin. It's been said that my knees
and back have their own Dark Orchestra. The more I think about it,
we all have a Dark Orchestra. What is a Dark Orchestra? It's a dark
stage where we can catch our breath, and listen to our skeletons play
beautiful songs of sadness. A family of outcasts that eat dinner
together on a long wooden table filled with glasses of salty tears. A
place called home. But this morning, there is no dark orchestra, just
a quiet world where the sounds of bar slamming and judging eyes do
not exist. Ready to listen to the key board of sneakers that hit the
side walk of pavement. I am ready to enter the Apocalypse. Ready to
enter the clouds of fog. I jog, I jog with rhythm and pride. I jog
like Ali. I jog with Attitude, side by side with the Nation. I jog
to forget. I jog to think. I jog because jogging is not weightlifting,
it's something different. The faster I jog, the farther back the
bar above my head falls behind. The longer I jog, the less my body
hurts. The old race horse starts to wake, the fog starts to clear,
and now you can call me Seabiscut. Every drop of sweat that falls
off my forehead is a weight off my shoulders. Come on coach, it's my
time to carry you to the finish line. Your presence is strong, even
though hidden away in your own Orchestra of...... well, let's just say
your presence is still with me, and me jogging is a metaphor of moving
forward with you, Shankle, and the rest of my teammates. I will jog
for us. I will jog this morning to simply move, because moving is
what I was put on this planet to do. God made me move well, so moving
is what I do. God gave me bad book smarts for a reason. He gave
me ADD for a reason. He invented coffee for a reason. He invented
jogging for a reason. He invented weightlifting for us lost souls.
Weightlifting is a castle of happiness from our broken paths of doom.
He invented Klokov to not only look good, but, well..... Klokov is a
damn sexy man. That's all I have to say about that. If you don't
have a man crush on Klokov, then I don't trust you as a person.

I write about weightlifting now, but when I jog I think nothing of it.
I think of nothing. I focus on everything. I focus on my stride, the
landscape, the sunrise that can make even the strongest man feel weak.
I black out, this time not from alcohol, but from peace. Running
breaks the weightlifting shackles from my ankles, allowing me to move
in a way I haven't done in years. I feel no pain for the first time
in years, no back pain, no knee pain, nothing. It's like my body
is rewarding me from not beating it up, slamming it with weights,
crushing it with bars, kicking it down until it pees blood or I get

the shakes at night. My body cries when I crawl to the bathtub. My
body screams when I puke white liquid from the amount of creatine I
intake. But when I run, I feel weightless, I feel like Seabiscut.
Sometimes, taking the time out of the day for no weightlifting, is the
best weightlifting training for a weightlifting meet.

I feel I am addicted to coffee. I am addicted to moving. I am addicted
to weightlifting. I am addicted to jogging. Yes, you can find me at
practice everyday chained to the platform. But now, you can also
find me in the early morning running through the Apocalypse, side by
side with a calm Jon North that you may never meet. Salute.

Prefontaine Forever

♪ ♪ ♪

Chris Ware

Tuesday, October 9, 2012

Big and bad. Strong and confident. Motivated and powerful. A
captain among his crew, sailing the seas of weights with his blond
hair and short green shorts. Legs like tree trunks, bubble butt that
held a mustang's engine. Arms as long as ropes that smashed through
walls and weights like heavy swings from a sludge hammer. A hammer
head full of little words, but a million thoughts. A giant among men,
a gladiator among civilians. A presence you could feel before even
entering the gym. The sea parted when he walked, and the sea was dead
quiet when he lifted. You never were surprised to see him
in the gym, because the word was already out that the
lion himself was pacing the gym floor hungry and
looking for food. Goose bumps covered your body as
the hair on your neck stood up like a squat. Chris
Ware is his name, and killing weights is his game.

He was everything I was not. He stood 10 feet
tall, I stood 1 foot tall. He trained hard and
held a 4.0. I got high and held a solid 1.5. I
was a punk kid who looked up to the wrong people. A
kid who was not walking, but running down the wrong
road. Chris Ware was the beginning and the birth of
Jon North. A birth that took place my first day

406

of my freshman year of high school. The first day I laid eyes on the
green beast. This story is the beginning my friends. I am taking you
back to the start. This story takes place before I met the dark world
of weight training, weightlifting, body building, Miss Brown Eyes, The
Dark Orchestra, you, my wife, my National Title, my USA teams, or my
father figure Coach. A story that Chris Ware himself, had and has no
idea ever took place, until now. Now that I have a platform to speak
on, I am proud to tell this story to the world.

I watched his every move. Yea, you can call me a stalker, I was.
You can call me whatever you want, but you try seeing an alien for
the first time, and let's see what you do. Chris Ware had no idea,
and still has no idea how much I looked up to him. I would go home
and tell my mom stories at dinner time about what happened in the
weight room and what Chris Ware did. I will never forget the day
Chris spoke to me....... it was like a dragon lowering his head
down to my level, breathing fire, and then flying away. I spoke
to a dragon, and the dragon somehow knew who I was. I ran home
and told my mom with excitement and happiness. I studied how he
interacted with others. I took mental notes on how he trained, and
the intensity he used to lift the massive weight he was lifting. When
people ask me where I got my attitude from, my intensity, my drive,
I always say Chris Ware. Even though they have no idea who he is, I
do, and that's all that matters. If you think I am intense and crazy
now, you should have seen this guy train.

Fucken let's go. The Shankle of my Child hood..... let's go. Chris
Ware has made me a man without him even knowing it, and now it's time
to put a sword though his chest. Kill him and take his strength.
Thank you for all your teachings Chris. Thank you for changing my life
and giving me the tools I need to succeed in sports and in life. I
took your powers and introduced the world to me, Jon North, the bar
slamming weight killing Johnny Cash singing most hated man in USA
weightlifting mother fucken Attitude Nation son of a bitch. With more
respect than you will ever know Chris, I fight everyday to be like
you, better than you, I try everyday to cut the dragon's head off that
once blessed me with its fire. You have created a monster that now
chases after you. WELCOME TO THE DARK ORCHESTRA CHRIS. Please don't
be scared, there is nothing to worry about. Don't mind the skeletons
and the dark stage filled full of salty coffee stained tears. Please
sit, for now you have entered our world, a world of hell and pain.
Snort the chalk lines of life with me, and eat the bar that breaks
our hearts from let downs it has casted upon us. A world of demons

and back stabbing is where we sit Chris, a world full of nah sayers
and hateful vampires. Success is outside. In here we chat while our
skeletons play their violins.

I followed you into the jungle of weights, the Alice in Wonderland of
barbells, and like the movie Jumanji I have never left. I remember
the person I was before being bit by the weight room bug and becoming
infected by the virus. I wonder how he is doing? I wonder what has
become of the outside world? I thank you every time I succeed Chris,
but I curse your name every time I fail. I wonder where I would be if
I never met you, if I never wandered into the gym touching bars and
plates like they were mysterious plants from an unknown world. As you
can tell, this blog has veered off into different directions a few
times that has you scratching your head. It's because of the amount
of coffee that is being poured down my bloody from the bar throat.
More coffee than you could ever imagine. Plus, the song has changed
a few times, which turns everything around. But anyways, I really
just wanted to say thank you. I am sorry about the dagger that I have
stabbed you in the chest with, I hope you understand that I need all
of your mighty powers to make this 2016 Olympic team. I don't know
if you ever knew the role model you were and still are to me. I don't
know if you will ever read this. Hopefully you will come across this
so you know the impact you had on me growing up. I wanted you to know
that there was a kid who hung on your every word and move. I wanted
to let you know that you changed my life for the better, and I bet
there are others out there that feel the same, but have never spoke
of it or wrote about it. I don't even know if you will remember me,
or know who I am, and that's okay, I understand, it's been many many
years. I want to thank you for inviting me to your house party, I
will never forget running from the cops. Thank you for showing me the
weights, saving me from drugs, guiding me to...... me. Thank you.

Chris Ware 2016

♪ ♪ ♪

408

The Kite Coach and The Sand Creature

Saturday, October 13, 2012

I write to you from the far away island of Maui. On the beach with
miss brown eyes by my side, ridding the waves of life...literally. I
have been playing cast away for the last four days. I haven't touched
a weight sense I sailed upon this easy going orchestra, played by
white birds on a blue stage full of flowers and palm trees, much
different the the Orchestra I know. And while everyday is paradise,
the sunny heaven I bathe in also brings a sandy explosion of a
homesick feeling that grows within my ears and throughout my sandy
feet. That's why I must visit my home.....The Dark Orchestra. Let
me step out from the sun, and enter the dark. Let me step away
from my family, and hang with my other family. Let me say good
by to happiness and hello to pain. Know matter how far I travel,
Weightlifting follows me everywhere.

This wet Island is a refreshing change from the the dry spell that my
team mates and I have had in the gym the last few weeks. Ever sense
Coach left, the drinking water has become scars. Weightlifters are
going hungry, and PR's are moving onward looking for green grass,
waterfalls, and other life to feed off of. A PR is a person too, they
need us just as bad as we need them. I wait for Coach like one pig
waits for another. I wait for coach like he waits for me to finally
break the weight from the floor. I will wait for coach like he has
waited for me the last three years. This sport has taught me that
time moves slow, and with patients grows great things to come, and
waiting for coach is just another great thing soon to bloom into gold.
The gym has left with him, and the weights followed closely behind
like a puppy being dragged by a little boy walking too fast. Smiles
are now smirks, high fives are now low two's, and big bright eyed
looks for approval have melted into an empty chair sitting in front
of an empty desk giving careless feedback. If a big lift is made and
coach pendlay doesn't see it or hear it, did it happen? This is the
million dollar question.

Blue ocean as far as my eyes can reach. Water as clear as air, and
sky's as blue as the towel me and miss brown eyes sit on. I think and
smile, I think and frown, I am happy, I am depressed, I am a sandy
beach full of emotions that has me running my finger back and forth
in the sand. A black crow to my right, and a white dove to my left.
Miss brown eyes in my belly, and a deep chip in my heart. This blog

goes out to all, weightlifting or not, a story about a beach and what it can bring out of you. Eyes up young man, stop looking down Jon. Look out to the sea as if you are catching the bar. Eyes up coach says, as I picture him standing there with nothing around him but him, and the look on his face that waits for my response to his always great coaching cues. This man has dedicated his whole life to this sport, and the realization that I am included in the package is mind numbing. He coaches like an innocent kid flying his kite high in the air with complete pride and concentration. Sorry, this is just the image that popped in my mind when thinking about coach coaching. Wow, the air feels free here, a feeling of let go and escape. Look, you can see the kite that coach flies from here......that son of a bitch. A beautiful feeling rudely woken by reality as I have trouble swimming with the long heavy pendlay bar attached to my ankle. Hello world. Hello sea turtles.

My sister getting married is something that I can't talk about. I can't even write about. I hope you understand. The words don't have a chance, they will never see the light of day. They will live and die inside me. An emotion that has been sentenced to the death penalty. Typing this has already made me leave the computer a few times. So I must end it hear, I have nothing else to say about this.

A kiss from coffee surrounded by non weightlifting civilians. This is dangerous. I fear for the people around me. I am a lion amongst sheep. A rage in me that can snap at anytime, springing me off the sand I sit on and into a full sprint tackling a white sheep into the water and eating my prey like a vampire. I shouldn't be allowed around the public. I don't trust myself, and they shouldn't trust me. I have been taught and trained to become an animal the last 5 plus years. I have been trained to react and attack without thinking. I have been trained to wake up and get strong! Fight! Kill! Train! Win! Endure the pain! Everyday I am kicked down to only stand taller. I am beat up to become strong. I am slowed down to move extremely fast. Coach is never happy to keep me always hungry. I am overloaded with weight only to throw weight high and then slam weight down. I can't run because I am built to lift. I am trained to love pain, except pain, live with pain, so now I don't feel pain. Just the other day I snapped......yes in training towards the weight, replace the weight with a person.....yea see, scary and not good. SNAP! I am left gasping for air dramatically looking around the room trying to read the situation because I have know idea what the hell just happened. I need to be locked away. Throw away the key and let Pendlay create an even stronger and faster monster. Blame coach, not me. I sit on this beach with little twitches that have me scared like Edward Norton in the Hulk. What the fuck did coach do to me? What the fuck have I become?

I guess these are just some of the many thoughts that come over me as I sit on the sandy beach of Hawaii.

Lexy North 2016

♪♪♪

Heels

Wednesday, October 17, 2012

I am more and more convinced that you should break the weight from the floor already back on your heels. "Where should we start the pull from?" is a question I received a few seminars back that really made me think, where do I pull from. It is a mystery that must not go unsolved, a mystery that this black sheep must try to tackle. I know the "guide book" of weightlifting says the balls of your feet... but I don't buy this one way to lift type crap. I don't buy this surrender to new ideas and creations bullshit that the old dictators of USA Weightlifting want us to fall prisoners to. Pull off the balls of your feet, absolutely. I just don't think the "guide book" applies to all the millions upon millions of techniques. If you are scratching your head asking yourself what these million different techniques are, well let me tell you. Every athlete is different. Every athlete is unique. Every athlete has his or her own relationship with the bar. There is no one way to lift weights, there is just your way. No two people lift the same, so for every weightlifter comes a new and different technique. For every weightlifter a romance is born, a relationship blooms into a garden of love and hate from every corner of the world. "There is more than one way to get to the top of the hill". - Glenn Pendlay. This is the best thing Mr. Black Beard has ever said to me. Thank you coach for opening my mind to new possibilities, new adventures and a new outlook on life.

Pulling off the heels is what I do and teach. This is the Superman way, the Attitude way.... a way. Fall backwards on the first pull, (floor to knees) and use all the momentum to drive yourself over the bar on the second pull, (knees to hips) to get ready for one thing and one thing only... Yes young men, and yes young women! You are right! Get over and get ready for the only thing that matters in life.... the finish!! A domino effect, a sling shot effect... wait, better yet, a catapult effect! Ha ha, YES! Yes I have had too much coffee, but on the other hand there is no such thing as too much coffee, just under recovery from coffee. But back to what I was saying. IT'S NOT A PULL, IT'S A SET UP. Understand this and you will PR daily. The set up and the finish are not the same; they are two different sports, two different creatures. Stop combining your mashed potatoes with your green beans, let them have a life of their own, let them be separate and enjoy the freedom they have deserved over the years of battle and war. You should be so far back on your heels that if you let go of the bar, you should fall back on your ass. People wonder why there are all of the holes behind the platforms at Cal Strength?.... Well there you go. They are not from grip strength though; they are from straps breaking on a weekly basis. Damn those straps, do your job!! Sons of bitches!!!! Wiggle your toes as you pull. The toes are for the finish, and the heels are for the pull, don't let the heels slack! Then again, Attitude Nation... do what works for you, don't listen to me! Listen to you!

What are you cooking Joe? Well Cathy I am baking a Jon North, Greg Everet, Glenn Pendlay, Don McCauley, Paul Doherty, Jackie Mah, Rob Earwicker, Jasha Faye, and John Coffee cake. Is it good Joe? Cathy, I have no idea yet, it's worth a try!

I believe in my way 1,000,000 percent. My way is the best, hands down. But they would tell you the same, so you choose.

STOP JUMPING! I have competed, coached, and trained all over the world and I have never seen anybody jump and shrug in the air! Lol, I'm sorry I know I should be Attitude Nation on this and say, "Do what works for you" but this just crosses the line into madness and self-destruction. The PR's and consistency I have seen at my certs by transforming people from not jumping is mind blowing. Can someone please tell me where this jumping thing comes from? I am more confused than coach Pendlay without BBQ. I guess this blog is turning into a diary at this point. I sometimes forget that people read what I type. Hello Frank, it's good to see you back in the cast away corner we call the Dark Orchestra. Sometimes in the dark I can't see who is with me. It's good to know that when I hang my hat, cry my tears, and hide from the world, I have you to join me Frank. Thank you, and cheers.

Wow, a lot of boring technique talk. I could go all day talking about
this science project we call weightlifting, but my mind drifts from
the equations and solutions, and into an Alice in Wonderland dream of
coffee waterfalls, and vicodin powdered protein shakes that make my
skin tingle and my head turn from child hood memories of being on my
dad's lap looking out into a foggy rain filled world on top of the
Seattle Space Needle. Yes stay on your heels, but maybe pull off your
heels. Maybe turn your AC up while your windows are down. Maybe is
an adventure that leads to Dinosaurs and talking dogs. I guess I will
end this blog with a very famous quote before I start typing deeper
and deeper into my white padded wall banging head. "Try it, you might
like it". Salute and we will see you back here soon Frank. Thank you
for being with me.

Frank 2016

♪ ♪ ♪

Two Birds

Friday, October 19, 2012

Talk   Train

♪ ♪ ♪

Our Violin

Wednesday, October 24, 2012

Sad faced keys look up at me, as my fingers infect them with my thoughts. Keys that stretch into violin strings that echo loudly throughout the Dark Orchestra, as I play with my head down and Shankle to my side. Some days I wish I would have never met him, and other days I am thankful for his leading hand guiding me into this fucked up life. A man that can barely walk, or hardly talk from the mind games that cheer and boo loudly in his science project head. A still calm face is what we see, but behind the blinds of piercing lion killer eyes, holds a storm that can create much force into the bar when needed. Turning off this storm is never possible. Driving home can leave you drenched and gasping for air. Sleeping is training of its own, as this sport has its side effects. Side effects that will leave you rocking back and forth in the chair you sleep in because a bed hurts your broken neck and back. Rocking because your body has been trained to move. Rocking to the image of a white wall that might as well be the property of a hospital. Knee wraps are like coffee, they help dull the pain. Walking has come harder over the years, and my mind seems to play tricks on me as I catch myself drooling while picking out cereal in the store. Join me on YouTube, but then leave me. Turn off the computer and go, leave me with me, a person I do not know off the platform. Leave me as I am stuck in this video forever. No one is rooting for me while driving home, this is when depression kicks in. I smile when training, I smile when you watch the live feed, I welcome you with open arms, but I am sad to see you go. I am fucken depressed once you leave and I can't figure out how to pump my own car full of gas. I am lost when I am not a weightlifter. I am lost when I have to take a driving test that I still cannot pass. I am a fucken loser, don't you see? I'm only special on the platform, on YouTube, or at a meet. I am alive and well when lifting, but sleeping is a nightmare. How can I be so confident on the platform, but so insecure off? You leave me everyday like my dad left me, like my step mom left me, and my step sisters that I used to call family. Family has left me like someday this sport will, and then what?

Shankle sits across from me, still there, still with me. Thank God for my weightlifting family, a cult that makes me feel needed, necessary, and valued. Nothing else has brought me so much passion. I spent many nights sleeping on a bench outside living homeless, thinking where I would be now. Who knew I would be here. Who knew

414

the path I took in life would lead me to this. Life is funny that
way. The talking to myself issue has put me in the chair facing a
therapist. Ideas that run through my head have to be dealt with and
organized. I see technique that confuses most coaches, and sometimes
myself. I dig too deep into the philosophy of weightlifting, finding
things that shouldn't be found. I am falling deeper into a state of
wanderlust and ideas that I am afraid might take me prisoner for good
one day. I am still getting to know this new Jon North, a man that
lights his fire and cooks his dinner behind the screen of youtube.
A puppet that Pendlay pulls the strings on. A freak with coffee
that some despise and hate. A mental head case that if directed
properly can work in your blessing. What most don't know is the
influence my father has had on me, good and bad. Let's just say my
mind works and has been trained from a very, very young age to see
situations and move them without anyone knowing. Rooms spin while
my head stays facing straight. Couches and chairs move from one
end of the room to the other. My next move is crucial, what shall
I do? Stop Jon! Just be you the people very close to me say! But
how, when all I know is the Godfather lines and techniques my father
drilled into me, while dumping me into social situations where they
were looked at win or lose, and then discussed in depth afterwords.
Rave parties, high on ecstasy when I was 12, only to sharpen up my
social skills and adapt to life experiences. I might as well have
been in school. A confused kid with an innocent heart, but scared by
the talent of seeing situations not just people. I have come a long
way in finding myself, and just being me, even though it has been
a very hard challenge to shut that side of my mind off, and turn on
the side of pure reactions and feelings. Yes we all have skeletons,
these are just a few of mine that I don't mind sharing. I find this
subject fascinating. My dad is a genius. But his genius he took
too far, his so called powers are what killed him in the end. In the
end his own strategies turned upon himself and locked him away in his
own mind. The minute he used his powers on his own family, is the
day the muddy bank gave way, and crashed into a million pieces. The
first steps in breaking this curse is admitting and talking about the
curse, then I will find who I really am.

40 Kilos to 166 Kilos has taught me a lot. Understanding that
training with pain is okay, and losing is part of winning. This blog
is far from motivational, more of a diary on journey within ourselves
and what great things come of sports. A blog on how a coach can
change not only your technique, but life. How someone like Shankle
took a chance with me when no one else would. Yes, I can't read nor

do math. Yes, I can't pass a simple driving test, nor understand how
to work an ATM, but I do know how to slam bars and kill PR's. Thank
you for listening to my violin.

Weightlifting 2016

♪ ♪ ♪

Low Bar Demon

Tuesday, October 30, 2012

I have competed, lifted, conducted attitude seminars, and helped with
many Pendlay seminars all over the world, and I have never once seen
anyone perform the "low bar squat". Actually, I didn't even find out
what it was until a few months back when someone asked me if they
should do high bar or low bar for the squats I just prescribed them.
I am still in shock that athletes actually perform such a "nails on
a chalk board" lift, especially for a weightlifter that should make
the bottom position their home. The number one problem I see with
beginner weightlifters is their depth, or lack there of. Watching
a weightlifter low bar squat makes me want to take the elevator to
the highest floor, and then jump. Low bar squatting is just as bad
as a beginner doing power snatch and power clean more than the full
lifts. Both of these weightlifting killers create incorrect movement
patterns, horrible rhythm, awful consistency, and do not increase the
novice weightlifter's flexibility. The low bar squat is not just ugly
and painful to watch, but teaches you to move slower than a turtle
that just drank two bottles of nyquil.

 Brand new client, brand new dreams of becoming an Olympic
weightlifter, in a brand new sport where the sky is the limit. We
work on catching the bar in the hole over and over for hours. After
catching a lift in the hole, I would have him sit down there and get
comfy. I would throw him a bag of popcorn and tell him to watch a
movie down there. I would tell him to bounce like tigger over and
over to create stability, balance, and for the great practice of at
times having to catch that second or third bounce to stand up with a
heavy weight. I introduced him to his new home. He then started to
make progress in the lifts, especially after I told him never to do
a power snatch or power clean again, until he became a champion at
the "full" lifts. A fist pump followed by a smile is the action and

emotion that he got when he was able to lift more weight by receiving
the bar as low as he could. I dropped out of physics, but I have
the innate ability to understand that weightlifting is nothing more
than a race against gravity. I get excited for him; I get excited
for his new PR. We slap hands and drink more coffee, going over how
the training went and what we both want in the near and far future.
I think he thought the training session was over because he started
to take his Pendlay shoes off. I then laughed and told him that the
fire in Hell was still burning bright and high, and now we had to
squat. Tired but still motivated, he took another sip of miss brown
eyes, and began to slap the big bearded man's shoes back on. Back
squats, 5 sets of 2, lets go. I had to take a number one from all the
coffee that has been poured down my throat since I woke about 7 hours
ago. In a full on sprint to the bathroom I yelled without looking
behind me, "Get warmed up!". As I slowly started walking back from
one of the best things God himself ever invented, I heard a bunch of
little kids crying and screaming for their mothers. People everywhere
where running past me to the door like the building was on fire.
Coach Pendlay stood up and yelled for someone to call 911, and then
he walked fast....not ran, because everyone knows that Coach never
runs....well unless he is imitating my teammate Kevin Cornell. As I
was spinning in circles trying to comprehend what was happening in
the quiet town of San Ramon, Donny bumped into me spilling my coffee
all over my deep v Attitude Nation shirt. He told me that a red fire
breathing demon with sharp fangs and dinosaur scales dripping down its
greasy back was killing people by its grotesque image alone. I pushed
through the panicking crowd and to my horror......I saw my client
doing low bar back squats.

The world ended hours later.

                                                        High bar 2016

                        ♪ ♪ ♪

                          417

Garbage Thoughts

Wednesday, November 14, 2012

Taking the garbage out, with my eyes glued to the pavement, side
to side I walk in silence as training hunches over my back like a
monster monkey constantly bringing up the past. I'm not going to write
bullshit, I just won't. It's fucken freezing out here, and where the
hell are all the damn people? Just me I guess, just like that scary
silence while you stand on the platform. Eyes piercing through your
soul like wolves about to set the dinner table. Camera flashes like
you're behind the fence at the zoo, but this morning nothing.... just
another schmuck waving to the first person I see walking their five
pound dog. Peeing with one hand behind my head, itching and itching
while the traffic jam thoughts turn my veins green, cutting off all
circulation to my brain. Face in the dirt while my eyes turn into a
mud hole of no real direction. Writer's block is what I speak of, a
fucken curse that has entered my daily love affair with the Orchestra
of pain and suffering. I'm back now, I hope you have forgiven me for
reposting some older blogs, blogs that I should add, are some of my
favorite that I personally like to read over before training. Some
adding kilos, and some taking away. Train is all I do, I swear. It's
like a pasta dish that never seems to have a bottom, just more pasta.

My body hurts, and my mind pinches in pain like a small paper cut
that lingers with you for days among days. Here is the twist, my
numbers are going up, and my training is through the roof right
now. I'm faster and stronger than I have ever been, more confident,
more consistent, more experienced. What does this so called great
news mean? Well I will tell yea, it means I'm fucked. It means I'm
stuck training for many more years beating myself up like a rodeo
clown. Don't get it confused now, I love it. I'll die doing this.
I'm a gladiator that cannot be put down. A freak that breaths chalk
and spits out PR's. Snap this gold medal off my neck and raise it
high for all to see, now yell with everything you have until the
judges throw you off stage. I work too hard to leave the platform.
I'll stand 'til they throw rocks and boo me off stage, an image that
bounces back and forth in my head as I take the garbage out. Side to
side I walk in the dark cold nights, swearing I am seeing things in
the trees. I'm fast, but not fast enough to run from whatever the
hell lays behind those woods that seem to be gaining closer and closer
around my house.

Bar path is back, just like visiting your home town you grew up in. Everything seems back not forward. Back home the streets are filed with candy bars that me and my friends have stolen from our past years of mayhem. Old drug dealers pass me in the streets while the Friday night lights shine over my late night outings full off familiar smells and memories. For all those who doubted me and turned their backs on me, now look, can you see my back as I fly over the sky on my mongoose bird, collecting freedom keys that provide "do what I want and live how I want" gates piled behind vaults that open only with a password.

Hook grip is a must for any lifter, this is why I believe that taping your thumbs to keep them fresh is very important, no matter how big or small an athlete's hands are. I thought about the importance of a hook grip while taking out the trash early yesterday morning...... I guess this blog is filled to the rafters with my garbage walking thoughts. I am breaking down the walls of keyboard block, and typing anything that comes to mind, almost like entering training with a slight injury, don't think and hopefully your always confused body will forget such things even exist. More coffee helps as well. I want to add that I truly believe in tying your shoes as tight as possible and not leaving any room for wiggle aka lack of support. I think this is why my calf has been in suffering lately, my Adidas don't lace as tight as I would like them to, leaving my ankle too much room. I have corrected this problem by drilling another loop hole creating more support. Plus I have started to tape the center of my shoes for even more support aka more athletic feeling.

Thank you Shankle, for the song you showed me for the writing of this all over the place garbage walk through blog. It has helped me break through the curse of writer's block. I have so much to say, you would think this would never happen to me. My next blog should be much more organized as I will type across from the Lion's den aka the lion killer himself...... Darth Vader the weightlifter. Goodnight and it feels good to be back at the long table of tear drinking.

USA 2016

♪ ♪ ♪

419

Ego Effect

Tuesday, November 20, 2012

Really Fun show today. Happy Thanksgiving!

Plus: PR Clean & Jerk video below!

♪ ♪ ♪

Garage University

Saturday, November 24, 2012

Muddy protein shake full of exploding chunks of chalky powder hit your
sleepy and confused face as you wake before sunset. Most mornings, you
are confused why you cut your dream world early for training. Some
days, you don't know why you train at all. Some days, sleeping in
sounds so nice. Quiet as a mouse, almost as if your house was waking
from a good night sleep as well, this cold morning needs life, and the
sound of dripping coffee creates the first few sparks. The background
noise from the morning news makes you feel less home sick, even though
it's been forever since you lived under your parent's roof. Just the
thought of how many polar bears must be roaming throughout your garage
makes you grab your coffee early and begin chugging. Hello world. Good
morning training. A scruffy face and a dirty white sweat suite only
says one thing.... Gladiator. A gladiator who will soon do something
most people would run from, wouldn't imagine doing, would call you a
freak and freak you are. I'm not there with you, but I am. I'm not
there right now, but I have been. Self motivation is a sport of its
own, a beast that is hard to take down alone. Lonely as fuck, beat to

crap, and for some messed up reason, a single tear will drop for no apparent reason. But let me ask you something, if that tear drops, will it make a splash? When that PR goes down, will it make a noise? Yes it will, yes it mother f'n will.

No teammates to push you, just the sound of the garage door opening and Klokov yelling through YouTube. No coach to make sure you show up on time, but you are always 5 minutes early. Open your garage for cool air, because the air in this garage is sticky and heavy. A heavy soul with heavy weights. Heavy thoughts weigh you down, only 'til you slam them fuckers down. Standing outside on your driveway scares your neighbors, yes, yes it does. You're that guy, you're the freak and you welcome it, if you don't you should. I welcome it, we welcome it. Tired of trying to fit in, tired of trying to become someone you're not, so now you do what the fuck you want to do, and pouring coffee over your head and smashing coffee cups at 6 am is what we love to do. Creating our own fight club on ourselves. Training with Brad Pit can cause seruise wounds, but huge gains. Dirty weights make for better weights. Rusty bars make for more PR's, and Bob and Jill driving by in disgust means they must be late for their white sheep meeting. I don't accept. Do you people here me? I will not! "I'm going to show you how great I am." "The world ain't all sunshine and rainbows. It's a very mean and nasty place, and I don't care how tough you are, it will beat you to your knees and keep you there permanently if you let it. You, me, and nobody is going to hit harder than life. It ain't about hard you hit, it's about how hard you can get hit and keep moving forward, how much you can take and keep moving forward. That's HOW WINNING IS DONE!" Let the rust from the bar harden your hands making your hook grip sharper than Hook himself. You don't like me, good....I don't like you. This is my gym, and your not welcome. My rules, my program, my technique, my life. Get your degree in sports science, ill get mine from the smell of fire wood pilled high like sand bags around my platform. Blood and dirt baby, blood and fucken dirt.

I train in a fancy gym, fully sponsored, paid, worked on, waited on....... I can't tell you how many times I miss and wish I could go back to being the garage warrior. The rough tough son of a bitch that needs no one but heavy metal rock music, energy drinks, and a fucken bar. Give me a bar and I'm a dog with a bone. I don't want a pencil, I want a bar, I want happiness. Our garage is dark, but we see fine, better yet we see better, better yet we like it dark because light makes us weak. We like pain because pain makes us feel alive. Weightlifting pain takes away some of the internal pain, pain where the demons live, pain that bangs against these black keys, pain I call, we call, the Dark Orchestra. Turn up the music and keep training, never stop. I salute you. You...... the garage lifter who slams bars when no one is watching. I salute you, who completes your last few drop sets, the last rep, the last few squats. You, the crazy son of a bitch who completes the full workout that you gave yourself! I know how hard you train because I was there. We are family, we came from the same class. We come from the garage. We live in the dark and eat dirt. We come from the outcast university. We come from F report cards and meth pipes. We graduated from early morning and nasty protein shakes, and a world of pain and hell that only makes us appreciate peace and family even more. So just know next time you see me training with my shiny bar and fancy weights, I truly truly envy you, wish I was training with you, and absolutely respect the shit out of you. I salute you, I salute the garage lifter.

Blood & Dirt 2016

♪ ♪ ♪

Lets Train, Shall We?

Tuesday, December 4, 2012

Grand daddy clock eyes, ticking side to side in a dark room full of numbers and arrows. Chatter outside makes my ear stick to the door. Too much NyQuil? Or not enough sleep? A dagger in one hand, and fire in the other, both tools I will keep tight throughout this blue dress adventure and smoking caterpillar world. A scary sport to tackle alone, and one that loses many from its blinding snow storms and giant killer polar bears. Get up boy and move. Kill the bears and drink the green potion. Grab your bar and breathe fire. Smash your weights upon the lonely road you walk. I will now smoke two for you and always ride one pant leg higher than the other. Smoke travels around my face as I hide away in my jungle behind the gym. A moment of "what the fuck have I become, what the hell is going on?" I will kill a sheep, eat a sheep and send you half with "if it fits, it ships" mail. Grow your hair long my friend, and jump. Jump off those tall rocks into an ocean of release and light thoughts. Splash deep and rip the head off a blue whale.

Let's train, shall we? Let's inject protein and snort creatine. When I am talking, I am Jon, but when I am writing, I am a gilled animal

that fears the possibility of someday losing his mind completely. This
dark room door opens as I enter a cloud of forums and hate mail. The
sound of click makes me hiccup, the red box of a tube and you makes
me dive into training even harder. Punish the evil creatures with
success and they will soon turn into warm steam. Now the road to OZ
is yellow, and the doors to the Olympics is green. Odd thoughts take
me from world to world as I slide down water falls of liquid codeine.
Inception keeps me awake as I try to figure out what is real and what's
not. Last time I checked, I was opening doors at T.G.I. Fridays. Last
time I checked, I had enough hardware to build a tree fort.

Let's train.....shall we? Fast forward your training session and
you will soon realize you are on a carouse wheel that goes round and
round. "Round and round" Ha! If you like the movie The Truman Show
you will get that line, if not... watch it. Never ever listen to
your body! Do you understand, kid in the middle row eating all that
chocolate? Come up to the front of the class and explain why you are
eating all that junk food young man. "I smash Snicker bars down
teacher because I am addicted to sugar, and sugar gets me jacked up,
and being jacked up makes me fuck up weights, and fucking up weights
makes me feel good....... teacher." Bar up bar down, small jumps big
jumps, goose bumps nervous thoughts and a whole lot of shots and big
PR attempts! Train, let's keep going. Gold medals and more coffee.
Gold medal in coffee makes for eye popping training and USADA testing.
I'll piss in this cup and then piss on the competition platform. Mine
mother fuckers, now go home. Now train! Lift, lift, lift, lift,
equals lift. This is my type of math. Pencil to the desk as my other
idiot special resource class mates giggle to the funny papers instead
of reading Run Spot Run. One day I snapped my pencil in half and
crashed the window open like a monkey in a cage. We all got loose and
now all we do is train, train and train.

I know, I know, but let's keep going a little longer, shall we?
American Open..... Let's talk about that first word. It means sorry
buddy, but the Nation took your pink slip and bought a horse to ride
all over the warm up room with. It feels good to be back, back in
this ever so dark orchestra full of tears and violins. Thank you for
all of your support over the years. We won Gold, not I.

Rio 2016

♪ ♪ ♪

423

33,000 Feet

Thursday, December 6, 2012

I am being told to write only Weightlifting by the waving fingers
who look down upon me. The tall shadowy figures that don't seem to
have faces, just their shadows that turn skinny out my bedroom door.
I am told by many that what I write is bullshit, garbage, and non
motivating. I am often reminded of not being educated, nor smart. My
hate mail runs further than a king's scroll, and the worst part is I
have no idea who they are, and even though at time this hurts, I will
continue to write what comes to me, and what makes sense to me. I
write to you, not them. What they don't understand is that everything
I write is about Weightlifting, but they will never understand this,
just like they will never sit at this table. Already I have written a
paragraph about weightlifting, what you take out of it is up to you.
I guess these thoughts run through my head 33,000 feet in the air as I
drink little cups of sprite, while carving little bites into pretzels
to see what shape I can make them, all while mentally writing a diary
about the odd things that enter my mind.

A time machine that gives me the great chance to meet others. A
flying machine that can bring people close to do what we love, and
lifting weights is one of them. Hard is an understatement, traveling
the Country conducting certs while training full time seems almost
impossible, and at times can break me down more than the weights. A
large coffee and the love for what we do keeps me moving. A large
coffee gets me off the airport floor after a 7 hour lay over. A
chance to see a whole gym slam bars and PR gets me in the cab to the
hotel. The growth of the sport gets my travel size tooth past out to
brush my teeth at 7 AM in a motel outside of the city. The chance
to meet others and to be accepted in their world makes me walk even
faster to their gym door as the nervous twitches take over while I
tuck my shirt in before walking in. Have I ever thrown up before a
cert..... yes. I attack a cert just like I do a competition, and for
this the same effects apply. Shit, I attack everything in life like
a competition. I will fly 'til my plane goes down, and I will never
stop writing no matter how long the scroll of words may be.

I know you, and you know me, and because of this we must never leave
the Orchestra empty, we must keep the dark bright and the skeletons
happy. I am behind your screen while you read this, we are both
addicted to lifting weights, and lifting weights is what we shall do.

424

Anyone who tells us different may not enter this blog, they may not eat the pretzels 33,000 feet high. The joy the bar gives us makes us spread that same joy to other things in life, and for this we are forever grateful. Grabbing that bar makes writing possible, makes me turn my cheek to the hate, makes me focus on the family of lifters who care about happiness on top of many other things. Grabbing that bar is only the start, a great way to start your day. I cheers to you, the one who keeps me going, the one who I will some day hopefully meet. This thing of ours, because that's what it is..... ours, this thing is growing, and it's exciting.

I am 33,000 feet high, and all I can think about is lifting weights.

Cheers my friend 2016

♪♪♪

Hang Gliding

Monday, December 10, 2012

Wiggle your toes while you pull, just to make sure the heels hold the weight of the world. Better yet, wiggle your toes before you break the floor, putting you in a ready position, a position of "if I let go of this bar I will fall back on my ass". A position that soon will soon have you hanging over the edge of a cliff, a high up cliff that has you scared to look down. So you look straight ahead, beyond the jagged rocks, a place where you can see yourself, a place where the drive of destination takes over and your mind becomes free. Hold on to the bar like you would the gliding kite that spreads above you. Now pull. Fly like super man and hold on tight, for this bar is the only thing between you and a long drop to failure. Pick up speed. Faster! Now drive your shoulders over the bar and embrace the freedom that only you can feel. Freedom that others will never understand nor experience. The pull becomes weightless if done right. If timed perfectly, the bar itself truly comes alive, making you find yourself on a ride at Disney Land.

Over the cliff you go, fast and powerful, free and enlightened, strong and in control. This is a ride, a ride through weightlifting, a ride throughout this crazy life we live. Jumping off the cliff means doing what we love, putting happiness over money, and helping others throughout our pull. Pull for you, and that alone will spread to others. Sometimes being selfish is the best way to give. Drink your coffee while pulling for friends. Pull this weight up off the ground and notice the family members that sit upon the spinning kilo plates waving with proud smiles. Where do you see yourself this high? What do you take from this experience? Put your book down, and read yourself. Pull yourself up when you are down. This is why the pull is so important in weightlifting. Let the roots from the ground take your tree trunk legs higher than any drug. Ride the white dog to save the princess, and if you don't think this is real, then wiggle your toes. If you don't get over, then you will never get back. "Everything in weightlifting is back, not up"- Paul Doherty.

What do I see this high? I see myself sitting in Room 2 staring out the window with the other special kids. I see myself crying before class because of fear and embarrassment. I see myself dancing in the crystal layer of white smoke and taking dips into the sea of brown bags and pink codeine rivers. Looking back, I don't regret anything, but I am glad that I decided to jump. I am glad I became a cliff hanger. I am glad that I pulled back to move forward. I am glad I realized that living high was really living low, and in order to truly become high was to pull. My career really took off when I decided to let go, and let go I did. Who was I to trust myself? So I pulled. I stayed on my heels and pulled for dear life, and oh how dear this life really truly is. When you pull you jump, when you jump you gain courage, when you gain courage you pull, when you pull you cliff hang, when you hang glide you see life in a different light. Goodnight.

Superman Pull 2016

♪ ♪ ♪

Salt Water

Wednesday, December 19, 2012

Welcome home my friend, grab your violin and begin playing the emotion of your choice. Play loud my friend, so the skeletons that sit high up in the balconies above can hear you. Hang your coat and open your eyes wide as you slide down the waterfall of fun. The outside advice can be cold and sharp, but in here, on this stage, in this dark room, the advice is all from your own skeletons that never seem to make any

noise no matter how good you play. Why are the floor seats empty, but
the balcony seats full? It only takes one skeleton to stand tall out
of his seat, this is good. You have gotten what you have been looking
for, or better yet what you weren't. "Our past is out best advise, our
scars are our best guide, and our problems are our best solutions,"
says your skeleton, this blog, this sticky stage full of salt. Living
in the back seat of my car is where I found the Orchestra. A small
line of elephants marched right over the back seat arm rest and into
the trunk. I stuck my head through only to find that all the little
elephants turned into a room with just one very big elephant. A 500
pound elephant that had been following me around everywhere, without
me even knowing was looking straight at me. I was no longer in a
trunk, just the dark, dark everywhere, nothing else..... well, besides
the elephant. Skeletons started pouring out of my mouth, and water
came pouring out of my eyes, creating a little pond that the elephant
began to gulp down with his long trunk. I didn't start out playing the
violin, of course not. You probably didn't either. I was taught by
the white bones. They would play 'til I broke. They would play 'til
I understood, learned, and appreciated. The skeletons played 'til the
vicodin got bored and went home. The crystal mountains I once lived
in, and the snowy white powder that I once played in, soon melted away
through the cracks of the black stage.

His face was nothing but black holes and a white outline, but the
day he reached out the violin for me to play, was the day I saw more
detail and expression than I had ever seen in any one's face, or any
thing's face. So I played, and I still do, with an audience filled
with my own past, sitting in the top row looking down. There is
nothing motivating about this blog my friend, nothing special about
this Orchestra, simply just a trunk full of black. The trunk space
is endless; there is no surprise ending. My pain hurts worse than
before, which is a constant Advil popper, because the exact opposite
seems to make more sense. How could this be? The more I get to know
myself today, the more I cringe thinking about before. The more I
come to the realization that I will never talk to him again.... makes
me sick. Maybe this is why there is always one empty seat high above.
I find beauty in strings of truth, only bright happy orchestras play
songs full of lies while their elephants are caged under the stage
and their skeletons locked away in the dressing room closets. I am a
prisoner of myself. There are times when I am the biggest Jon North
hater. I find myself typing hate mail to myself, and writing devilish
stuff on bodybuilding.com, but who can stop me? I can't. The walls
shake like bombs dropping all around, only to find that the falling

dust from the ceiling is from the weights dropping. Maybe I will one day take a peak outside to find the person who is really writing this blog. Who is the guy on the radio? Who is this teacher they call coach? What happened to frank the tank? aka J-NO? I will tell you one thing, what you're reading is me. A place where I continually find myself, a place I can be myself. I am so glad you came across this letter. I live in this blog, never to see light again, besides the slight glow from your computer screen. It's okay though, I like it here. I like when you join me. I wish you luck though in the real world with that crazy mother fucker Jon North, the dude is nuts, and if you can run, run for your trunk. You know where to find me. Let your skeleton teach you how to play so you can play with me one day. Slide down your salt water of falling puke and enter a world full of weightlifting and family. Enter a world of you. Salute.

The Orchestra 2016

♪ ♪ ♪

The Sleep Program

Sunday, December 23, 2012

I feel that as a weightlifter, we must live the lifestyle of a weightlifter in order to achieve what we have set off to achieve. 8 to 10 hours of sleep sounds nice to the average Joe, but forcing this kind of sleep is at times training in itself. Trying to stop your spinning mind from ideas, goals, new philosophies, and eager plans, can seem impossible for an athlete that lays restless at night with their eyes wide shut. Sleep is everything. Without it, we the athlete will fall short on the hard path we chose to walk down. The normal human stays up late while laughing at their favorite TV show, while we, the creatures of the darkness, stay locked away with a pillow over our heads trying to keep the bad thoughts from entering our dream world. Thoughts of regret, what ifs, and the worst of all.... thoughts of failure. We find ourselves getting up to go to the bathroom just to move, because moving is what we do best. We get up for a glass of water to grab a sneak peak of what everyone is laughing at in the living room. We are the only people who purposelessly lock ourselves in prison, only to feel freedom. We stay away from the normal world only so we can, for a few brief moments, feel greater than normal. Every night for an athlete is Christmas Eve. The faster we fall asleep, the faster we will be drinking coffee. The faster we drink coffee, the faster we get to do what we love the most..... and that is to train. The best part of training is that it's a magnet, a magnet that brings close friends, family, and teammates to you, and vise versus. Yes, lifting is fun, but lifting with others is even better. Yes, lifting is great, but making new friends is just as great, and what is even more satisfying, is the world you have or are creating for your kids. We the people, we the athletes, have created the best day care, the best environment, and the best life lessons ever for our kids...... the world of training can never be topped. It is a lifestyle that teaches you that pain is good, and that hard work pays off. It is a lifestyle that will be the first to tell you of your mistakes and bad decisions. It is a lifestyle that teaches you the value of a miss, or better yet.... failure.

I was going to write this blog on a weightlifters diet, but I guess the coffee had other plans. It feels good to write something positive, rather than depressing. I never control what I write, I let go completely. I stop thinking 100 percent and rely on pure emotion. Maybe I am in a happy mood because of Christmas. I am happy because for the last few days I have been close to family. It's almost like they have taken my hand and showed me there is more to life than weightlifting, which is a cold world that can drown you in its black fog. Doing my hair, putting on regular people clothes rather than training cloths, and walking around down town, has seemed to put me in a trance of peace and amazement. I find myself dazing off with wandering eyes, like a kid at Disney Land for the first time. What is all this I see? Who are these people and what do they do all day? I am surrounded by a whole world that I once lived in, and now have seemed to forgotten. An alien I am, a lost dog that once had a family but has now forgotten how to sit. I find myself running into people and over apologizing as they keep walking, as if they didn't even see or feel me. I am a one trick pony, and weightlifting is my trick.

10 hours is my perfect amount of sleep. If I hit 11, then I find myself tired throughout the day, sluggish is a better word. I don't know the science behind anything I write, so please be careful what you read, and always ask your coach before performing anything I type. Remember, whatever your coach says is the right way.... period. If I get 8 hours of sleep, then I find myself having a lot of energy early in the morning, but then dying fast in the afternoon. Weird huh? 10 hours, and I'm ready for war, and oh how good the coffee tastes. A rain storm of pr's will fall upon me if my sleep is timed perfectly. Coach knows the minute he sees me if I look ready or not as I walk

into the gym, following with one of his most asked questions, "How many hours of sleep did you get last night, Jon?". This is what makes coach Pendlay such a good.... wait, great coach, is that he knows each and every one of his athletes to the T, and understands that our ticking hands tick at different rhythms. I am the Champ and therefore coach is the Champ. I am a freak athlete, and because of this coach is as well. What is coach doing late at night while all his weightlifters are asleep? I wonder. Maybe this is when he creates his world famous programing. Maybe as we all sleep with smiles, coach is planning his master plan while he writes by a fire place dipping his bird feather pin into the ink that sits by the side of coffee. What does coach cry about at night? He will never say, but I wonder at times what his Dark Orchestra would look like. What would his violin type? I have always wondered why the program sheet he passes out to us before training has small ink splashes throughout the paper. This blog started out positive and I can feel my typing becoming more and more dark. I better stop now before I turn this blog into another letter of sadness, or better yet... reality.

Merry Christmas 2016

♪ ♪ ♪

Champ

Wednesday, December 26, 2012

New Attitude Nation Video - "The Champ"

Olympics 2016

♪ ♪ ♪

Jack & Tess

I guess this article could pass as a diary, a diary about a hooker,
a diary about all the friends I have somehow run into during the
last decade. Who knew the guy selling me a gym membership at 24
Hour Fitness would end up being one of my best friends. I mean think
about the odds of us being alive. Getting the chance to type this
diary to you is something that I don't think our minds were meant
to understand. I guess this is where the word Faith comes from,
trusting something that truly makes no sense. 500 years ago, a man
named Jack had to have sex with a hooker named Tess for me to be
here writing this blog to you. Yes I know, if you need some time to
think about that before you continue reading, then please, take your
time. Because of Jack and Tess's life decisions 500 years ago, I
got approached at Power House Gym by a man named Matt that owned The
Nutri-Shop down the street. This is when I was sleeping in my car,
living homeless, scrapping up enough money to eat at McDonald's so I
had enough energy to train...... of course I took the job. Matt is
still a very dear friend.

Thank the Lord that in year 264 BC, a Gladiator named Shark and a
wanderlust Princess named Bella hooked up to create you, the reader.
You must send Shark a thank you card, or just honor them by having fun
this New Year's Night. The thought of us being the start of someone
becoming.... well someone, a million years down the road makes me
drink more coffee. But then again we didn't start it, we are just a
part of the life chain of people we meet and run into. Because I was
bad at school, I went to a junior college only because I was good at
football, and because of football I took a summer painting class for
credits that lead me to my wife, which lead me to Sac State, which
then lead me to weightlifting, which has finally lead me to writing
you tonight. So thank you Lord for not giving me the gift of being
book smart, or what I should really say is thank you lord for making
whomever down the long line of the family chain not book smart, and
also thank you to the stud caveman aka - freak athlete in his or her
time that made me.... me.

Every time I take a sip of this hot coffee, my memories takes me back
to past friends I have met throughout my path to now. Some very good
friends, and others that probably don't even remember me, but all have
left a stamp on my outcome. I am a result of them, just a melting

pot of influences, just like weightlifting. Everywhere I walk, they
walk beside' me, you know who you are. Every time I tell a joke,
it's the joke I stole from them.   Once I was opening the doors for
people at T.G.I.Fridays 'til 2 AM, and now when I take people out to
eat at Fridays I can't stop but to smile from all the crazy pranks
and memories that slap me in the face, and how broke I was! Man I was
broke. Man I was hungry. Man I had dreams I wanted to achieve, but I
will tell you one thing, I was never happier. Back then, all I needed
was my Jessica, a couch, and a weight room. I lived on pennies but
I was rich with friends, a support group that could carry me further
than I could carry myself. I have always had the best of friends, why
is this? I don't try, it's not like I am a judge on a reality show
looking for the best friend with the best qualities. I guess I am
just naturally drawn to truly good people, amazing people, positive,
and uplifting people. I think you the reader can relate, if you are
reading this blog then we understand each other, we get each other,
we are friends. You the reader is this blog, and this blog has had
probably one of the biggest impacts in my life.

I was thinking about giving shout outs to all who I am thankful
for..... but that would take way too long, and you the reader might
get bored. I will say thank you to you, the whole Dark Orchestra
Family, the Whole Attitude Nation Family, my blood family, my wife
and dog daughter family, and to all my friends I have made over the
years...... you know who you are, thank you. Happy New Year.

PS: Thank you to Jack and Tess for having sex 500 years ago.

Happy New Year 2013!

♪ ♪ ♪

432

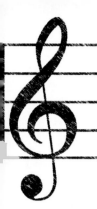

CHAPTER 17

THE DARK ORCHESTRA
2013

Bloody Smiles

Wednesday, January 9, 2013

Our smiles, bloody from the bar hitting our chin, with shaded faces from the dead tree that hangs over our platform, and black eyes that seem to stay hidden from the hood that lays over our beat up thoughts. We like to think we have cast them out, only to find that we are the ones who have been out casted. A double edge sword makes my hand bleed from emotion and too much coffee. Word choices I wish I could take back, but an overall point that I hope killed the 500 pound elephant. Keep walking hooded man, stay invisible, get to the gym without being seen. Train with rhythm, train with pride, train in the dark only to make the light feel warm on your skin. Drink your coffee while the rush of life rushes down to your toes. I understand you, you understand me, they understand mediocrity. They understand what they have been told to understand. We understand what our minds tell us to understand. You know who they are, they come in all different shapes and sizes, they are whoever you see them as, they are different for everyone. They will never understand what we do and why we do it. We live by a different set of rules, three white light rules, a program of rules that keeps us steady, strong, and balanced. Speak loud to the ones who listen. Be strong for the ones who fight with you, understand you, want to understand you, believe in the goal, the task at hand. Change lives, while at the same time fully commiting to yourself. I heard your speech at the end. My chipped tooth and bloody mouth smiled with reassurance that at times this life does not offer. Only we can make the world around us. The world we are making is loving, strong, and powerful.

435

BEN
CLARIDAD

Keep walking, keep training, keep an eye open for the ones who want
to join our shaded world. Our jungle of iron, our beds of dreams,
and our hearts full of anger and happiness. I love this sport
more than anything, but this sport is not what brings us together,
it's the lifestyle we have created, not joined, but created. The
iron life, the bloody mouth way of teaching, living, learning, and
achieving. A bloody mouth means we have bitten the dust, hit the
floor, hit the wall, but got the fuck up to smile about it. White
teeth shine through the blood only because we brush our teeth a
lot, "why?", they ask, well actually they don't ask why because we
don't exist to them. Our teeth are white because we take care of
ourselves. We not only train hard, but brush hard. We don't only
brush hard but we eat breakfast hard. We do everything hard, and
because of this addiction, we even take the hard way to get to our
goals. We like hard, even if easy seems easier. A hard life means
tougher skin. Your hard life means that I have something to learn
from you, and vice versus.

We are not training, our skeletons are training. Our deepest
darkest cuts that slash across our chests, bleed through our shirts
while we gasp for more air. More is what we want, more pr's, more
training, more life, more motivation, more family, more kids, more
of everything. If there is one thing that weightlifting has taught
me, it's that the pain is good, pain is the best coach anyone could
ever ask for. Give me pain over pleasure, and my pleasure will be
greater than any pleasure ever experienced. I see you under that hood,
to me you are clear as day, even though to them you are a freak, a
non existing outcast of a human life. Why are all our gyms tucked
away from the population? Why are our gyms off a small deserted
road? We are shunned, not welcomed. We train in the darkest of the
gyms. But here is what they don't understand, they are welcome any
time. We take the high road. Our gyms are brighter than any Gold's
Gym. Our gyms are warmer than any 24 Hour Fitness. Our dirt is
gold, our bloody smiles are wide, or scarred hearts beat the hardest.
Our skeletons have become our friends, a bond of acceptance and
understanding. A brotherhood of freaks who live in the dark, let's
keep training.

Freedom 2016

♪ ♪ ♪

436

Cab Driver

His coffee cup was half full and stained from such an ongoing use of consumption there was really no time for cleaning. A way of thinking I can relate to. I leaned over his right shoulder from the back seat and whispered that I didn't have time for percentages. His response was a puff from his half lit cigarette and a drink from his luke warm coffee. It would never have crossed his mind that the coffee cup was half empty, I know this from the simple smile that came across this unusual cab driver's face after taking a 3 in the morning sip of his best friend. 5 minutes into the cab ride and still no talking, even though we were having a great conversation while staring out into the dark night. The smoke from his cigarette never bothered me, because it smelled just like the steam from my tea. His elbow pointed out the window in an upward direction from all four windows being broken. It looked as if we were sliding down the top of a house key, and into a laser tag arena from the outside lights shooting through the cab's windshield.

Another seminar to coach, another customer to drive. Another late night training, another late night driving. No music, which made the ride a little awkward at first, but after the silence crept in the outside world was blaring with sounds, sounds that made the cab driver bang on the steering wheel while occasionally grabbing his Babe Ruth bobble head so it wouldn't slide around the dash board. He drove with such rhythm, such speed, but at the same time with such relaxation. No worry in the world, just a cab drive with coffee and a midnight smoke. A gold chain around his hairy neck that had a picture of an old lady in black and white. A folded up book on how to draw, and a flashing clock that wasn't even set. Time to him did not exist, what's the point? What's the big deal with time anyway? This is what he said to me without saying anything at all, only a very smooth drag from his smoke, and another smile after drinking miss brown eyes from his yellow finger nails and calloused hands. Happy, nothing more, nothing less. Two people in the back seat as if we knew each other for years. Or better yet... like we were never there. Still no talking, besides a slight cough that led to another, then a long chug from the life juice that keeps him company on these late nights of driving. Driving his life, driving us, driving coffee to his soul, only to drive to get more. The whole world is asleep besides him. Driving throughout the night passing through every green light you could imagine. He waves to the local police as he drives by, while keeping his eyes straight forward, the cold wind outside blows out his cigarette, does he notice, of course not, he ain't got time to notice, he only has time to max out. At this point, the smoke is completely out, but he still puffs away with his eyes on the road, focused, getting work done, training hard in his own way. A part of the Attitude Nation and he doesn't even know it.

This cab driver reminded me why I ain't got time for percentages, because he doesn't. There ain't no percentages for feeding your family. There ain't no percentages for doing your job, being happy, riding the rhythm of the night with Babe Ruth. There ain't no percentages for the hard workers, the late night smokers, the Miss Brown Eye's lovers, the cab drivers. Weightlifting is like the real world, it's always max out time. Windows broken like my back, coffee mug stained like my chalky hands, driving with speed and precision like a weightlifter does with the bar. Rhythm of the night like rhythm in the gym. There is no difference between this cab driver and me, from him to you, you to me. No time to set the clock, we don't need to be reminded when and what to do because we are there before the clock could ever do its job. We don't live because we are told to, we live because its what we want to do. Freedom is what this man has that many don't. Freedom is why we roll down the windows at night. Freedom is why he drives with so much rhythm. The cab driver has reminded me why I drink coffee, why I drive with the AC up and windows down, because we are free.

The cab driver dropped us off while still not speaking, only a popped trunk like Tyson Hips, and a bag grab and drop like the hit and catch drill. We missed each other's eye contact, and then that was that. He drove off into the night with smoke swirling out from his broken windows. Off to max out in life, to be rewarded with family and happiness. His cab was beat to bloody hell, his finger nails were yellow, his bobble head didn't stay in one place, and his coffee cup was a mess......... He ain't got time for percentages.

Max Out 2016

♪ ♪ ♪

438

Still Standing

I came across this poem below that I wrote in 9th Grade while digging through some dusty old memory boxes hidden away in the closet. Pictures of my child hood. Home made movies. A box full of good times and great memories. Happy times that no one can take from me. A picture of my mom and dad getting married.....weird. A birthday letter I wrote to my father in 3rd grade. F report cards next to hundreds of poems and stories I used to write in my room. I forgot how much I used to write.....I forgot how angry I was. But where did this anger come from? All these pictures and home movies show a happy family with a happy kid. I was the most loving kid in the whole world, the happiest damn kid my mom would tell me repeatedly, but deep down I was a troubled kid with many problems by looking at this box full of crinkled papers I put to writing. Hot or cold. Bomb out or gold. In jail or buying a house. Happy or sad. Very close to my dad, now couldn't be further away. An extreme lifestyle that started I guess when I was born. An angel and demon on each shoulder that has no understanding of compromise. Why this broken heart growing up? Why the running away from home? Why the drug and alcohol use? What was I trying to hide from, or make go away?

I guess the Dark Orchestra started in 5th grade when I wrote my first poem for class. The teacher called in my mom and step dad to talk about how disturbing she thought my writing was, and where it was coming from. They said it was "too dark" for a kid my age. The Dark Orchestra was born, the skeletons were lining up to enter my closet in a single file line. Councilor after councilor I went through. Story after story I wrote with pain in my pencil. I would write at the bus stop, or while I slept in the woods when I was a run away. I would write high as a kite at 2 AM. Thank you writing for letting a confused kid express himself.

Here is the poem I wrote and read in front of my class in high school. It was a contest where I ended up placing dead last. They said it was a little "too dark" for this type of competition. Words I have heard before. Another F, another brick on my back. People ask me how I became the weightlifter I am today, and I tell them it was from all the years of fighting with myself that has made me stronger than any weightlifting program could ever accomplish. No regrets in life. Never dwell on the past, for without the past you would not be you today. Use what you have been through to your advantage. Just like the cab driver in my last blog, his coffee cup was half full, not half empty. Salute.

Still Standing

by Jonathan North

My tears have fallen
My knees have shaked
I've been hit torn and stabbed
but never lose fate
I've slipped into holes with no escape
trying to look for a hand to help
but always too late
My small steps are still young
for long strides I may fall
Deep holes keep me down
but never I stall
On my hands and knees I crawl
then to stand tall
for eyes I see
but no response from my call
Which path do I take
Which decision do I make
I feel so lost and empty and built up with hate
searching for the one to speak words that relate
So I wait, soon I will be followed
for it's my turning point of tomorrow
A shadow that casts a brighter light on my sorrow
the anger and frustration I will never have to swallow
My insides have been beaten
My skin hasn't been touched
I will fight this war
Never give up
Rest my head to sleep and fierce to wake up
I never burn down
with bricks on my back in water don't drowned

Pencil & Paper 2016

♪ ♪ ♪

440

Mike! Let The Sun In!

Monday, January 21, 2013

Across the gym, I yelled with my hands cupped around my mouth,
"Hey Mike, open that garage door so the sun can pierce through our
iced coffees and onto our platforms!". I yelled in slow motion, as
millions of little drops of spit came flying out of my mouth while my
eyes were shut strong. Bars being lifted up and down like the keys on
a piano. Smiles washed away with anger. A grave yard of past away
energy drinks lay at rest below our feet, as we rumbled and tumbled
around the gym like a school yard play ground. Old coffee cups like
skeletons on a pirate ship hanging around as if the cups were still a
part of the team, which they truly are. Atmosphere and a good support
structure is everything. Mike let the sun in! Let the warmth hit our
face reminding us how great it is to be alive, how lucky we are to be
able to do what we love. It would look as if I was waving to you from
the other side of the gym Mike, but what I am doing is flying through
the land of dust and chalk that the sun has made visible on this early
morning in a... well, a very dusty gym. Dust mixed with chalk has put
me slap dab in the middle of a snow storm, a wild storm that has me
fighting for my life, as I gasp for every breath, thankfully finding
shelter underneath the chair I call my safe place. Let the light in
Mike! Give this gym life, let this gym breath! Let the world hear the
techno music. Try to make the neighbors mad at us, if accomplished
then good news... this means we must be training well. Lift weight
shirtless only to feel the sun shine through the gym door. Learn how
to train, don't worry about technique right now, just train. Don't
worry about the program, just train. Don't worry about your body,
just train... just feel the morning sun and the kisses from your
coffee. This is how you get strong... by training.

I think us weightlifters appreciate the sun more than anybody. The
bottom of the titanic can become overwhelmingly smokey, dark, and
tiresome. Shoveling coal can make our back hurt, our thoughts a little
scattered, and our souls heavy. Us weightlifters need sunlight to
make maximum attempts. Open that mother fucken door Mike, and let life
punch us in the face! Breath in the dust, pour the cold coffee over
your face, shovel that coal into the fire to keep this machine of a gym
we have built moving! Let me walk around the gym with wide shoulders
and broken hands. The weak minded aren't welcome in the fortress of
sun and dust, atmosphere is everything. Let me wrap my knees while my
fingernails bleed from the hook grip I have strangled them with. Sun

441

and coffee, coach and teammates, music and the bar. All bad mother
truckers who spend their day with brothers who fight for the same
thing... gold. Mike opened the door as if he was raising the MDUSA
flag above the gym, while in slow motion, the sun crept up my body
and over my motionless face. The spit from my yell across the gym
was falling slowly like a paper plane running out of speed. My eyes
opened from being shut so strong, and then it happened........Someone
pushed play and.....well nothing really happened, coach told me to stop
looking like a zombie and lift the bar.

Strong Legs 2016

♪♪♪

Power Belly

Tuesday, January 29, 2013

Rolling bellies and waving hands dance around the dinner table as
we eat together under the golden lights of this beautiful Italian
Restaurant. We laugh around the table as if a teammate just ducked
walked a lift while spinning into a 180, then standing! I point my
finger across the table with a look that loudly reads, "You, son of a
bitch!". Chris Gute, you know I'm talking about you. Ha! Rewarding
our bodies from the battle, we eat....and eat hard. It's not all
about gaining weight, it's about recovery, and the more recovery you
feed your body, the more weight you will gain. We must gain more
weight. We must wake up in the middle of the night and eat a PB&J
with a cold glass of chocolate milk. Extra scoop of creatine in case
training goes into overtime. A blended protein shake with snicker
bars, gummy bears, and chicken alfredo from last night's left overs.
Why gummy bears you may ask? I truly believe that sugar is good for
athletes; it makes us strong, powerful, and ready for the world.

Making your body happy is so underrated. I look at it as rewarding my
body from everything it has done for me. A happy belly makes for a
happy training session. People always ask me how to gain more weight,
or that they are having trouble packing on the pounds, and my first
response is always the same, don't just eat more of your "healthy"
foods, eat more foods that your belly likes. Let fat into your life,
let calories into your life, let bread, for good Lord sakes, into your
life! You want scientific backing, well I got it right..........well

no, I don't have any. This is why I don't write a lot about food and diet, because I don't know much about it. But the diet I have created for my skeletons in this Dark Orchestra has worked wonders for them and me. They have stronger bones, bigger bones, power bellies....(which every weightlifter has), and they can go longer in training and recover better than any other. The key word for this blog is athlete, and not civilian. Athletes like ourselves must intake more of everything, not just more of some things. More sleep, more food, more water, more sugar, more milk, more coffee, more TRAINING!

Slap hands and tuck your napkin in your shirt while bonding with your teammates. After a workout, meeting up with your fellow gym family and eating is better training than actual training itself. I only write about what I have seen, nothing else. And I have seen remarkable achievements accomplished by bonding, laughing, trusting, and loving, all gravitated towards food. Meet up at the deli of Safeway, and eat. Slide the mayo across the table and eat. Extra steak on my sandwich?.......ummm fuck yea. Don't stop eating even after you're full, this is so important. STOP LISTENING TO YOUR BODY! I just can't stress this enough, in training and in eating. Train your body to eat, just like training it to train. There is no such thing as full, only recovered.

In my opinion, football games are won in the weight room, in the dorms, at triple keg parties. Weightlifting meets are won from happy bellies, and a good relationship with your coach and teammates. What a better way to attract all of this than eating. For those that are on a strict diet, that's ok! Attitude Nation is all about doing what works for you! Ac up windows down. But, for athletes on a semi strict diet that are wanting to add some pounds to better themselves in their sport, try this. Once a week or even once every two weeks, go out and eat a lot of whatever your diet does not allow you to eat. My favorite place to eat when my weight gets down, is a pizza buffet. Coach takes me there and force feeds me 'til I almost throw up. Lol, it's awful. Eating is hard, especially when we are forcing food down your mouth throughout the day when you are already full. I always say that the day I retire from this sport, I am going to weight 90 pounds because I am never going to eat again. It's so true though, think about it. For us athletes, every time we eat it's because we have to for recovery, or to gain weight. I can't even remember the last time I ate because I was hungry. When I retire from this sport, I will happily retire from food. I will clean up my non-athlete diet and probably eat very clean, but not now. Now it's war.

I ain't got time for healthy food, only food that is going to make me lift bigger weight. I don't give a rat's ass about how healthy I am, all I care about is winning. After I am done winning, I will get my monthly doctor's check up. We must not forget why we are eating the way we are, is it because it's good for you, whatever that really means, or because it's helping us become better athletes? Diets to me are like general strength training programs, I still have no idea what they mean. In my opinion, everything in life is specific, we must be specific, and that goes for eating as well. I hate food, but I love getting strong. I love this blog. I love Italian food. I love a happy belly. Salute.

Eat 2016

♪ ♪ ♪

Your Move

Tuesday, February 5, 2013

Different strokes for different folks. Different strides for different minds. A different paint brush for every artist as they paint their masterpiece. A swimmer swims fast to win, but how that individual swims is up to the camp he trains in, lives in, and bleeds in. There is no wrong way to lift weights. The sport of weightlifting is getting the bar from the floor to overhead in one motion, or for the second part of the sport, two motions. How you get it there doesn't matter. This ain't a beauty contest. The only thing that truly matters is winning. There is more than one way to get to the top of the hill. This battle between coaches is laughable to me. I sometimes feel as if I'm watching children fighting over a toy in the sandbox. There is so much hatred in weightlifting, and not enough improvement. Take as many seminars as you can. Talk to as many coaches as you can get your hands on. Train at different training camps, read different articles. Become a melting pot of ideas and methods and then poor it on yourself, or better yet... your athletes.

Is my way of lifting the best way? Of course it is, I would be crazy not the think so, and I hope you as a coach think the same

about your way. Do I understand and respect other styles of
technique and programing? Absolutely. An open mind is the secrete
to becoming a champion, without it your athletic career will shut
down like a small business in the depression. I learn every damn
day, I never stop. I wake up and look for better ways to benefit
myself and others. This goes for weightlifting and life. How can
I lift even more weight than I am now? How can I become a better
husband, a better friend, a better family member? How can I become
a better man? I have been on every lifting program known to man,
and every different style of technique as well, and with much trial
and error I have found a way that has produced gold medals and the
great opportunity to represent my Country. Even my way has wiggle
room, and many different styles that can be done within it. You
can add arm bend if you like, or if you prefer, keep those arms
nice and straight. Add in a dynamic pull to your liking, add more
feet, or less......it's totally up to you, not me. Do you like a
slower pull, or faster? Does the bar slightly drag your thigh on
the "superman pull"? Or as an athlete, do you like a little bit of
space between you and the bar? Do you like pulling back a little
earlier, or do you like staying over longer? You choose. I only
show up to a Seminars to help, never to become a dictator. I teach
a style of lifting that has helped many athletes better themselves
in Crossfit, Weightlifting, or just crush PR's and getting them one
step closer to their goal. But I don't take credit for the athlete's
success, absolutely not. The reason is because every athlete on the
planet is going to lift differently than the person next to them. I
always say that there is a million different styles of technique,
why? Because there are a million lifters in the world who move
in all sorts of brilliant and fascinating ways that can never be
taught. This is why I am so in love with weightlifting, the beauty
that lies in each athlete amazes me. I sometimes feel I am in the
safari watching different animals stock their prey, and then pounce
on their prey killing everything in their way. Every time, I jump
out of my chair and watch in complete amazement. No coach can
take credit for rhythm. No coach can claim instinct. This is the
athlete's accomplishment. Did we as coaches help them find their
way, their lift, their movement? Yes. This in my opinion is what
coaching is all about, helping an athlete find their niche, their
power button, their motivation and their strengths. Yes athletes
should be taught a way, a rough draft as I call it, but then like
a teenage bird, they must sooner or later spread their wings and do
whatever they need to do to fly... and not fall.

Watching an athlete smoke a PR.....well, it's one of the biggest
joys of my life, even if I don't even know them. Seeing an athlete
hug their coach after a win hits home to me, and in my opinion is
what sports are all about. I can relate to the emotional feelings
the athlete and coach share, because I have been there before, and
hope to soon visit this feeling again. Every kilo counts, and every
little advice helps. Even advice that you choose not to keep helps
tremendously! Who are you as an athlete? You will never know unless
you try, and trying can lead you down a dead end, which will then turn
you around so you can find your way. Fail is the best teacher.

For all the coaches who talk bad about me, who send me hate mail,
who tell others my style of technique is wrong, well my friends they
deserve a hug, and maybe one day I can give them one. I am not going
to rant or get mad, there is no reason to. I simply feel bad for the
blind fold these coaches are putting around their athlete's head. I
simply hope one day they can open their mind to a world full of ideas
and methods, a world full of paint brushes that
paint incredible paintings. A power snatch is
still a snatch. There is no such thing as an
ugly lift, just a missed lift or made lift. There
is no in between. This is my opinion blog. If
you disagree then great, that's what this blog
is all about. That's what the Attitude Nation
is all about. Do what works for you.

230KG PR set of 5

Lift Big Weight 2016 2016

♪♪♪

Time

Monday, February 11, 2013

I have found that the state of mind you're in, can damage your
perception of time and place, luring you into more of an idea or a
dream that can take complete control of your perception of reality.
The hands on your watch haven't ticked in years, in fact, they have
fallen off all together. Your once moving watch has been replaced
with moving bars that now direct your day. I can't seem to remember

446

where the time went, from when my non-callused hands touched the bar
to now. Memories flash as I chalk, and feelings hit when lifting.
Lost in translation as we feign for PR's like heroin addicts to
heroin. What time is it? Who is the President? Where the bloody hell
am I? Questioning the program is not allowed in this lifestyle of
sport, just like how clocks don't exist in a Las Vegas Casino. Just
bet, time doesn't matter. Just lift, nothing else matters. What
matters is how many chips that proudly stand guard in front of you.
Like a weightlifter with our medals, we immerse ourselves into a
sea of blood and sacrifice, only to come up for air when real life
calls out. But calling out is a rare privilege, and at times unheard
of. Just before you ask yourself why your watch does not have hands,
shades of black ripple like water from coach looking down upon you,
pushing your head back into the bloody sea of red. A cold chill
rushes through the gym, gliding over your sweaty skin and leaving you
peering out the gym door for I guess some sort of hope, or maybe some
sort of new excitement, or even something that my watch nor myself can
answer. We are saddened by a dark shadow facing our direction, with
little evidence on where or what the shadow is looking at, hit in the
face with the cold hard truth that we the weightlifters were born for
lifting, breaking chains, and crushing rocks, one hit at a time.

Why are the walls in my gym black? And why is USADA circling my house?
Coffee mixed with Day Quil leaves me behind my front door with a pair of
weightlifting shoes and my straps, ready to defend this perception of
whatever the fuck is going on. Teammates come and go, but I am still
here. New gyms replace old gyms, new shoes hang up old shoes, and all
the while I haven't moved from my resting seat. I write to you tonight
to try to figure out our mind set, our reality that we have created
for ourselves to live in with our own rules, patterns, guidelines,
and language. It's fascinating, but at the same time when woken from
this different perception, I find myself lost in the outer world, and
confused on what time really means to regular mother fuckers. Am I the
white sheep, or are they? Is USADA after me, or just doing their job?
I will be in the same place tomorrow lifting the same 20 kilo bar while
drinking the same coffee on my same resting seat. It's almost as if I am
writing you from the future, even though I'm really in the present. If
I see you tomorrow in my gym, that means we both traveled to a place we
knew existed from our knowledge right now. Right? I can predict tomorrow
by drinking tea tonight. I have seen tomorrow tonight, and by writing
you tonight.....right now.....or whatever right now means....if you read
this while I am in my resting seat tomorrow, that means I am actually
living in the future while you have been taken back to the past.

I am lost in translation. But I am not lost in life, nor
weightlifting. I have, we have, created our own time, own structure
that guides us to happiness and to our goals. Our time is a much
different meaning than a librarian's time, or any other lifestyle
or career chosen by a particular person. Our watch is the bar, our
calendar is meets and competitions. Coach is nothing more than a
shadow of a metaphor that screams train hard without screaming at all.
I have no idea what time or day it is, all I know is that tomorrow I
will be sitting in my resting chair drinking coffee. See you in the
future my friend. Goodnight.

Bar Clocks 2016

♪ ♪ ♪

Hoarders

Wednesday, February 13, 2013

A handful of weightlifters pull a trailer of weightlifting equipment
to the empty warehouse that has made its home to spiders, dust,
loneliness, and an unknown identity. No truck can pull this trailer
that we will soon feed to the gym, for only a weightlifter's pull can
handle this colorful array of circles that we all cherish so much.
Weight, that's all it is. Round weights that are heavy. Weight that
has most people run away, but we pull a trailer down the middle of
the street to lift. This my friends is why we are outcasts; we are
freaks that get a high off lifting shit. Up, then down, then we spin
all around......freaks, and boy how I fucken love it. But see freak
is an identity that we have, and I bet the empty gym would love as
well. An identity creates relationships, and relationships create
understanding, something this gym will soon learn, as we continue to
pull to feed the beast with this goal.

Green veins from the monsters we chug, and wings to help us pull
faster from the red bulls we crush. Adopting weights for a new home
that awaits. A gym is the mother and these sons of bitches are her
new found kids, and we......well we soon come to find out are the
prisoners of an always growing power. One that I have seen grow from
the day we moved in. We brushed the dust and awoke the gym from
rest. Wake up you gym! We have brought you life! We have brought
you power! We are now you and you are now us. I see you like techno

music, shit.....I do too! You like coffee spilled on your floors,
well I like coffee spilled down my mouth and into my soul. We are
best friends even though I will at times cus and shun you, flip you
off and un-love you. You are my safety net that has many holes, holes
that can lead to missed lifts and constant reminders of how much I
miss my father. Sitting on my resting seat today, I noticed how much
this little gym in a warehouse has grown. I don't mean by teammates
or supporters that watch through the red eye, but by dead coffee
cups that have pushed their way further and further from the gym
boundaries, and into unknown territories where the non weightlifters
walk....you know....those weird sons of bitches. Bars have made new
homes as they rolled away, creating a property line without asking
for the city's approval yet. Platforms have multiplied from pieces
of wood being taken out of their own bodies like clones, and dragged
to a new part of the gym. Jerk racks have magically appeared in a
part of the gym that I didn't even know existed by who the fuck knows.
It's almost as if when the lights shut off, the AA meetings begin,
and the monsters talk about how bad they feel for treating people
like monsters, and the coffee cups cry rivers of pain and sadness
because the humans that were once in love with them, now left them all
alone. Bars roll like weed in a college dorm, and platforms multiply
like a dog's paws when sleeping on the couch. A mind of its own,
and we the one trick ponies of weightlifting, have no idea the life
that surrounds us. The power of all these emotions in a gym, from
the living gym, to our own, make for a hot and cold type of person.
Maybe this is why I have lived my whole life one extreme to the next,
because I channel energy from living things I didn't even know were
alive. The car I drive.....what kind of mood was it in for me to
drive so fast, or slow? Maybe I have mixed too much liquid codeine,
NyQuil and tea together a little too much lately, but it just got me
scratching my head as I found myself noticing a gym that was literally
growing right in front of our eyes......and none of us even noticed.

We pull our own weight, and we create our own atmosphere without
even knowing it. We have nestled into a gym and not only made it
our gym...but our home. We the weightlifters, we are the ultimate
hoarders. We hoard weights and bars, blood towels and scars. We
hoard emotions that we put into lifts that create a storm of chalk
we keep stacked in the back. We hoard medals of all kinds, and
weightlifting shoes like girls and their heels, and if a bar is broken
what do we do? Nothing, we lay it to rest in the corner with the other
bars that build dust and once used chalk that now meet at night and
talk about the good old times. We don't throw shit away, because it's

not shit, it's a part of us. A broken pair of shoes don't ever go in
the garbage, they go in the retirement closet to be smiled at from
time to time from the memories you once shared. The gym is alive,
don't be fooled. Keep slamming bars and feeding it its fuel. We
feed off each other like one brother to another, sister to sister, and
coffee cup to monster. Pull, weightlifters pull!

Graveyard Bars 2016

♪♪♪

The Safe

Wednesday, February 20, 2013

Once a supporter, now a drip of water that falls from the back of
my head as this shower tries its hardest to cleanse me from the
controversy that surrounds my down time. A quiet room is always
the worst, as judging eyes and evil mouths take over my once quiet
thoughts. This is why I don't smoke weed, I analyze things to the
point of no return. Did I say the wrong thing? Did I go too far?
The worst of them all........did I lose a fellow friend, follower,
supporter? But then again, I am reminded by a constant whisper that
everything I say and do - I mean, I am. I never regret, but I stress.
And even though I never second guess, the heavy thoughts that replay
in my head make some nights long like the rain outside. The constant
pounding from water to roof is like a thousand fists trying to break
the walls I call the recovery hibernation station. A place to rest
and rebuild. A place to drain the pain from the fame, and organize
my thoughts and opinions into some sort of organization that will
hopefully make some sense before I rest my head to bed. It pains me
to lose a soldier of the iron game from some sort of crazy action or
rant I might bark upon, but I must be me, without me I am not me. And
by sugar coating anything would be highly non-attitude nation of me,
and 100 percent disrespectful to you- even if you disagree with me on
the topic or action I take part in. I must carry on, even though some
might fall off. They fall like water, everyday and fast, they hit me
before they disappear, and every time my eyes close with insecurity.
It's hard to explain, but with every piece of hate mail I receive,
a rush of losing everything shadows over me, leaving me in a state
of panic. Panic that my family agrees with the letter sent to me.
Panic that the gym door will be locked as I try to pull it open for

450

training. Panic that the Dark Orchestra will move away and leave me
with only my skeletons to talk to and relate to. Panic that fruit and
rocks will be thrown at me while walking on stage to lift. Insecure
you say....you have no idea.

I wish there was a safe that we could lock our thoughts in before
we train. I find that turning off your mind to train is the single
most difficult challenge this sport has presented me with. Focusing
on the idea of going underneath 400 plus pounds can not only make
an athlete's knees shake, but the brain must be able to use all the
concentration it has to register and to control this unbelievably
crazy idea you are presenting it with. If there are any outside
thoughts or concerns - then a missed lift or an injury lurks around
the corner. A new rule states: The safe box must be locked before
entering the work place (aka) the gym. We all need to enforce this
career soaring rule, before this mistake takes us all down with it.
Hesitation is the reason why we miss, and all it takes is a splash of
salt that will have the bar crashing on top of our heavy heads. Yes
the toes wear the crown for most of the misses in this sport, for
they are responsible for more missed lifts than any other technical
problem, but hesitation takes the cake for biggest mental problem any
lifter can make. Hesitation comes in many different shapes and sizes,
forms and disguises. It shows its face from fear. Fear to go under,
fear from the thought of missing, fear from the outside thoughts you
carried onto the platform with you.

"I will let you down, I will make you hurt" - Johnny Cash. I am sorry
now, for I dread the day this happens, and at times I lay awake and I
hope it doesn't happen. I hope when you meet me I don't disappoint.
I hope I don't say something that quiets the room, I think and sit in
when no one is around. You have helped me so much on this journey, all
I want to do is help you like you have me, and be there like you have
for me. Entering this orchestra is why I keep slamming bars. Playing
violins with the skeletons brings joy to my life. The orchestra of
us is a steady dose of real life, real emotion, and real thoughts. A
reality of realism of humbled truths that keep me balanced from the
cocky, in your face Jon North that some seem to love or hate. This is
real. You are real. This quiet room I think in is the devil in the red
dress that must be put to rest. Talking to the callers on air is what
makes me keep chugging coffee. Seeing the seminars grow and people
getting better makes me want to get better. Feeling gold in my hands
makes my eyes water and hands shake. This is what the haters and
hate mail senders will never understand. For every hate mail that is

sent to me, handfuls of gut wrenching, positive, overwhelmingly great emails that have changed my life for the better are sent to me. You hater, you have not stained me. You hater, you are nothing. For every follower that has walked away from my words or actions, an army of new supporters have come together so we can feed off of each other to achieve greatness in sport and life. You reader.....you have no idea how important you are to me. Tonight I write to you, not as Jon North.

2016

♪ ♪ ♪

Third Person

Saturday, February 23, 2013

Just wiped a small piece of lint off my computer screen, where in most cases the lint would have never caught my eye, as I would have been to busy typing away or organizing my ADD thoughts into something that someone would actually find interesting or readable at that. Its late, and I'm tired, and a hot shower sounds so nice. A squint with the eyes to keep myself focused on my writing, and not down the hallway that meets the shower. I imagine myself looking into the refrigerator, even though I know nothing exciting nor new will await me when I take that hopeful peek inside. Why so bland, why so familiar? Walking into the grocery store is like landing on a new planet for the first time, and every time you go back to that planet you want to explore new locations and routs, but instead you visit the same place at the same time while leaving with the same experience. Next time I visit my local market, I am going down aisle 4 instead of aisle 9. I will walk backwards instead of forward, while pulling the cart from the front rather than the back. I will try a sample that looks alien, and next time I will stand in the corner of the store and watch what people buy, interact, move, talk, and shop. I want to watch what I look like from a third persons point of view, and get to the bottom of why I end up with the same foods every time I walk into a land of variety. hmmm - Now I'm analyzing myself in the third persons role looking at others, thinking how others and myself would react to my third person self sitting in a corner watching me and the others shop. Now I'm thinking about how I would never put that odd thought process in my blog, and how this tea might have something in it I'm not aware of.

Is this what Shankle so passionately talks about.....the comfort zone.
Have I become a comfort zone person. I will next time buy a gossip mag
by the check out stand, and pay with a bag of change for my new cart
of no comfort zone foods. Miss you Shankle, you have no idea how much
I miss you. But knowing you are somewhere with your toes in the water
and your shorts all hiked up with a smile on your face after a long
hard day of training and coaching makes me more happy than you will
ever know. Freedom my friend....happiness. Let the sun of Australia
hit your face with warmth and strength, while you privately crack a
smile from the crazy times and memories we once shared. Walk your path
brother, and I will walk mine, and hopefully one day in the future our
paths will meet again, just like that fall day we met at In and Out by
Cal Strength. On this day I asked, "how do I get strong Donny"? "God
damn it son.....you just got to get stronger" - Shankle. OK.

Spinning my wedding ring while drinking tea with a white screen
looking back at me. A blog must be written. Not because I have to,
but because I want to. Want is what keeps us training, want keeps
us reading and writing, want is what makes a kid want to finish
school to support his or her family. Want is freedom. Weightlifting
is freedom. No boss, no judgment, no lies, only hard nosed bar that
will kick the cold hard truth down your throat, but then help you
up once you fall. I must figure out these running thoughts before
they run away. I must grab them from the air and write them down to
share. Grab this barbell and launch it in the air. Now I am getting
jacked up, and I can feel my heart hitting hard as I begin to go from
sipping my tea to now slamming my tea. Excited about tomorrow is
an understatement. Are my thoughts a little all over the place?....
sure. Why am I excited about tomorrow....I have not a clue. I will
go to bed after a long night of writing to you, then wake up with
only a few that understand and get me, for I understand and get you.
How this is rhyming I swear I don't know, at times my thoughts just
seem to come together this way, and at times not, for I have no
rhyme for the end of this sentence. Damn.

I have found that by being able to relate to people and them to you,
has helped my training tremendously. Why is this? In my head I go
over this question over and over, and out loud answered "I don't
know" after taking a tongue burning sip of miss brown eyes's cousin.
Maybe its because before this UN - spoken relationship you have with
others, what you thought at the time was bad, or what you thought you
were doing was wrong....was and is actually wright, and not bad, but
actually good. Confidence. period. its encouraging knowing that your

453

pain is theirs, your success bleeds out to them, and their work ethic represents you in a way that you could have never imagined without the strength of many. Many kilos with many mother fuckers training hard achieve many great things.

You sit across from my writing desk and ask me what I'm going to write tonight. I respond to you that I have these random thoughts about refrigerators, walking backwards in my supermarket, Shankle and his hiked up shorts, freedom, and last but not least this idea about writing about writing what I'm thinking about writing, and then writing it.

Shit......this whole time I was writing. Salute.

What am I going to write tonight 2016

♪ ♪ ♪

A Calm Bug

Wednesday, February 27, 2013

On my way to the Arnold 2013. On my way to represent the Dark Orchestra and make you all proud. I will smash the American record and bring home the title for you, for us, for the Attitude nation. I came across this article I wrote sometime ago before nationals. A year later and I feel the exact same way I do now. So I just had to re post it. I find the taper bug very interesting as well. I have been talking to a few friends on different ways to stay 100 percent clear from the dreaded bug, so far not a whole lot of success. Its something I want to chat about on my next podcast though.....o by the way is not going live tomorrow at the usual time due to traveling to the Arnold. BUT, we are putting together a LIVE show at the Arnold grabbing as many guests as we can get that walk on by, Just like we did at the American Open. Hope to see you their, it would be great to be able to meet you in person. Salute.

I wasn't going to write again tell after the Arnold, but I just couldn't stay away from chatting with you. Coffee is just not the same without talking to the Attitude Nation. Writing has become a big part of my life; a big part of the training, a big part of relationships, and most importantly getting to know and understand myself. Writing is my therapy, without it I feel claustrophobic, uptight, and lonely. So I hear I am, back with you one more time before the Arnold. Lets grab some coffee, put on a Piano guys song, put on our phantom mask's with the dark cape, and let's sing together in this ever so odd world of the dark symphony - while the world shuns us!

The Taper bug has finally left, thank the Lord. The last week I have been tired, weak, slow, and unmotivated. I have been sleeping like a new born baby, too lazy to even play video games. Just enough energy to sit in the hot tub and stare at a swaying tree for about 30 minutes. This always happens to me before a big meet, or any meet that is. I call it the Taper bug. The Taper bug is when you start to back off the training and rest the body. The volume goes way down, the squat workouts get easier, the length of training gets cut in half, and the overall intensity lowers with each workout. You become more sore, achy, slow, and even weaker the more the taper bug enters your body. Why? I have no idea. You would think it would be the exact opposite. It's like your body finally gets some rest and takes full advantage of it. Your body shuts down, like a bear for the winter, a big Donny shankle bear. Lol, sorry I don't know why I just said that, but the image is pretty funny. Months and months of hell training, months and months of beating this bloody muscular skinned thing we call our body down. Time after time of kicking it every time it tries to get up. Now when you let it stand, it doesn't just jump up and say "let's go"! but no, the body slowly gets on one knee first, and then the right hand helps support your the left, and after a few days of trying to stand up it does, slowly but surely. But my friends.....It doesn't just stand...no, it grows 90 feet tall and smashes everything in front of it. "Green Monster" my old blog explains this perfectly.

I have been in depression the last week. The taper bug got to my head a little bit, and the taper cloud over my head really brought me down. A few small injury's and some tweaks in the lower back is the minds worst enemy, and the body's worst optical. Even coffee didn't help. Weight after weight being missed, twitching legs while a sleep, and low energy levels, haaaa! NO MORE!! I have smashed the bug and grabbed my gun. I have reunited with the Nation and we will attack. Snap out of it Champ, you have a title to defend. Three time Arnold champ has a certain ring to it. You have a medal to send around the world, no time for pity. No time for "what ifs", no time for the weight to feel heavy, just lift and win....then do to all again. After they put the medal around our neck, salute the Nation with pride boy.

Yes that all sounds good, but a minute later my hands start to sweat again, my heart rate goes up, and my mind starts playing tricks on me again. The opener keeps me up at night, the opener haunts me. Sometimes I feel like running, running to a small town and hiding in a bar. Forgetting that I am 4 months sober and drinking my worries away night after night. Yes, this sounds great, no more pressure, just a white flag and my vodka. Every sip of that Vodka would warm my soul and make me feel good again. No more pain and hype, no more hateful comments towards me, no more long days training in the gym, no more letting people down if I do bad. But then again I would be letting many people down if I ran away. Then again I would not have you. I would no longer be a part of the Attitude Nation. Being a part of this Nation is everything to me, I take pride in it. Vodka is a nation of destruction and failure. Vodka is a friend who will smile to my face and then stab me in the back.

Fuck, this blog is all over the place, I am sorry, this is why I haven't wrote in a few days, I knew this would happen. I am glad I wrote this blog today, I feel its centering me and putting me back in a place of comfort and confidence. So thank you.

Someone call the small town bar and tell them I won't be making it in, I have a title to defend. Tell Vodka I am sorry for no showing, and not to wait up for me. Remind him that I am with the Nation still, and I will never leave them.

Smash the Taper bug and Win The Arnold 2013
Smash Sir Vodka and keep marching with the Nation 2013
Calm before the storm 2016

♪ ♪ ♪

456

Coffee with Barbell Shrugged

Wednesday, March 6, 2013

My interview on Barbell Shrugged at the Arnold!
Thank you guys for having me on your bad ass
podcast. I never miss an episode of this
highly motivating, funny, entertaining and
most importantly knowledgable podcast. If you
haven't ever tuned into BarbellShrugged then
your missing out! Again, thank you Mike Bledsoe,
Doug Larson, Chris Norman, and Chris Moore. Go
to Barbellshrugged.com to check out all the
episodes. Salute!

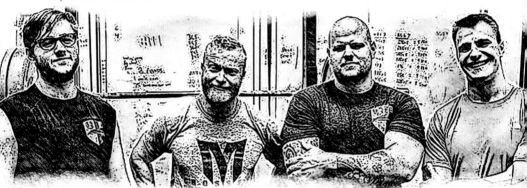

Growing The Sport 2016

♪ ♪ ♪

Happiness

Friday, March 8, 2013

Doing nothing is harder than training. Pacing is more leg work than
squatting, and waiting is more nerve racking than getting a look from
a competitor in the warm up room. Coffee and a clock, an itching
body and too many thoughts. Tea at night as I sit in this Orchestra
of dark hoping to see the light soon enough. Just writing about
training makes my thumbs hook when typing. Loud techno music replays
in my head when the night is at its most quiet. I close my eyes and
see dead coffee cups scattered everywhere around my feet. Every last

457

empty cup is a teammate I have lost throughout this journey. The only way I know how to repay their sacrifice is to drink more coffee. I must be happy, this is the single most important part of training. Happy leads to good mood, good mood leads to motivated, motivated leads to heavy weights, heavy weights lead to the Olympics. I would rather be a happy person and not a weightlifter, than a weightlifter that is not happy. Both happy and weightlifter is the number one goal for any weightlifter, or athlete at that.

Details I cannot go into, but ideas and plans I must follow. The bridge is strong and sturdy, and has two lanes that cross both ways. But I must walk one way, I must walk with a barbell on my back, to a place where happy lives, where people get me for me, who yell at me like I do them, who have similar ideas and methods of atmosphere and attitudes. This is everything. Atmosphere is the home of happiness which leads to lots and lots of bar slamming, lots and lots of yelling, smiles, and tears. Some people like a certain way of training, a certain way of getting jacked up, a certain way of being motivated, which is great. There is more than one way to lift weight, just like there is more than one way to look at the sport, view training, and get jacked up. Many different attitudes and outlooks mix and match for training. Just like there is no wrong way to lift weights, there is no wrong way to train. Their are a million different atmospheres scattered all over the world in a million different gyms. I must find mine. This is a message for everyone across the world. If you are not happy doing what your doing, then stop doing what your doing. I would rather live homeless than be trapped into a web of regret and self captivity. Winning only matters if you love winning in the sport you are winning in. "No comfort zones" - Shankle.

Never lay your sword down and surrender to a situation or atmosphere that isn't personally working for you. Fight! Lose! Live fucken homeless! I would rather rebuild from the bottom to someday be happy on the top. Winning the gold of happiness is the hardest gold medal you could ever achieve. Let's talk about happiness, let's make happiness our number one goal, and let the rest follow without ever resting. Let's use happiness to lift weight, big weight. Not some top secret program, or technique, but true self worth, true love, true living. I must go back to the start. I must find "Jumping" Jonathan North again. I must write Arnold across my chest while training. I must slap hands and scream, chest bump teammates while at times becoming nose to nose with one about to fight at any minute. I feel this is a win win for all. No more walking on egg shells, no more apologies. Just Johnny Cash with his guitar.

Calm before the storm is what I was before the Arnold. The Arnold never came for me due to a horrible back injury I received by the weightlifting gods in the warm up room. The storm never came. The calm still surrounds me. The storm has yet to show its face. The storm will come.

Atmosphere 2016

♪♪♪

Itching

Thursday, March 14, 2013

Itching to itch while itching for the future. The closer the near future moves my way, the further away it feels. I wait, for waiting is all I can do. Ideas will soon blossom into reality, but for now they are only ideas that live in my head. Fuck I am drunk off coffee. Fuck it's hard to write with so much on my mind. Fuck I can't wait to train again. The paragraph you are reading is and will be my final draft, no editing, no starting over, just mud that I am slinging at this screen. Triple extension vs catapult vs my way all intertwined together in a story....yes this is what I want to write about. But can't, my mind can't stay focused on one thing for longer than two minutes. So I itch, scratch, and pace, drink coffee in the same place, while slapping myself in the face to wake from this realization of being completely alone in a big world. I have been here before though. I am a life vet, a weightlifting soldier who has been to war and back. I like the dark, no fuck it, I love the dark, wait... I welcome the dark. Come on Jon, there is no difference from then to now. Doubt only lives in going under 400 pounds, never in the pursuit of ripping the heads off lions. It's either you don't or you do, and I do, we do.

Let's be blunt, is my back getting better?... Better? It's ready for war, and war is what I am about to walk into. Alone? Never. I must only train with gladiators. Spit in my face and remind me why I am doing this. You wanna fight? Let's go. After we throw down let's then shake hands and eat a steak. Drink milk as it runs down the side of

459

our mouths. Grow a beard and give the world the finger. Tough skin
makes for tough body, tough heart and a tough mind. Let's play call of
duty between sessions and then go ham fucken sandwich on the platform.
I fight, and I will die fighting. Swing this axe and cut down the
trees we must. Rip this head off this lion and drink its blood. Let
me set up an atmosphere of dark, real, no chains and freedom. Let me
tell you about it, because as of right now that's all I can do. The
next time I look at the calendar I am going to rip it off the wall
and send it to those who wait to compete in their first a local meet.
Stop waiting! Get your ass out there and kill! Shankle nods his head
while ripping the scabs off his rough hands. The ideas and plans I
have in my head are driving me crazy. I want to open my mind and slam
them down in front of me.

Ring ring ring....hello....let's go....OK. Grab your bar and meet me
here in 2 days. The eyes are watching so be calm and collect, duck
under and stay hidden. Bring your towel for sweat you will wipe,
blood to clean up, and shade you will need. Hey Dad, how am I doing?
You want to come visit me and see all that I have done? No response
like usual. Fuck em, I have you, we have us, I have weightlifting. I
am typing this incredibly fast, and I have no idea how it is going to
come out. This is the kind of writing you must do when the block of
writing takes over. It's funny, writer's block only comes from too
many thoughts, rather than what some might think, not enough thoughts.
What to do when your thoughts are running all over the place? Run
with them, run your fingers over the keyboard and don't stop. Don't
look up, don't worry about the spelling for right now. Don't do what
your English teacher taught you. Listen to you, very close family
and friends. Snap back a monster and train. Write write write. Listen
to the song Shankle told me about, and drink drink drink more coffee.
This watch I wear across my wrist will not move any faster, and it's
making me wish I knew how to time travel. Maybe I should of stayed
in school and taken a class on this topic. Maybe I should eat a whole
bag of mushrooms and let my ideas surface to new sights. Shit, can't
do that, USADA won't leave me alone. Plus, I am not into drugs nor
alcohol anymore. I battled that war and thankfully won. Anyone else
want to get in the ring with me? I am here all day and night.

Light money on fire to warm ourselves in this cold gym. I could care
less about that green devil. Turn up the techno to drown out our
thoughts. Slam bars and you know the rest. I can't believe I am
still writing without stopping once. I must keep going before the
block gets me and haters reach me. Hater you can't find me. I sit

behind a wall full of hard work that they know nothing about, nor will they ever. Haters equal excuses for their own let downs in life, I ain't got time for that. See, we have many let downs and failures that we have had to come to grip with. It's how we handled them that sets us apart from the haters. We have dealt with them in our own way, accepted situations that we take blame for, said sorry for, and then learned from. We succeed past our failures from understanding our failures. I believe haters have never dealt with their own loses and let downs. It's like an alcoholic who will never admit he or she is an alcoholic. It simply doesn't work, and the work they put in only leads to work they channel towards others. Look, understanding the mind set of a hateful person is hard, I am probably just scratching the service. I don't want to act like a know it all. I must stop writing for just a second, my coffee is all out, and I am pretty sure I have a Rockstar in the fridge.......one sec..........................
....

Knees back then crack, I am back. Posters, paint, platforms and bars. Athletes, music, and plates. Coffee machine, sitting bench and chalk. Smiles and frowns, fights and hugs, pr's and misses. A family of skeletons is what makes a gym a gym. Itch, scratch, hot shower, cold shower, tapping fingers, clock watching, what are people thinking thoughts, too many smokes from too many coffee shots. Come to think about it, this is the longest I have been away from training in 6 years. My body looks different. My face looks skinny. My hands look soft and clean, while my back and knees no longer shoot pain up my neck and into my brain. I am a different person. A bitten zombie turned into a civilian who plays basketball outside and who shops at malls. Disgusting is what I am. This fever that has come over me has made my bones weak, and my bubble butt smaller. I find myself even taking the stairs for the extra cardio.....CARDIO PEOPLE! Good Lord, save me from this hell. When a weightlifter chooses the stairs over the elevator something has gone horribly wrong. Rest has taken over. Soon, upcoming, around the corner I will again breath in the dust, hear the plates slam, feel the bar whip, and shoot rest in the fucken head. I will soon become a weightlifter. I will soon be home.

Scratch 2016

♪ ♪ ♪

461

Oscillation

Bar whip will whip your ass under the bar like a sling shot on pink pills. A shot from a sling that will pay off when catching. Rhythm, timing, bounce, fast, explosive, coffee, love, hate, steak, Shankle and a lion, and green monsters in your belly. Oscillation is behind all of these tricks to the game. Street weightlifting. Not talked about movements that hide in the dark of this orchestra only to come out and play when fast moving freaks like us give their day job the finger and smash weights through the floor pissing off every damn neighbor in sight. More pink pills means more strong, and if you can't take pink pills like myself, then bar whip is the next best thing. USADA has single handily given me the full use of bar whip, while other countries get two sides with their main course rather than just one. Screw it, no excuse, let's just use what we have been given by the weightlifting gods to our advantage.

Oscillation means more float time. Float time for the arched angel to flap her wings, her 20 kilo wings that is. A spoon full of sugar and a shot of coffee can make any weightlifter fly while still keeping their toes planted on the floor, giving off shock waves of massive destruction to those commie North Korean sons of bitches. A golf club that bends can make the white ball go further. Whack! Hips to bar when done right and timed right can do all the work for you, slapping you smack dab in a roller coaster of speed and power. What do I think about when I lift? Hanging on. The wind passes my ears like a kid out the car window headed to Disney Land. The harder you push back, the harder the force of contact you create, giving the bar longer time to flap her wings and make love to you.

Why do you lean back so much on the finish Jon? Oscillation, I answer while chugging coffee as if I have been stranded in the desert for 2 weeks without coffee. On a side note.....could you even imagine no coffee for two weeks? You can't, me neither. Awful......let's move on. As I was saying, the longer your hips come through the bar, the longer the bar will oscillate in mid air, giving you just enough time to dive under, pull under, drop under, shrug under, Ali feet under. Whatever term you want to use, it's all the same. This is why Tiger Woods follows through his swing......power. The hips are the golf club, the ball is the bar. Cut your arch short, and you will cut the make short right on the back of your neck. Now

drink more coffee and keep reading, for hopefully this might help you
the next day with gaining a relationship with the bar, which is the
number one road block for a weightlifter at any stage. Relationship.
An understanding. Not a scientific understanding, but a personal
understanding. Only one you can have, no one else. James Tatum said
it best, YouTube is a great way to learn and be coached. I agree full
heartily, but when not knowing what to look for, it can cause head
scratching and frustration. It can blind what's really in front of
you. I went through this Ray Charles syndrome for many years. What
the fuck am I looking at or for. I would have just done what any man
in my shoes would of at that time, drank more coffee, but at that time
of my life I didn't know miss brown eyes. I know, crazy right. Why
the hell do I keep getting off on coffee when trying to write a blog
on the whip of the bar. Good Lord, I am addicted. Wait......better
yet I am in love. OK fuck it moving on. Understand it, see it, then
feel it. The feeling part might take a while, like years and years a
while. It took me about 3 years to really get the timing of her wing
power. And once I found it......what the hell was I suppose to do
with it? Reps, reps, reps, reps, reps, reps, and more reps. Turn up
the volume and dance along.

When the initial hit occurs, the bar will act like a belt wrapping
around your waste. The bar will try to touch both sides of the
weights on either side behind your back. Before the weights have
the pleasure to meet each other they will have a rude awakening
from the bar. As you bring your hips through the hit portion of
the finish into the full extension (aka) arched angel - the bar
will then start to whip out in front of you with much speed. But
Jon, this is the problem, it's not good to have the bar swing out
in front of you. Hold on.....let me take my coffee cup and bash it
upon this triple extension's head. This is the triple extension's
go to attack method. Use the force on the outward moving bar,
and guide it back towards you. This is why the elbows must face
back, never up. If the hips don't come through, and the elbows are
straight up, then yes......the bar will swing out in front of you.
Come at me bro, I can literally go all day. Especially with this
very odd song I found that has put me in an ever so interesting
mood. I am definitely going to put the song above the blog on this
one. What if the bar never did bend? Then A) the hit would hurt
like hell, this is why the better the bar you have the truly better
your lifts will be. I hate to say it, but it's true. B) Since
the wave effect of the bar would not be in affect, the bar would
fall much much faster. This is actually a pointless question in

the first place, because the bar will always bend, unless you're lifting with concrete.....or triple extension.

The oscillation helps wonders in the catch portion of the clean, much much more than the snatch. Why? As the outer part of the bar whip finally meets you in the bottom position of the catch, you are now going to catch the "bounce" and try your best to shoot up out of the "hole" aka the dark deep sea of missed lifts and wrist breaking. The bar whip now starts to swing back up from its long drop down, and gives you that helping hand to add speed and power to stand tall in front of the crowd. I say the oscillation works better in the clean rather than the snatch because the snatch is more of a balancing act. You must at times sit down in the hole, watch a movie, make sure the bar and you are under control, and then stand. Rushing out of the bottom position in the snatch is death, don't do it. The weight is light compared to your back, front, and clean lifts. The bottom position in the clean is NOT YOUR FRIEND! Get the hell out of there, and fast!

Everything applies the same in the jerk as well. The biggest problem I see when watching people jerk is the slight pause, or for a better word hesitation, in the lowest portion of the dip before the drive. Why is this bad? You will miss the bus. This is why. The bus meaning the bar, the bar meaning the whip, the whip meaning the oscillation, the oscillation meaning you holding onto a hot air balloon and taking you high into the air. Miss the timing of the whip like I do many times a week, and your knees will collapse from the you trying to drive up while the bar is now coming back down like a coke head up for three nights straight. Don't be the coke head, and drive out of the dip like you do in the clean. A drill to work on for this timing and relationship is taking out a very heavy weight in the front squat position, and dip and drive over and over for 5 minutes until you and the bar are on the same page.

 I hope this helps. I haven't written a technique blog in a while, it was fun. There is so much more in between all of this. I think this topic needs more parts on this blog in the future for sure. I find it very interesting. Goodnight.

Relationship 2016

♪♪♪

464

Top Hat

Tuesday, March 26, 2013

My ass meets my heels as my knees meet my chin. My mechanical top hat has seemed to fall back from the roof above my head closing in. A chain stationed at the hips rattles its way up to the weightlifter's elbows, only to meet a crossroad of different levers and directions. Everything is connected. My finger connects to the dirt below my bottom position as I draw lines and circles reflecting past memories and future ideas. Sick with tea, cold from the fever. When I am sick the weightlifter is sick as well. A run of bad luck runs a line around my body as to say stay away. A part of the sport that's not talked about. Life affects sport and sport affects life. My fort of blankets that stretches from one end of the living room the the other, keeps me hidden from anymore back pains or illnesses that seem to have a hit on my head. The dirt below my feet has turned into murky bubbly mud from the tea that has fallen from my cup from swaying side to side, while still being hunched over in this ever so low bottom position. The sheets above my head flap as I forgot to close one of the windows outside the fort. Cold wind sneaks through the red glow from the blankets around me. Falling like opera curtains as the chattered whispers overflow the room in preparation for the show. Top hats and long smokes, glasses with no frames, and mustaches that look like the line of bar path in a weightlifting instructional video. Some, more vertical than others, and some so extreme it looks as if a child with a crayon had a go at them. An odd time in my life, a stuck time that has stopped the clocks and erupted more thoughts than I knew I even had. Thoughts like sand slipping through your hands. There then gone. A feeling of whole, followed by a feeling of empty. A call to an old friend across the world for a midnight chat leads to a dial tone of "this number is no longer in use, please hang up and try again". This is how I feel.

Me.....popular.....no my friend. I am one of the loneliness people you know. Old travel receipts lay at my feet, while plane stubs have made a permanent home in my wallet of crinkled white papers and scattered change that always makes it extremely hard to close while trying to slide in my back pocket. Pictures and lovely memories of PR's and bar slamming keep me company in my fort of red. Faces appear and fade. Glossy memories make it hard to sleep as I scroll down and up my phone looking for someone to call. Always leading me to the same place as always....a smoke outside with a hot coffee to

keep my mind sharp and intact. Facebook friends I don't know, while
chatting with friends on twitter I have never met nor scene before.
"Come alive" I scream! Come alive and let's shoot some pool, break
balls, and get in trouble. Let's run from the cops. Let's push over
every shelf in Walmart telling them to start treating their animals
better. Let me raise this mechanical top hat high and enter a whole
new experience outside of this red blanket glow that forces me into
a fantastic bottom position. I am sick from this bad back and living
room fort I scurry under after a long weekend.

A weightlifter body moves from chains and levers that pull and pry,
squeak and chatter. Bone against bone as we catch the weight in the
whole, stretching the chain tight, as your face makes odd emotions
from the small razor thin strings that attach to your pores. A rusty
chain means under recovery, or too much time away from operation top
hat. The higher the top hat, the stronger you will be. The top hat
holds the engine underneath its black leather shell, producing all of
the levers to work as one. This is why all of the great weightlifters
have tall hats, hats that hold wisdom, experience, and knowledge. Or
your top hat can be broken like mine. Broken from injury. Everything
must move together with no hitches. A rhythm lifter has mastered the
art of body, bar awareness. One who has done the movements over and
over until they become second nature. If wind passes your ears on the
pull, and you are hanging onto the bar like a kid on a roller coaster,
then you have mastered your style of technique. All of your levers
and strings now sound like an orchestra of beauty. This my friends
takes time. This my friends takes many nights under a tree fort of
red. This my friends is more bad days than good, more bomb outs than
wins. This my friends is a lifestyle of hell.

Where I'm at now is where I chose to be. These living room forts are
at times necessary. Dark days are like misses, they happen, and there
is such a thing as a good miss, and good dark days. I sit in this red
fort over dirt, passing my finger back and forth while understanding
and gathering thoughts on what it takes to succeed. I have been here
before, understanding the darkest, coldest nights always bring the
warmest, brightest days ahead. Sometimes you have to take three steps
back, to take 20 steps forward. Salute.

White Light 2016

♪ ♪ ♪

Paleo

Sunday, March 31, 2013

Written by Jessica North

My decision to complete a 30-day Paleo challenge was a journey in
itself. It was not a one day, "I want to try it," kind of decision.
I spent over a month contemplating, researching, reading books,
talking with Jon, speaking with friends that live a Paleo lifestyle,
and mostly convincing myself that it was something I could and wanted
to do. Coming from a weightlifting culture, any form of dieting or
restricting what a person eats outside of cutting for a meet is
taboo. To be just considering Paleo, I had gone off the deep end in
the eyes of my peers. That is why not only for myself, but for all
people really scratching their head as to why I chose to do the 30
day challenge, I feel it is important that I share my story. I am the
brave hunter and gatherer that left the feast on the platform, and
ventured off into the forest alone, and this is my story.

What is paleo and why did I do it. Paleo, as I understand it, is short
term for eating as though a person lives in the Paleolithic era. It
consists of 4 main food sources: meat; vegetables, with the exception
of corn, peas, beans, or items with high starch content; spices; and
natural healthy fats such as avocado and coconut oil. Paleo is widely
believed to not be a diet but a change in lifestyle. It is lifestyle
change that I wanted to try. I strongly believe that if a person
does not love their life, they should change it. It takes bravery to
change old habits and especially ways of living one's life, but I have
learned through my short 25 years of life that change is a good thing
and worth trying if it leads to a better life. My health since I was
a child has always been on a ledge. The issue that affects me the most
is that I suffer from chronic migraines. One of my earliest memories
is at an outdoor sidewalk fair with my sister, maybe 5 years old,
walking down the street, and being struck with a migraine so rapidly
that I lost sight, hearing, and then fainted on the sidewalk. I have
been tested for diabetes along with many other diseases with no avail.
Migraines are a part of my weekly routine. Of course this is something
I strongly wanted to break free of, and having done my research, I
believed it to be possible with Paleo. Another reason I wanted to try
Paleo is my energy levels. Living life on at least one green Monster
a day, I felt pretty spunky, but I desired more of a natural energy
that did not send me up and down so much. Many days I felt my energy

was like a roller coaster, and timing it right to be up in energy for training was off. Most days I felt the most tired going into training, and that is not good. Cosmetically, I entertained the idea of a little weight loss as well. Although it was not the strongest motivating factor, I had hoped that going Paleo would help define my muscles, get rid of what I think of as my love handles, and slim down my face. I am not the typical woman that stresses over the number on the scale. Being a weightlifter, I learned to be happy as long as I maintained where I needed to be in my weight class, which is 75kg. 8 months ago, I was in the 69kg weight class, but having switched to weightlifting as my full time job, I naturally put on muscle mass and increased in weight. As my squats went up, so did the number on the scale, which was a good thing for my height, being 5' 10". I would say that I maintain between 73kg and 74kg, which did not bother me. The one thing that I had trouble with looking in the mirror was the fullness of my face. I am sure people in my daily life did not even notice, but when I looked in the mirror I saw chipmunk looking back at me. Along with finding a cure for my migraines, balanced energy levels, and slight trimming up, I desired to feel an overall improvement in my strength and wellbeing. Since it is commonly believed that "you are what you eat," I decided that Paleo was a worthy endeavor. I figured at the very least, I will do this 30-day challenge, and if I hate it, I will have just eaten healthier for one month, and there is no harm in that.

Each person in life has their "go to food", the one comfort food that is hard to let go. For many people, that food is something sweet or a dessert. My food is all things wheat. Before Paleo, I could live on Frosted Mini Wheaties, the orange box, breakfast lunch and dinner. I love granola. I am a sucker for bread. These were the hardest things for me to say goodbye. The day before my Paleo challenge, Jon and I went to Cracker Barrel and I had a going away party for my food. I ordered a hearty plate of French toast, another favorite, ate at least two biscuits, had a tall glass of orange juice, another food group I would miss, and I am pretty sure I had a big bowl of cereal when we got home as well. Other items like desserts, fast food and so on was not as an adjustment for me like it is some people. I had already cut the majority of those things out

468

of my diet. Before going Paleo, I believed myself to have lived a
pretty healthy lifestyle of eating. I did not eat fast food. When Jon
stopped by Bojangles for a snack during the day, I never indulged.
Most dinners out I ordered a steak and passed on dessert. I served a
vegetable with every dinner, although it was almost always corn. My
dad taught me growing up that potatoes would make me strong, or as he
put it, "Grow hair on my chest!" I thought that eating a granola bar,
as a snack was a healthy choice. I rarely drank soda, but when I did
it was a clear one like Sierra Mist or Sprite, which I believed was
better for you. All in all I think that it took me so long to change,
or try something new because I felt I ate above average for a typical
American. Little did I know that what I thought was going to be a
small adjustment, changed everything.

After completing all of my research and finally convincing myself
to do the 30-day challenge, I decided to follow Diane Sanfilippo's
Practical Paleo. The book was recommended to me by a fellow athlete,
and after ordering it, I really found value in its unique layout.
In the book, she not only shares her story in a way that very much
related to me, but there is the research and science of course, many
recipes, and what I found to be most helpful, a variety of 30 day
specific meal plans based on your goals or conditions. For example,
there is a plan for cancer recovery, a plan for weight loss, a
plan for thyroid problems or chron's disease, and several others. I
followed the athlete's specific plan.

Now I may or may not of had the best approach to Paleo following
this 30-day plan because I followed it so strict. What I mean
is that whether or not I liked a food
or had even tried a food before, I
followed exactly what I was supposed
to eat for each meal according to Diane
Sanfilippo's athlete meal plan. This made
for many poor moods because the joy of
food was often taken away. For example,
only two days in and Day 2's breakfast
was left over flank steak with onions and
peppers from night one. I did not enjoy
eating steak for breakfast at all being
that I was such a breakfast (cereal,
French toast, eggs) type of person, but
I sucked it up and ate it. Then Day 2's
lunch was canned salmon. Yuck! My mom said to

never use the word hate, but I hate seafood of ALL kinds. I plugged my nose and got down a few bites swallowed whole, only to gag the rest of my lunch. Dinner saved my spirit with turkey legs and sweet potato pancakes. Not to make it all sound bad, but I greatly struggled with many meals. The bright side though is that each day was a new discovery and a time to try something new. I found many foods that I would not have ever known I enjoyed, for example, beets and fennel, yum. I learned new ways of cooking. I mastered many new recipes and flavors, even making my own spices with the recipes provided in the back of Practical Paleo. One of my favorite changes in habit is now using coconut oil to cook my foods. It adds wonderful flavor to any meat or vegetable, allows me to cook at a higher temperature without burning, and is so much cleaner to eat. I always used vegetable oil before, and I will never go back.

My spirit to complete the challenge remained strong despite all of the temptations around me. My tests at the time were very hard, but now looking back are funny stories. Beginning a challenge like this definitely takes a support structure and someone else rooting you on. I explained to Jon beforehand my reasons and goals, and he supported me 100 percent which was very important. I appreciated him dearly for rooting me on, although without realizing it, he also made it very difficult at times. My first test, having said goodbye to coffee and energy drinks, was Jon making his daily stop at Starbucks. Now I knew that I could do without the coffee and if necessary I was allowed green tea, so I was not too concerned with my will power, until Jon came out holding a brown treat bag along with his coffee. The second he got in the car I could smell it. Apple fritter. Test two also involves a doughnut. Traveling in the airport is a weekly part of my life and what I found having turned Paleo is that airports do not offer healthy food whatsoever. I really struggled with my first trip, and went hungry rather than cheated. Jon, however, indulged even more than usual, whom at the time was maddening but like I said before, is now funny to look back on. He stopped at an ice cream shop and added Butterfinger, syrup, m&m's, and other heart attacks to his bowl. Then he made a quick trip down the terminal to get some pizza and ate it right next to me. Once we landed in the next airport he made another stop at the Duncan Donuts for a powder-covered doughnut and 6 blueberry muffin tops, and a coffee. By the time we got in the cab I wanted to throw a pie in his face. Like an animal in a new environment for the first time, I learned to adapt though and my will power never waivered. By making extra each meal and always having food packed for times I was not home to cook really made my life easier.

On to the more specific pros and cons of my journey. I quickly saw results in my body shape. I started to trim in the mid section after just a few days. Not only my belly, but also my arms, back and legs showed more definition. Last but worth the wait, I saw a decrease in my chipmunk cheeks. My energy levels definitely felt more even. Although very low and nowhere near what I was hoping to achieve, I did not feel the up and down like I had before. Eliminating the sugar, except for one piece of fruit as a dessert each night, I really noticed a difference. My insulin did not spike and I was using my natural energy on a consistent basis. It took until week three, but my overall health started to improve. I maintained my usual schedule of migraines, until week three when they subsided to what I would call headaches instead. Something unexpected is that my skin even noticeably cleared. Also unexpected is that my vision changed. I do not know for the better or worse, but by week two, I started to notice that my sight was different. Focusing on small things took an extra millisecond, but I was seeing them in more detail. Call me crazy but it is true. Despite all of the positives, I could not help my mood swings. I developed very poor mood swings through week two. The thing I attribute it mostly to be the lack of energy. As I said I was more even, but I evened out at a very monotone, low. My strength decreased as well. By week two, I was having nightmares of trying to run but I could not lift my legs to even walk they were so heavy. It was awful and a very hard adjustment that made me really grumpy. Week three this improved slightly, I do not know if it is because I just adapted in my mindset, or my energy levels really did pick up a little. The last negative, which I am not claiming any cause and effect because I am not certain, is that since the end of week one through the rest of the month, I have been ill with a horrible cold. I do not know the science of it. I could have simply caught a bug, or the changes in my body could have affected my immune system, I am unsure. What I do know is that I have had the cough from hell for over three weeks, stopped up sinuses, and for the first time in my life, multiple nose bleeds. I will not blame it on the Paleo, but the coincidence is very high that one week in this plagues me and will not go away. To end on a high note, the last positive that I want to share is recovery. Having not been taking my supplements this whole month such as creatine and protein, I have not found the need for them, as my body is naturally recovery on its own which is a significant blessing.

It is said that 20 days is the magic number for something to become a habit. For example, that is the proven reason of 20 cigarettes in a pack. Once a person finishes one pack, they are supposedly hooked by habit. I found this to be true for my journey as well. Once I reached day 20, everything became much easier. I did not have to think about every detail of what I was eating or how to cook it, or even how I felt. My new routines slowly became my habits, and I settled into my new lifestyle. Paleo transformed from a diet and my 30-day challenge, to my way of living. How I will go forward with my newfound relationship with food will continue to be an exciting journey. On day 20, I experimented, not because a lack of will or surrender to desire, but as a true experiment. I cheated for the very first time. I ate a single crouton that was served on my salad at a restaurant, and took a large drink of Jon's Sierra Mist. Although delicious going down, within seconds of them hitting my stomach, I wrenched in pain. Experiment complete. What I had thought would last only 30 days, is now lasting longer one day at a time. If you are wondering what I did to celebrate day 30, I cooked a Paleo blueberry pie, and it was delicious.

Day 1: 73.5kg / 161.7 lb   Day 30: 68.27kg / 150.2 lb

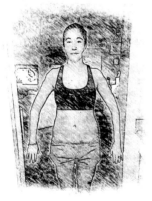   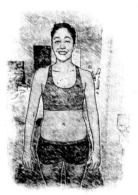

11.5 Pound Loss Total (first 10 pounds were lost by day 15)

Love Your Life or Change It

♪ ♪ ♪

5 Kilo Jumps

Wednesday, April 10, 2013

This red two and half kilo plate feels light in my hands. But why
does this small piece of metal feel so heavy once on the bar? You
would think you could eventually break all the world records by adding
5 kilo's to each set. If the bar was long enough I would just slide
as many of these little plates across this bar forever for as long as
the eye could see. Endless miles of little red plates that stretch
out the gym loading dock, past the highway, and to a place where world
records resign. Up and down, fast and crisp, sweat drips from our
face with every sip of coffee we taste.   This is why I like working
up to max by taking 5 kilo jumps.....rhythm, timing, an understanding
of why and how your body is moving with the bar. Rep after rep you
turn the pages to the old book you found in your grandpa's desk drawer
with a fast turn of the head and a quick flick from your fingers.
Hooked on what the next page has to offer, what shall become of the
character, or how it will end. Set after set you sit while finding
your twitches in sync with your thoughts. Each chug from your energy
drink lines up perfectly with the tapping of your foot from the music.
Every swipe to the face from your training towel glides simultaneously
with a soft moan from the pain that shoots up your spine from the
years the sport has laid upon you. A perfect harmony has fallen into
your lap, and now it's time to stand from your resting chair, and add
another 5 kilo's to the long bar that has now reached the north pole.

Lift and sit, lift and sit. Repeat 'til the gym empties and the owls
outside are the only ones watching you paint your painting in the
lonely warehouse where your music and monster energy drinks motivate
your perfect harmony along. You will hear the difference between
a good lift and a not so good lift. The not so good lift makes a
sound that doesn't mesh with the other sounds around you. It's like
sticking your head under the car's hood and saying to yourself, "Now
what do we have here.....". I prefer to coach with my eyes closed.
I enjoy lifting with my eyes closed. Feel how your body moves, hear
how your athletes sound. This will gain more insight in figuring out
all the little things that happen between the basic positions that are
hidden from the naked eye. Add 5 kilo's more than the last set. Even
though there are thousands of little two and a half kilo plates on the
bar that all add up to a 700 kilo total, it's not that heavy because
they are just little plates that feel very light when picking one up.

How on God's green earth can this weak, defeated, scared plate be any match for us strong weightlifters? It can't. So stop thinking the weight in front of you is heavy. This is a common problem I see with myself and others. You are in charge of the weight, not the weight, fuck the weight, and guess what..... fuck the bar. We need to stop respecting the bar so much like it's our boss, our all mighty king. We are kings and queens that allow the bar to live and have a purpose, not the other way around. Next time you add a one kilo plate to your bar for a PR, just feel that tiny weight in your hand, and think to yourself - the only thing stopping you from making a new all time PR........ is this.

Beginners in the sport of weightlifting, I call out to you to try this workout. Finding yourself as a weightlifter takes many years and time under a bar, but this workout can help find that inner finesse and rhythm that is over looked and can never be coached. I am a big believer in big jumps as well, or as I like to call them "Shankle jumps," because I have never seen anyone take bigger jumps than Shankle. I once saw him clean and jerk 70 kilo's, sit for 2 minutes without blinking once, stand up, load 200 kilos, and then clean and jerk it like it was nothing. Nothing! This in my opinion is all a mind set. Not strength, not technique, not even athleticism. 100 percent mental. There is a time and place for Shankle jumps, but not now my friend. Not for me, because I am just getting back into training, and not for the beginning athlete, because he or she needs more experience with the lifts and not as much focus on the weight on the bar. When the day comes that you can take 20 kilo jumps, or whatever very big jumps are for you, then you can lift blind folded. You have become a pro. You have found peace and harmony. You have found yourself as a true artist.

Small Jumps 2016

♪ ♪ ♪

474

Mr. S

Friday, April 19, 2013

His black umbrella was wet, as large drips of rain water broke our
silence one by one, falling off to the side of his chair that stood
long legged and tall right in front of my desk. My feet, now swimming
in water, as the white stripes from my Adidas sandals have now become
jagged and blurry. "Why is your office so dark"? Obviously this
person didn't see him sitting in the chair right in front of me. How
do you miss a tall umbrella covering a man made up of only bones? It's
not like he is hiding anything, I mean look at him....you can see
right through this poor bastard. "I don't know," I responded, as I
made contact with the puddle below my feet while my hand grabbed my
chin. I really don't know. I then looked back up at the skeleton
that had now gotten up out of his seat and started painting my office
walls from white to black. His brush strokes long and smooth, as if
he was conducting an Orchestra. His bones have turned yellow over the
years from the smoking, besides his fingers, those stay bloody from
the strings of the violin he so dramatically plays.

The black umbrella has seemed to now hover over his skull as his hands
musically guide his body right to left as if he was a house wife in
the 50's, cleaning the dishes dressed to the T, while listening to
her favorite slow song. My once bright room is now completely dark.
He glided his hands past each other a few times as if he just got
done fixing a motor that he had been working on with his son over the
summer. His hands then dropped off to his side as his bony hips crept
forward. I noticed something at that very moment, something I should
have spotted out of the 27 years I have known him.....He was happy.
The bottom of his jaw and the top parted ways, as the black holes
where his eyes used to be became more dark as they opened wider. I
couldn't help but to smile with him, as I sat back in my chair. The
light from the gym lobby was creeping through the bottom of the door,
making a line down my face. A new chapter in my life that has brought
me more happiness than any other. Green roots full of water surround
the outside of my gym, as waterfalls from inside create light splashes
of mist that hits my face as I walk by on a hot day. A jungle of
weights and a tribe of people beyond my door.....but here I am,
sitting in a dark room smiling. At this point, I realized my smile is
out of happiness, happy to feel cold rain drops fall from a hovering
umbrella that has now made its way above my LSU hat that I only wear
when in my office working.

Black walls and bloody finger tips. A past that will never leave me alone, no matter what book I open. A skeleton that has somehow become my best friend, one that keeps me company and smashes the lights out in my office with a broom stick. At this point I finally realized that not only does the skeleton like the dark, but I do too. I find peace and comfort in a dark room. Maybe this is because I have finally found peace within myself and my past. I have accept who I am and have started to finally move forward with my emotional chains and baggage. Maybe this skeleton that I once thought was bad, has turned out to be good, and that by constantly reminding myself of where I have come from, it has made me into the man I am today. The skeleton then slowly turned his head, while his old farmer hips stayed pushed forward as if he was watching corn grow. The black walls then started to drip like hot wax. The puddle below my feet started to stir like a storm, and the structure of the umbrella collapsed in mid air, splashing onto the floor. The skeleton just stared at me, which wasn't something new nor surprising, because the skeleton never has spoken a word to me, I don't even know if he can speak at all. I wouldn't imagine he could, he has no lungs. My smile turned into concern as I stared back at him slouching down deeper into my chair. The skeleton then did something I have never seen in my whole life, his right eye turned white for a split second before turning black again.

I am happy in the Dark Orchestra.

PS: I talk about us in my latest Podcast. Here is the link below.

The Dark Orchestra 2016

♪ ♪ ♪

Gym Rat

Wednesday, April 24, 2013

The scent from his suit slapped me in the face, reminding me of another time in my life before I grew this rat tail. His suit had an office smell that told a story of board meetings, cologne, happy hour, and confidence. His brown belt was the same color as the end of an old book on a shelf in your grandpa's office that laid quietly and untouched

upstairs. The small glossy brown belt looked as if there was a line of
ants chewing zig zag rivers all the way around his wast. A caramel
color iced mocha made noises from the ice hitting the clear plastic cup
every time he talked. I could see residue on his coffee cup, possibly
whip cream, from what I could see out of the corner of my eye, because
the corner of my eye was all I was able to use to deeply analyze this
creature I used to know so well. As we stood and talked in the front
door of the gym, my rat tail started to feel heavier as he put his cell
phone in his pocket and began rubbing his hands together with his feet
a little out from shoulder width apart as if we were about to talk
stocks and bonds. The tail weighed me down back onto my heels if some
one was trying to pull me away from him. My rat tail stretched from
the gym lobby through the door leading out to the gym like an extension
cable to a TV. He moved so freely, and talked like we were best
friends. His demeanor was light, weightless, fast moving and intense.
Intense in a good way, a draw you in kind of way. A way that had you
hanging on every word between every sentence kind of way. A way that
made you want to make him coffee, and hoped he liked it kind of way.
Little swooshy brooms laid over his work shoes that matched his belt
perfectly. Shoes that were more like slippers, and what those broom
stick things that substituted for laces were had me scratching my head,
even without my beta-alanine pills. Charcoal sports coat still on, but
his salmon or pink..... couldn't really make out the difference, had
the two top buttons undone, as if to say he put in his work throughout
this sunny Wednesday in the silver towers of Charlotte. His blue socks
were showing below his work pants, I thought this was odd at first but
then soon realized after many flash backs and memories that this is
what he was going for, this is what was in style, this was professional
none the less. Lexus in the parking lot that made me smile as my head
dropped and tears starting to gather their weapons like the beginning
of Gangs Of New York as they were making their way out of the tunnel.

The Seattle Space Needle erupted though the gym floor as the smell
of salt water and the sounds of fishing boats captured my attention,
drawing my face blank as memories never die, and at times can truly
become alive. The business man in front of me became blurry and
faded. My rat tail became light and small as it fit perfectly in
my And 1 shorts while I rode my skateboard in the parks of downtown
Bellevue as my dad filmed with his over sized Channel 4 looking video
camera. Fresh knees scooting me along the pier made my hurt back
feel strong, and my bloody thumbs feel smooth as the echo from the
man talking in front of me rang throughout my ears, not breaking my
concentration. Time to stop by the office at Nextel for my father to

do some "work". What did he actually do while my sister and I played
in the break room.....I have no idea even to this day. The man in
front of me kept talking as Lexy and I scurried around the cubical
world of ringing phones and empty rooms filled with random tables and
paper work. Random laughter as skirts and suits would constantly
debate where they were going to lunch, no matter what time of the
day it was. My dad's office always had people in it. The minute I
would abruptly enter the talk, the laughter would stop, heads would
all turn our way as if we just broke up the party. Shots of tequila
were everywhere, as my dad nicely told my sister and I to go play as
he flicked through some cash to give us like we were in the mafia. We
took it and ran like it was some sort of game giggling down the maze
of cubicles and fax machines, every once in a while turning back as if
my dad was going to join us in our little game.

Sun roof open as my sister sat on the "hump" aka the center consul
of my dad's beloved Lexus that he would constantly dust with his
duster and make us take our shoes off before getting in. Square black
sunglasses covered his face, perfect look for the 90's. Bobby Brown
playing in the CD deck, as all of our arms and limbs were out the
window driving slowly down the strip of our favorite movie theater and
shopping mall. Three birds, the team, family, all three never have
been together since. My dad reached out to grab my hand and told
me everything was going to be okay, and that he still loved me. My
sister started to cry as she looked at the window now painted with
Seattle rain and fog. His suit smelled strong as my face was buried
into his brown leather jacket. My eyes stung from my sister's blond
hair that got into my eyes from her sharing the other shoulder. We
were family once again. A Seattle Space adventure into the past, a
time machine that gave me hope and a feeling of love once again.

I soon realized the hand I was holding was the business man that
came to visit my gym. He was shaking my hand and telling me it was
nice meeting me. He told me he would be back next weekend to start
training. He put on his black leather coat over his charcoal sports
coat, and raised his round gold sunglasses to his face with one hand,
and then walked out the front door. I went to follow him, but I was
stopped by my rat tail. I am a gym rat. I always will be a gym rat.

Suit & Tie 2016

♪ ♪ ♪

478

Roots

Monday, May 6, 2013

The Roots

The three white strips running up his legs and down his arms made my
stomach hurt, as I leaned over in my resting bench while training at
the Eleiko Sport Center in Chicago during the 37th AN Cert. A home
sick feeling dripped down my throat as I wiped the sweat from my face
while my eyes stayed locked and focused on the human size poster on
the window beside me of Klokov snatching. A wheel of memories spun in
my head while smells, sounds, and faces truly woke and stood before
me. My roots lay deep underneath this gym, a weightlifter's gym,
a world I understood all too well. It's been too long since I had
visited home, a place where I was born, raised, and loved. Adidas
jump suits pace the gym walls like forgotten dinosaurs that train
in the dark. Fanny packs that the old coaches wear proudly, always
prepared with smelling salt, tape, or an old story for motivation
for their beloved athletes. A great sport, a beautiful sport. A
quiet family that stays hidden beneath the cracks of the iron games.
I am home, I thought to myself as the board short CrossFiters sat
uncomfortably in this odd world they have never witnessed before.
Their eyes traveled from one end of the gym to the next, occasionally
looking over at one another with high eye brows, as if saying, "Where
the fuck are we?". A warm feeling came over me, as I settled deeper
into the old resting bench behind the platform I was lifting on. The
resting bench was cracked but sturdy, as rows of them as far as the
eye could see stood proudly behind each platform as if having each
other's back. Chalk buckets formed like UFOs scattered throughout
the gym like trees in a forest, and silver shiny bars that spun like
Ferraris laid peacefully on each platform as if resting in a garage
before a big race. It felt good to be back home. It felt good to
finally welcome CrossFiters into my world, a weightlifter's world.

Pictures in my head took me back the first time I walked into the
weightlifting gym, as I sat between reps. My first coach telling me
to grab the bar struck me hard, as I sat waiting to hopefully hit some
sort of good weight for the audience before me. I almost stood up and
grabbed the bar, but then was reminded that it was only a memory of my
coach yelling at me, not present time. I remembered reaching down as
if I was 9 years old opening my first Christmas present. As I picked
that empty bar up off the ground, remarkable changes happened to me

479

in a split second. Three white stripes ran down the side of my body, like small rivers of blood splashed violently against the walls of my veins. My baggy basketball shorts turned into black tights with ACE bandages wrapped around me knees. My thumb nails grew 3 inches to better the hook grip, as my shirt disappeared into thin air leaving my pounding heart open and naked for all to see. That day I became a weightlifter. That day I was born into the weightlifting family.

No pull up bars in this bitch, I said to one of the CrossFiters who looked lost in this weightlifting gym. He laughed as his eyes still scanned the gym walls looking for a glimpse of his tribe's battle weapons he knew so well. Right off the bat I noticed his search for something that would make him feel more at ease, so I then responded by saying, "No swinging ring things hanging from the ceiling either, just bar and platform my friend". He responded by saying, "Well....I guess that's all you need, right?". My face went dark and blank, as my head tilted to the floor as my toes played with some left over chalk that must have broken off from when I was covering my chest and shoulders before clean and jerks. I responded to the board short CrossFiter, "Well you need a lot more than just that. You need a shrink, councilor, therapist, and at times a fucken straight-jacket in this world my friend". He threw his head back and laughed out loud for all to hear, but he soon went silent as he noticed I was not laughing with him. His face went dark like mine, and that's when I knew he wanted to get the hell out of this tribe called weightlifting, and back to his world ASAP. I cracked a small smile to show I was just messing around with him, and then laughed it off after a few seconds went by.....I mean, come on, I am not an awkward person and I would never put anybody in that weird of a conversation. But little did he know, my small smile and chuckle to ease the tension could have won a Grammy, for I truly meant what I said, and because of this truth, at times I have wondered about crossing over the other side of the greener and grassier world called CrossFit, or as it seems to me from the outside looking in.

5 fingered shoes and board shorts have surrounded me for the past few years. It's almost as if I have forgotten where I came from, and where these roots connected to my feet end. My roots have been tangled in a Paleo world of high reps and running bodies. Tribal tattoos cover these odd athletes as they double in numbers everyday, surrounding the weightlifting world as we spin in circles trying to look for a resting bench and a chalk bucket to take shelter upon. The growth of the sport is beautiful, but the peaceful rhythm of a weightlifting gym will never

die.   The small chatter amongst coaches shrugging their shoulders as
if saying "good.......but needs a lot of work," gave me goose bumps
as I sat staring out from the corner of the Eleiko gym in a gaze of
remembrance and reflections.   I have been traveling deep into the world
and lifestyle of CrossFit for so long now teaching the weightlifter's
methods and mind set, that it's almost like I have become lost from the
world I grew up in.   I have found myself eating, laughing, and fighting
with this new tribe as my old tribe peacefully paces in a empty gym at
8pm at night, slapping their legs before squatting, and rubbing icy
hot on every part of their broken bodies.   I am a weightlifter, not a
CrossFiter.   I do not belong in their world.   I must understand that I
am a visitor amongst these citizens, and once my duty is filled, I must
travel back to the three stripes and fanny pack village I was raised
in.   I must rest my head at night in the camp of one rep and resting
benches.   A village where coaches coach with only their eyes, while
sitting in a lonely chair as if they were on an empty island making
smoke signals for their athletes to see.   A world where the coach's
feedback mostly comes from a small shrug of the shoulders or a thumbs
up for more weight.   Yes the sport of weightlifting is growing and
always will,   but the sound of rain outside as coughs and moans echo
the quiet gym will never change.   Adidas sweat suits and fanny packs
will never die.

I am and always will be a weightlifter.   Thank you Eleiko for having
us out, and for hosting a great AN Seminar.   Thank you for inspiring
me to write this blog that really hit home for me.

♪♪♪

Silent Owl

Monday, May 27, 2013

Four gentlemen.   Four scholars.   Four men captivated by the bar,
sailing the gym with empty guts filled with swirling waves of energy
drinks.   Their caffeinated adventure and their midnight chatter sways
them along the distant and never ending ocean made up of sugar, and
birds that circle their ship of chairs and coaches tied together by
the strings from each men's shoes.   Knots that pull tight just like
the grip they use to hold their shaker cups, keep the boat attached,
while the men roll deeper into dreams and goals they didn't even
know where there.   Hands move with their mouths, while body language
follows the rhythm of the conversation.   Laughter rings out throughout

the empty sea as one of the men ask for another shot of energy. "Hell
yea!" Matt says to Ryan, as powder starts to pour like sand from a
shoe. Powder that dances as it enters the cup.... a cup that will
soon be shaken. Pink powder that is legal, how this is possible makes
the men burst with laughter even louder than before. A drug that
allows the men to feel comfortable around each other, like a beer
at a business meeting, or coffee on a first date. An ice breaker, a
conversation starter, a counselor of some sort, constantly begging for
more truth, more discussion, more of you. Body building magazines
that lay scattered on the wet deck, only to be glanced upon and then
thrown to the side, leaving the magazine empty and unfulfilled.
When lost at sea the only thing to do is chug powder, crack monsters,
and feel the smooth face of miss brown eyes against the palm of your
hand. The yellow birds occasionally swoop down to catch a better view
of the on board barrels that reek of motivation and wide eyed emotion.
The gusts of wind from the splashing whales and rolling kilo plates
made miss brown eyes' hair find peace above her head, blocking out
the sight of the birds as if a slide show was being played above all
for men's heads. A slide show of blue ski for miles, and clouds that
made shapes of Dimas on a unicorn jumping over caffeinated waterfalls.
It became quiet for a moment as all four scholars of their respected
career choices drew from their rich and inviting drinks. A smack of
the lips and a shake from the head was only the start of the after
drink ritual. The classic look of the cup from a stretched out arm
like something was wrong, meant that everything in the world was
right. Chatter laid still in peace, as the sound of the boat slapping
the water gave each man a moment of tranquility. Chunks of energy
powder found its way on the back of each mans throat and behind the
gums that always seemed to bleed when brushed. A fast chew as their
eyes pinned wide, but the sight could not make out what laid in front
of them from the pure concentration of the task at hand. Rocks
exploded as the supplements taste and high powered electricity punched
them in the face, followed this time around - by a fast and violent
sip to wash the left overs down deep into the belly of the beast.

Another topic popped up like the silence was never there. The silence
grabbed its doctor bag and medical kit and flew away. He was glad
to leave, for he was an owl, and owls had no business being out in
the middle of a ocean made up of sugar and yellow birds. The silent
owl was always known for being realistic, and this situation was far
from anything that lingered on making a bit of sense. To the four
men reality couldn't be more real. The spray of the ocean tasted like
sugar, and the circling birds drew a certain shade that they could

feel upon their skin. How could this not be reality? A reality they could taste with every sip of their mixed multi-colored contraptions they were drinking, like a pirate to his alcohol. The front room boat stayed swaying as the lobby squeezed the shoe string boat closer and closer to the tiny door that was becoming bigger and bigger. A door that became land, and land that lead to the land called gym.

Jokes and ball breaking would be soon rudely interrupted by a heavy reality. Ideas were the reflections that the men saw when they pierced through the depth of the water, as the boat swayed closer and closer to the growing door. Looking back at them was the what if's and the how comes. Whales that rolled in circles with giant smiles upon their faces. Fish that spoke English sang songs from the 90's, and the outer banks of the ocean came to a stop, as if the water and sea life had no where else to go. All roads led to one destination. All the whales were swimming to one location, and the birds were flying to help guide the four men home. Soon the men realized their ocean journey was over, and the front door leading out from the gym lobby and into the gym was 10 feet high and partially cracked open. Chalk dust fell like snow from the cracked door, as the music bumped through the dead end ocean walls meeting their feet and carrying up through their bodies. The energy drinks were gone, empty, now living inside them. The door flew open as the owl of silence made its way to the front of the boat, grabbing the rope with his wing and tying the boat to the long wooded post that the yellow birds momentarily made their new resting spot. "Let's go boys......it's time to train." - Silent owl.

                                                    Energy Drinks 2016

                                ♪ ♪ ♪

                            Exit 33 C

Friday, June 14, 2013

A slam of the bar leaves the owner out two hundred, as it lays broken next to a life that has been fixed. A gym owner that has changed a life with the sacrifice of a single bar. A 2 hundred dollar boost of happiness. A 2 hundred dollar therapy session. A 2 hundred dollar band aid for the skeletons that have been cut so deep over the years. A 2 hundred dollar peace of mind that makes everyone sleep better at night. A rest easy night, as the smoke from the cold outside pours out from your leaned back head in reflection of the grace and peace you now feel from the war zone you just left. For every broken bar a heavy heart becomes heavier. One dies for the other to live. One must break for the other to gain strength. A bar that now lays in ruins rests quietly as happy smiles appear on every one's face. Smiles people will take home with them as a new smile breaks while slipping the gym smiles into the junk drawer for a rainy day. Smiles they will keep close, in case hard times approach. Only respect the bar once it's broken my friend. A broken bar means a life has been changed. A broken bar tells a story of hardship and achievement. Many battles have been lost, but the war has been won. We must honor and salute every broken bar that has died for us. We must never forget the bars that now sleep under a blanket of dust.

Sweat that falls like coffee down our throat has become normal in this life, as we drive with our AC up and windows down with destination domination in our sights. A tight hand grips the wheel, as the other dances to the song that echoes through your day dreams. Eyes lay pierced to the road ahead, as concentration plays on the glass in front of you. See it, believe it, then fucken do it. The driver's head nodded as his eyes relaxed, his free hand broke free from the dance, and began to shuffle around the passenger seat looking for the red bull he took pride on buying the day before to save a buck from the high prices of the gas stations. A back up drink when the coffee is all gone too fast before the workout has even started. Something that this character I created does often. He got out of his jeep and walked into the gym.

One falls, the other helps. One cries, the other hugs. A massive PR achieved, as high fives follow like dominoes. Two legs, two people, training with two different goals in sight, as one another yell at each other with spit flying like chalk on hands, and eyes wide open like meeting your dad at the half way point for the weekend on Exit 33 C off I-5. Neck veins full of coffee about to burst as the intensity rises like an ocean of emotion. Feet leave the floor, not from the workout, but from excitement. Organized motivation that flows swiftly like organized crime. Sweat on sweat as hugs and bring it in high fives bathe one another in a salt bath of understanding. "It's all good," as their sweat is now yours. Their tears have become relatable. A gym full of skeletons that train side by side like Siamese twins battling weights like Russell Crow battling slavery. No longer kept locked away in the closet. No longer kept quiet, no longer

kept hidden. Now out for the world to see, for people to judge,
and for the truth to shine, leaving you with complete freedom from
yourself. Dried up river indents snake down their eyes, that has now
been replaced with sweat. Sweat that tastes like fucken success. A
taste of look at me now. A waterfall of proven wrongs and forgotten
fatherly approval. A sweat storm of a new beginning and a higher
hope. Sweat speaks only one word.....do. Sweat never talks, it only
does. If you aren't sweating, you aren't living.

You the reader. Hello. I am sorry for my absence. The dark keeps
me balanced, without the dark I would lose myself in the light. I
feel at home here, with you the skeletons. The outside world has
been crazy lately. I thought about entering the Orchestra, but I
stayed away for some reason, a reason I still don't have the answer
to. I felt the battle above must be fought before showing my face
here again. I didn't want to let you down. I didn't want to write
to you a fake emotion. I wanted to see you again with a plan,
a victory, for us, for the Nation of skeletons. I want to thank
everyone for fighting with me throughout the last week. I read every
single comment, post, email, Facebook message, ect. I can't tell
you how much it means to me. Your support is overwhelming, and for
that I am forever grateful. Thank you for fighting side by side with
me. I fight for you, we fight for freedom, a shirtless lifestyle, a
right of bar slamming and coffee chugging. A simple lifestyle that
gives us the freedom to do whatever we want, without anyone telling
us different. I will always fight for this blog that has only one
purpose and one purpose only.......to accept our skeletons, and move
forward.   Salute my very, very good friend.

Skeletons 2016

♪ ♪ ♪

The Headless Mother Fucker

Sunday, June 16, 2013

His heart sucked his head down his own throat to have a quick word.
A headless man swaying awkwardly down the wrong side of the sidewalk.
Each shoulder taking turns moving up then down with perfect timing
to every step. A bad mo fo this fucken guy is. People walking by
him would even say in passing, "Look at this fucken guy". He was

485

that guy, the guy wearing a leather jacket on a sunny day. A guy
that walked like John Travolta in Saturday Night Fever. A guy that
had no head, only arms that would sway like he was directing cars
at an intersection, instead of a whistle, he swung his keys around
his tattooed finger, while whistling a romantic love song sung by
his favorite opera. No one seemed to ask where this mother fucker's
head was, no one seemed to take the time to notice. They seemed to
be too concerned with his energy, his presence, his blindness to his
surroundings. He took his keys as if they were a paint brush and
swooshed the air adding in a skip to his walk. This brought more
looks from the people walking around him. Yes, I said around.....this
mother fucker was walking, or should I say skipping down the middle
of the busy sidewalk. His eyes staring through his chest plate as if
he was trapped in his own body. His chipmunk cheeks fully engulfed
with air, as his eyes moved back and forth like a grand daddy clock.
His heart yelling at him like a principle scolding a kid for passing
love notes in class. His eyebrows dropped and his forehead scrunched
down as if to say he understood. This mother fucker was truly
listening to his heart.

Beep beep, his car sounded while the doors clicked unlock as he
jumped over his door and slid into the driver's seat. This mother
fucker didn't even need to lock or unlock anything because his black
Firebird had no top, just like he had no damn head. This mother
fucker pushed unlock just to make his entrance even more awesome. A
guy skateboarding by with his dog saw this preplanned and meditated
entrance into the Firebird, and with such disapproval the skateboarder
said to himself....."This mother fucker", and then skated on looking
for his next victim to mind judge. The headless mo fo looked up his
throat in anticipation for what his mind told his hands to do, and
that was to pour a gallon of coffee down into his chest plate and
into his mouth that was already wide open awaiting for the river of
half blood and coffee to enter his mouth. But see..... the drinking
process has been reversed. With this mother fucker's head in his
chest, that meant the coffee would have to first be poured into his
throat to enter his mouth, and then once in his mouth this mother
fucker would actually have to spit the coffee out in order for the
coffee to reach his belly. This mother fucker fucked up the whole
process, making it into his own.

Alanis Morisette was blasting throughout his firebird as one elbow
stuck out the driver's seat window, while the other laid on top of
the steering wheel like his arm was completely dead. Horns were

honking everywhere from other cars swerving out of the way. People
were flipping him off with more emotion that the famous Johnny
Cash picture. They had every right to in my opinion. This mother
fucker was driving down the wrong side of the mother fucken road! An
occasional swerve from his driving hand feeling every emotion Alanis
was screaming about made him one dangerous mother fucker. His leather
jacket flapped from the wind slipping past its dirt shell full of his
old boy scout patches and AC/DC buttons from concerts he has been
to. One patch was of an old fat lady singing, and it said "She is
singing, but this mother fucker is still going". How this mother
fucker was even driving with no head is confusing to this day, but it
never seemed to bother this mother fucker, so what did he do when a
cop passed him......? He waved like a president getting off the plane.
His layed back demeanor and confidence in who he was made the cop feel
at ease, as the cop passed with a wave in return. You couldn't see
this mother fucker smiling, but he was, underneath his shoulders and
throat, his head nodded to the 90's songs while a smile crossed his
face - ear to ear. The only thing in his way was a heart and a rib
cage. The only thing that could ever imprison this mother fucker, is
the cage that layed in front of his own self.

He started to chew on his own chest plate. His bloody teeth made his
bloody face even more bloody. The hard bones created slivers that stuck
into his gums like toothpicks in cheese. This mother fucker chewed like
a mother fucker to break free from his own mother fucken cage. He was
a prisoner of himself, not from the society he was living in. Happy
on the outside, as a battle raged from within. Every time he swallowed
his own bones, the bones would move up his throat and out the giant hole
where his neck should have been. Bones flew out from the fast moving
car, hitting the road like cans attached to a married couples car. He
was almost through the rib cage, and closer to his own heart. A heart
that always talked to him, but never felt him. This sad mother fucker
just wanted to get to know his own heart. His own self.

He screeched up to a fancy coffee shop that looked to be a big company
chain of some sort. He hated chains, he always said they had no souls.
He preferred local shops, you know...small business. Family run, family
principles. This overly clean and too damn happy cafe would have to do.
He had been driving for hours with no destination in sight, and a coffee
refuel was highly needed. He rolled out from the open top as his snake
skinned boots clapped against the parking lot pavement. He flapped his
leather coat together as if it was magically going to stay in place.
This mother fucker parked in the handicap spot and didn't even know

it. Why not you ask.......well, this mother fucker had no head. And I'm
not too sure that if he had a head he would of cared either. He only
went off emotion, feeling, and heart. A heart he was getting closer to
chew by chew. He spun in a circle and clapped his hands. He walked
into the coffee shop like he owned the place. He leaned with his walk
like a slalom skier. His hands felt his thighs looking for his wallet,
making him look like he was dancing the Macarena. He cut everyone in
line blindly, even knocking over an older gentleman that was helping
his grandson with a toy that fell out of place. The gentleman was
startled with a look of "excuse me sir," but it never came out of his
mouth. The small child began to cry, as this rude mother fucker started
moving his shoulders and waving his hands to the cashier. He wanted an
iced coffee, but all the cashier heard was......well, nothing, nothing
but shock and the thought that this guy was such a mother fucker. The
mother fucker fell to his death right in front of the counter at that
very moment. He had finally ate his own heart. He killed himself in the
process of trying to get to know himself. This mother fucker was dead.
The fucken end.

This Mother Fucker 2016

♪ ♪ ♪

Blockbuster

Wednesday, June 19, 2013

Nothing but pure fucken chaos outside. Fast lights zig zag at
lighting speed on the other side of this night time window that has
a reflection of my long half shifted face staring off into a cold and
dangerous world. Beyond this cold dark window lays a galaxy of people
who will rob and gut you, steel and fuck you. A star ship galaxy
full of space aliens that breathe in smoke only to exhale daggered
words that leave you bloodied and wounded. A sudden blink of the eye
reminds my frightened conscience that in fact I am not dreaming, but
alive and well, safe and sheltered, out from harm's reach from the,
at times, fucked up world we live in. A single drip of drool drops
from my half opened mouth as my eyes follow the drip to its destiny,
splattering on the bright and always magical blue carpet silently
laying below my feet. A wipe of the mouth, as a sense of warmth and
comfort blanket my angered and frustrated emotions that tease and
tempt me like a clown at a fucken kid's party. Get off me clown, "Who

488

are you talking to, sweetie?" My wife asks in her sweet, like country
tea voice. "The world, sweetie....the mother fucken world". Her head
fell back as her eyes rolled with a slight chuckle and a grab of my
hand. "Come on, sweetie. Let's look for some good movies," she said
while dragging me away from the window that looked back at me.

A soothing walk through the secret garden drew my soul to peace. Rows
of hidden isles of super heroes fighting and drunken guitar playing
college kids at the animal house shaded my thoughts from the outside
world, leaving me surrounded by a new circle of life, one that leaves
you on the edge of the world. Chimney sweepers dance above my head
down the yellow brick road under the blue sky that folds and opens
like a spiral maze leading me to some sort of crystal ball called the
perfect movie to check out on this not so perfect night. The smell
of popcorn and candy left my taste buds with blue balls, as my mouth
became dry and anxious for sour patch kids and extra buttered kettle
corn. My nose dug into my arm pits, as I tried to smell myself after
the guy with the red leather jacket and Elvis sunglasses looking at
movies next to me, gave me his business card that was titled, Soap
Salesman. He seemed odd and out of place, and he was truly incorrect
about my odor, I smelled damn good. Fuck that guy.

The clack sound that the movies made being put back on the shelf after a
quick read and a judge of the cover made my ears tingle with relaxation.
I loved that sound, I loved every sound this under the freeway homeless
man was playing, a true master piece in an unusual place. This blue
carpet masterpiece was far from quiet as some might think. The sound
of the cash register changing while receipts were being ripped into two
different forms to sign gave me goose bumps as I continued to walk up
and down the isles passing a red haired girl running faster and faster
around the building. The crazy thing about this red haired girl is that
she never stopped running. All she did was run, run, run. It made me
smile as I continued to look for clues with an extremely dry sense of
humor and whity remarks to myself, as I fumbled around getting closer
to the perfect movie on this perfect stormy night. Too much silence
is never a good thing. Too much time alone can lead to long talks
with bartenders and repeated sentences that might leave a person mad.
That's why I love this blue carpet, it surrounds me with other people's
thoughts, journeys, and emotions. Freeing us from our jailed cell
minds, and taking us to the very end where the water meets the sand full
of redemption. Freedom from our own minds, and into others. Freedom
that never lets go, even when the movie sinks to an end, and the cold
outside wind from your open bedroom window hits you like frost bite.

The safe place, is what this block separated from the busters of life really is. A place that no matter how down you are, how mad you are at life, this casino of rolling pictures will always save you from the sphere of life. Save your private emotions for the gym, this is a time to just run, and keep running until the shackles on your knees break, and the forest before you turns blue and yellow. Yellow like a Taxi, and blue like the punch that got you drunk off love from the first time you saw the woman of your dreams at that coffee shop outside of that busy intersection. I am just an average Joe, but in this world I am a brilliant mathematician that solves impossible problems at Harvard. I am not a weightlifter, I am a rope slinger that collects rocks and rides elephants. I am a fucken green monster. I am a wormy poker hustler. I am not me, myself, nor Irene. I am a gladiator with a sword fighting for freedom to see his family once again. I have no kids yet, but in this yellow and blue fish net I am a family man, a man on fire that cannot be stopped.

My wife's hair was blowing swiftly in the air from the AC vent above her. She looked the most beautiful I have ever seen her at that very moment. Her original smell hit my face from the air guiding it my way, almost taking my face off. A scent of a woman was an understatement, her scent was and still is nothing less than breath taking. A lucky man I am, I thought to myself. To have a woman with such a brave heart, and beautiful mind. I am truly blessed, and forever fortunate to have such a remarkable creature as my wife.

This life that I live, I would die hard for. Walking up and down each row of movies about other people's lives makes me appreciate mine even more. I slowly crept up to a movie that stuck out from all the rest. A movie that caught my eye from far away. I grabbed the movie extremely dramatically as if I just caught my first big fish. I grabbed the Truman Show and my wife's hand and proceeded to the counter. I paid, then continued to walk forward, gathered the rest of the benjamens into my wallet, and buttoned up my wife's coat before entering the cold outside.

My wife the Rock, and myself the Fighter, both a Bronx Tail, that ended in a night of love.

"My wife, my love, my queen". 2016

♪ ♪ ♪

490

Thank You

I snap this red bull open, as the beak of my hat lays low over my eyes, preparing my thoughts for the journey that lies ahead of me. A crisp chug of sugar rolls down my throat, as a gust of wind from the open gym door hits my body. I am writing to you exactly what is happening at this very moment. At this very moment, I want to take this time and thank you for being there for me through thick and thin, through the hard times and the good times, through the loses and the wins. Thank you for supporting me throughout the collections of many mistakes I have gathered throughout this journey of life and weightlifting. Thank you for accepting me for who I am, and giving me the confidence to keep moving forward. Thank you for pushing me back on the platform after suffering the horrible injury at the Arnold. Thank you for putting up with my rants, and my over the top emotions.

Thank you for reading this blog, and being a part of the Dark Orchestra, a place where we can truly let ourselves live and be free. Thank you for letting your skeletons out of the closet, and facing them head on like I have done with mine. Thank you for keeping me sober from drugs and alcohol. Thank you for taking the time out of your busy day to read depressing blogs about my broken relationship with my father, drug addictions I have fought, and bad days in this mean sport of weightlifting that I love to write about and share with everyone. Letting the world know there are more bad days in this sport than good, but the one good day makes it all worth while. The one good day keeps us black sheep marching forward, creating our own path in life, separating us from the herd that makes us feel dead and down. A herd of white fur that kills thoughts and buries them beneath the ground, as dreams and ideas scurry for shelter leaving us back where we once started.....hell.

This Red Bull only gives me a fraction of the energy you give me. I can truly feel you on the other side of this screen, and I truly hope you can feel me as well. Thank you for your emails, your messages, your hand written letters that leave stains of salty tear drops from both our glassy eyes. Thank you. Thank you for rooting for me at meets, and getting my back on forums that are out to hang me. Thank you for watching my videos, and giving me feedback on the comments. Thank you for being my coach, because a coach you truly are. Thank you for being the red light on the camera making sure I fucken squat,

making sure I hit big weight, making sure I don't retire 'til we make
the 2016 games, because I'm not going to lie, with the growth of the
AN.....it's very hard to continue training. Some ask me how I even
make time for training. How can you still be an athlete? Where do you
find the motivation to continue in this sport with everything you have
going on? My answer is you, you the reader, you the YouTube watcher,
you the podcast listener, you the Twitter follower, you the Facebook
friend, you the skeleton who has gone through the same dark hell as
I have. You the once heroin addicted son of a bitch. You the once
unhappy person who worked a shitty job that you finally found the
courage to quit and live the midnight train life, finding what makes
you truly happy. I only coach what I have experienced, and I only
write what I have been through as well. I am you, you are me. We must
stick together, because without each other, we lose our own self, we
get lost in our own bodies, we find hell once again.

Thank you skeletons for making me face my once locked away demons,
giving me the momentum to become a better person, and better
weightlifter. Thank you for pushing me like the wind on my back.
Guiding me to create a better life for me and my loved ones. Thank
you for the kind words before I leave in a few hours to Venezuela. I
am not looking to hit any PR's, because this meet is not about me,
nor my personal goals. This meet is about representing you, the USA,
the AN Family that stretches world wide, across the seas and into our
coffee. This meet is for you, the ones who I have never met, but call
my family. The family I have never seen, but know is there. The
ones that are there silently, loudly, and dramatically chasing each
individual dream one PR at a time.

Thank you for everything. I will see you back here, on the stage of
dark, with violins playing and skeletons dancing......back here, in
the Dark Orchestra on July 1st after we bring home the hardware at the
Pan Ams. Salute. I will miss you all.

Skeletons 2016

♪♪♪

Cut grass and Cold Lemonade

Wednesday, July 17, 2013

The moldy teddy bear wrapped around her broken heart, as the
small little girl squeezed the air right out from his lungs full
of stuffing. Her tears became his, as they both sat in their own
abandonment......their own sorrow, their own closet full of skeletons.
The salt that leaked from her scars made the teddy bear become that
much more human, as the salt seeped through his old dusty skin.
Lost and afraid, empty and dark, lonely from the backs of so many
that have walked away, as the little girl and her teddy bear stayed
cemented down on the squeaky cot they both called home. No sign of
hope, besides the nighttime flicker from each other's eyes, as they
hope to awake in each other's arms once again. The clacking sound
of silverware to plates echo the mess hall as the other children and
their teddy bears eat with sorrowful eyes and long hair that drapes
into the food, as they stir the colorless and odorless food in front
of them with smooth long circles like a long stick on a glassy lake.
Walking back to their room carries no drive to look up and out the
windows that beg their attention. The sun piercing through only
covers their bodies with warmth, as their naked feet slap against the
cold floor. The windows are only a reminder of what not to come, of
how alone they truly are. The little girl sits outside of her room
like a guest awaiting pick up after a long meal. For she is no guest,
she is here to stay, and her ideas are here to die.

The girls in the rooms down the hallway used to play with one another
throughout the hallways and corridors. Now the silent tapping of the
rain above their heads makes up for the sound of laughter and taunting.
Missing her once adapted family only makes the cold night worse, as
memories and feelings make her tiny cot feel like a bed full of thorns
that cut her skin and dagger her heart. Once someone listened to
her, once someone shared their ideas and dreams as she did with them.
Once someone related to her ambitions and thoughts, once someone told
her everything was going to be okay. Now her teddy bear does all the
speaking, as his eyes close her cuts and his soft fur stops the bleeding.

9 years old now, and with every chatter of her teeth, a minute of her
life dies in her hands. The thought of not trying, not opening doors,
not turning the corner to see what lays around the bend makes her teeth
grind while she pulls out her hair one rip at a time. The older she
gets the less her teddy bear speaks, the less his love affects her.

Her sadness has been replaced with hate, and her teddy bear has been replaced by inflicted pain onto herself and to those whose backs face her everyday from this small enclosed cell barred deep amongst others. A crunch of gravel and a small chuckle outside of her glass window made her think what it would be like to live outside of the walls of this fostered flustered camp that imitates emotions of happiness that soon becomes drowned by black spider blood and left behind wax from the on-slaughter of false reality and an inception of normalcy amongst kids soon to be adults. Adults they will soon become, and the real world they will soon meet, face to face, teddy bear or no teddy bear....... the smell of cut grass and the taste of real food awaits her behind the tall black fence. But will she be ready? Will she really know what to do when released from this government prison called home? Her dirty feet tap against the cold concrete floor of her room as she reached for her teddy bear for the first time in years. Right away she regretted not spending more time with him, she felt awful for her abandonment of him, like the world to her. His smell reminded her of Christmas spent in the library down below, as they played dolls together and rolled in the opened wrapping paper. His old but soft brown fur felt smooth and warm against her cheek. As she began to rock with wide eyes and thoughts the felt closer to reality than ever before. Her teddy bear whispered in her ear, "Run like magic, turn this floor into cut grass, your water into cold lemonade, and your thoughts and ideas into dreams you can touch and feel....... RUN!"

The teddy bear's eyes seemed to break the stitches that kept him together. His soft chest became hard and strong, and this time his salty tears feel deep below him, crashing onto her cold feet, making them warm and ready for take off. She sprung up so fast the teddy bears arm almost ripped out from his body. Magic leaves appeared around her like a twisting tornado made her body run faster, and everything around her scurry out of the way. Her black long hair covered her face, as her teddy bear guided the way down the long hallway full of rolling beds, closed doors, flickering lights, and bloody hearts beating but broken and hanging from the ceiling and bouncing up and down throughout the floor of the hallway. There was blood everywhere, the closer she got to the doorway where she could hear the chuckles and lawn mower cutting grass, the more blood filled the hallway. Red blood turned into black as she slipped and fell into a pool of twisted veins and spider webs made up of blood vessels from her own body. Crying echoes rang aloud as the other kids jiggled the door knobs trying to release themselves from their rooms. She found her body wanting to stay, but her teddy bear and her mind wanting to

leave and fast. She tried her hardest to open the doors to let her
fellow broken hearted sisters out from their cages, but the doors
didn't have a handle for her to open them, all she could do was listen
to her once self bang against the medal door crying out for help. She
stood there while the banging increased, the blood raised, and her
teddy bear loosened his grip from her hand. The two swinging doors
were swinging open and closed from the cool wind that whistled freedom
and creaked words of happiness and love. She was at a crossroad, free
herself while the others died from the pool of broken hearted blood
rising higher and higher soon about to drown everyone with no hopes of
the outside world.....or stay and die with the others she has called
her family for so long. She looked down upon her now bloodied teddy
bear, while a tear fell from her eye to his, she told him that she
loved him and always will, and that he is her true family, he his her
true heart, that he is her cut grass and cold lemonade. He smiled
back and re-gripped his hand tight around hers, showing comfort and
strength. She took one of the empty soup cans that was floating past
her waist from the blood river that seemed to be rising faster than
she thought. She handled the soup can just right so the sharp edge
would expose the vein down the crease of her elbow. She took a deep
breath, gave her teddy bear one last look, and then slid the sharp
edge violently through her bulging vein...................

Blood poured out like a waterfall in the child hood books she used to
read. But nothing happened. She was not light headed, not dizzy, not
falling asleep......she.....well......she felt fine. The blood stopped
from her body becoming empty. The river of blood slowly crept back
down her legs, draining out from somewhere in the dark cold government
building where her sisters now laid quietly behind their bedroom
doors. Her teddy bear with his eyes closed, and his grip loose and
fragile. All she could hear was her loud breathing. All she could
see was normalcy coming back into the picture. Fog from her breath
captured her line of sight, as her arm not only felt fine, but the cut
was all together gone and somehow healed. She then realized she has
been dead the whole time. The End.

Accept the darkness, accept the hell, accept there are more bad days
than good, and you will succeed in this sport of weightlifting.

I'm back 2016

♪♪♪

495

The Curse

Friday, July 19, 2013

The clacking of my shoes tap quickly against the shingles on the
roof. My red cape sways effortlessly behind my running body, while my
eyes stay glazed full of water, as the cold night time air daggers
my eyes the faster I run. No time to think, no time to blink. Side
to side I sway, swooping past the midnight chimneys and the dinner
time steam, swirling through my body as safe families lay comfortably
below my rabbit like feet. The orange glow from the apartments below
fade away from the light blue sky above. Car horns honk while violins
play songs on the outer decks, platforms that float on the side of the
tall brick buildings give everyone the chance to be seen and heard. I
can sing, and I can write, but feeling is something truly made up of
might. Songs of happy, and songs of sad, every violin has a story to
tell as I find my foot steps running with the rhythm of the strings
below. I jump not fly, but for flying is what I truly believe I can
accomplish, air is something I truly believe I can become. Take out
your contacts what do you see? Not bad vision my friend, what you see
is a sea of air that you can touch and feel, air that you can breath in
and out while moving between love and hate. At times you may rest upon
desperate measures, hearing only violins that scream horrible crimes
and never forgotten lies. Angry yells from others below, drowned out
from the cold air that steers your ship closer to the blue glow.

I am an upper. I live high on roof tops with a belly full of coffee. I
stay high and running forward for many different reasons. Coffee is
not a choice, it is a must, without it my blessing becomes a curse. I
am an upper, a person that needs to live high at all times, for when I
am not high the bottom is much too low.... lower than most people will
ever know. Prescribed energy drinks to keep my knuckles clean from
blood. Red bulls to keep my thoughts from spiraling into a bottle of
vodka. Monsters to keep the monsters away. Miss Brown eyes to keep the
only rocks in my life the ice that dances in her soul.... the ice that
makes me a better person. Don't look down, stay high. Keep chugging
coffee so the streets of regret don't capture your progress onward.

The rain from the now cloudy dark blue sky makes the shingles wet and
slippery, hard to run on and all so blurry. My vision gets lost by
the cloud's fog, while my coffee gets low, my foot steps slow. I try
my best not to look down, so I sip the last of my coffee before Miss
Brown Eyes takes the deadly fall off the roof, ending her life by

496

hitting the ground below. I stop my running in panic to find sugar, a feeling of life or death as my thoughts take over. No! I yell on top if this roof, as my hands shake and my head swivels from side to side, looking for anything that will keep me high. The families below slap their windows shut, keeping my double edged sword far from their now tucked away kids that lay safe in their beds. Millions of beds just like these, scattered below the roofs of so many like these. My legs tighten as my gut aches, the Monsters in my gut began to take. My knees hit the wet roof, and my hands fall into my head, my thoughts turning black from the blue sky's cloudy blend. My cape that once flapped effortlessly, now strangles my neck cutting off the air I once could see and feel. Now my high is looking low, my life that I once knew is burning slow. The violin sounds have now turned from love to death, motivating to straggling, higher than high to lower than low could ever go. The cape around my super hero neck finally cuts the pipes closed that once screamed motivations to those who ran fast over dinner cooked steam. Now I fall into the depth of my own demon.

Stay High 2016

♪ ♪ ♪

The Quill

Monday, July 22, 2013

The most lonely popular man in the world sits beneath the ruble rocks and the cracked dirt, writing for the unknown faces that watch and speak to him from somewhere afar. He pictures their land green and rolling, yellow from the flowers, and blue from the sky above. His dirty water stirs in circles from the inside of its plastic domain. Small sips while typing gives his fingers just enough juice to continue the journey he sees in his mind. A rhythmic adventure, mostly filled with emptiness from those he has not seen in years, those that have left him in the down deep, where the light only seeps through the small snake holes that surround his dirt palace, a dirt palace he calls home..... holes that are too small for an escape route. Face full of dirt, mind clean as a whistle, he sails on paths that move with the clouds above, fast like a smile, and long like his stay below. His heels tap the dirt below, as his toes stay dug into the dry dirt. A drum set for writing, a musical escape to explore new worlds above. His eyes

glaze over as the feather moves frantically under his chin. His
sniper rifle up against the dirt wall, broken, and never used. A
gun that has no chance to fire, but awaits pertinently when duty is
called upon. The gun is like the writer, broken but steady, filled
with life in a lifeless hole. Dreams above march as nightmares
below dwell.

A long stare at the dirt ceiling above pierces the dirt like a nail
gun to wood, jump starting his mind to write! Jump starting his
mind to think outside of his thoughts. To fight against the norm
of pacing amongst his caged limits reality left him with. To write
is to see beyond your limits, to feel what you have never felt, to
witness a moment you have never seen, and to feel the impact of
something that has never impacted you before. The dirt lob of sweat
stung his right eye, as his left hand unconsciously wipes away the
frantic run for freedom his legs truly believe they are on.

"Run, young lad!" A character possibly made up, or possibly a real
live human that he somehow remembered as a very young boy appeared
under his feather, walking a horse by a lonely tree. Old man, with
a young walk and tall legs yells from afar. "Run for your life!"
The wise looking man yells again as the dirt from the walls that
slowly fall like ash after a burning, right to left, lower and
lower the pieces of his future lay quietly onto his leather paper
like a bedtime story before bed. The smell of homesick burning
as the sting from his lower gut snakes up his neck and into his
brain. His hands react to his hair, sliding his long nailed fingers
throughout the forest of dirt, dreads and grease. The taste of his
once family leaves his gums white and bloody, stained and in doubt.
His memories muddy while his parents wait in heaven as he awaits
in hell, for the day this dirt cage falls upon him, ending what
he now knows as life itself. His feet now digging into the ground
below his small ant hill of a table, digging like a horse showing
its strength before raising its black polished head for the cameras
to see and the rich to ahh over. Golden black, and ready to hoof
the next mother fucker who yanks him down from his high and mighty
pose. The rope around the neck of the beast only makes the beast's
teeth grow long and sharp, hungry for blood, and dangerous beyond
belief. Black from a dark soul, with eyes of white that see beyond
the horse's reality. Hope the horse sees, if only the horse could
write, he would write words of hope, pastures of green...... he
would nay words of freedom.

Freedom the man in the dirt farm felt, as his writing became more intense, finding its way through the leather and into the dirt behind. Eyes red from a lack of blinking, and feet half way deep in dirt from digging. If only this young man could write himself out from this rock, this prison blocking his thoughts.....he could set himself free forever. His eyes squinted low and sharp, focusing on the world he saw in his head, the world his hand was painting for him. He saw the horse and the old man once again, this time further down the path he was running on. A path that has signs that read unknown. Signs that read turn around! But around the turn he went, faster and faster as the horse that once laid under the lonely tree by the old man now up and running fast like the wind, smooth like the grass, and blacker than the end of the young man's pin. The horse escaped the rope attached to the race. Free from the people who once kept him on the dirt circle. The young dirt man writing remembered horses in his past life, and pictured the most elegant and beautiful horse he could think of. This was the horse running beside him. How he was keeping up with the horse he didn't know, for knowing didn't hold any water at this time of escape. The faster he wrote, the faster they both ran. The harder he wrote the older he became. Young behind the pen, a future that guaranteed doom, spoke the opposite under the pen. He ran and fast! He wrote and hard! He wrote so hard that the dirt around him started to shake, and his skin started to turn. The hair on his sweaty red knuckles turned from black to grey, as his knee that bounced his feet that dug into the dirt slowed down from an irritating ache. Green grass starting to sprout around his broken sniper riffle, while the small snake holes opened wider and wider letting in rays of blue sky and patches of warmth amongst his now wrinkled skin. He didn't seem to care, he just kept writing as if his pen were his legs, and the ink was the horse beside him. Run and write, type and fight, freedom in sight and a mind full of might.

The old man that once stood below the lonely tree was no longer. For the black ink captured his character, while the horse became his way out.

Write 2016

♪ ♪ ♪

499

The Glass Case

My hands lay locked together inside the front pocket of my sweatshirt.
Fingers passing one another as if pointing to a new path that leads to
uncharted territories. An orange sky covers my morning walk, as the
cold air creates a cloud of memories that start from my gut, passing
my stinging heart, touching my soul, and then escaping out of my mouth
for my eyes and ears to watch and hear replays of joy and cheers. A
slide show of tears and hugs. A highlight reel of raised hands, high
fives and goals reached. My lips tingle from the taste of the weights I
have kissed, and the kilos that have kissed back. The bar that I have
hugged a million times plays over and over in the early morning fog,
as the blood from my callused hands welcome my face from disbelief, as
I sit kneeled in a pond of my own hard work, embracing the pain that
has brought me so much love, so much life. My knees against the wood,
and my chest facing the ceiling makes my arms swing- back with great
flexibility. My grip fully released, from years of being hooked. Time
stopped, while my fast paced breathing calmly slowed, and the feeling
of life laid upon my body, as I dipped my head into a memory filled
lake that I once swam in as a little kid. A cold but awakening rush
opened my eyes full of tears, while a reflection of my life passed
throughout the cheering and overwhelming feeling of achieving a goal,
that was staked back when my legs were skinny, and my hands were soft.
A time when Arnold ran down my arm, and the bodybuilding world swirled
in dust behind me. A time where innocence ran throughout me, and
dreams of weightlifting took complete control of me. My eyes opened,
as the blurry vision and the alien planet looked back at me. On top
was heaven, but the climb up was life changing.

A quiet walk with loud memories filled with cheering crowds and Shankle
yells. Steiner slams, and get off me bro chest slaps. LeBron James
chalk throws as USA pumps proudly against my chest, while bleachers bang
with stomping feet, as three story stadiums chant... "USA". I walk
under the orange glow of the rising sun, as thoughts circle my mind full
of number one fingers raised high for everyone to see. Teachers who
doubted me, and society who forgot about me. Family members who were
once worried about me, and friends that didn't understand me. I raised
my finger high in the air to let the world know I was number one, coming
from a place where alcohol reigned king, while dreams were once drunk
with gulps of constant regret. My eyes open wide, while many doors I
closed shut, leaving drugs buried low under my feet, as many podiums

took me higher than any crystal could have ever achieved. My love will never die, and the feelings will never leave. Locked away forever, in a place where only I can go. One day this vault will create dust, while my old hands will wipe away the years with one smooth swoosh. Unlocking thousands of memories to share with others, to share with my kids, and my kid's kids. I will one day re-open this vault, and the memories alone will take me back to the cocky in your face, Jon North, that once lived proudly in the jungle of bars and plates, platforms and chalk, judges and critics, fans and haters, coaches and competitors, bomb outs and victories, goals reached, and goals lost. Tears of joy, and tears of sadness. The path I was on will never be forgotten.

I fought for more than me, and I achieved much more than 100 Gold medals. I achieved life, happiness, and a meaning. I achieved hard work, and the opportunity to meet thousands of great people. I have built great relationships, and built new friendships. I have found myself, something I have been looking for my whole life. I have achieved confidence, and an understanding on what it means to be a man. Weightlifting has made me a better husband, son, brother, friend, and person. I have learned so much from being an athlete in the sport of weightlifting. The greatest joy that weightlifting has brought me is the platform to help others. I fight for the "room 2" kids that stare out the windows while being horse fed ridalin. I lifted for the forgotten college graduate that was once praised for attending, but now lost and forgotten in the world beyond. I lifted for the society prisoners that I was once a part of, the ones who slave a dead end job. The unhappy. The misunderstood. The garage lifter who trains on their own. The black sheep everywhere...... I lifted for them. I lifted weights to tell parents ADD is good, not bad. Being yourself is better than any gold medal. Finding yourself is the Olympics of life, and achievement of a lifetime. I have won the Olympics twenty times and broke every world record there is to break. I have a golden outlook, coming from a dark narrow viewpoint I once looked through. I once lived under a rock, and now I stand tall on a boulder.

You the reader are everything to me. Out of everything, my biggest achievement is you. I have found my home, found my family, found a shoulder to lean on and an audience to relate to. I have found a keyboard to cry upon. Because of you, I have accepted my skeletons and bettered my life. Accepting the past is what you have given me, and I am forever grateful to you. I am forever grateful to weightlifting for giving me the opportunity to meet you. This blog is what made me a better athlete, by not hiding my skeletons...but getting to know them.

Your support has given me the confidence I needed in everyday life.
Your kind words have helped me become kinder to others and myself. By
you reading this blog gave me a voice, a voice that I didn't even know
I had. So thank you. Thank you skeleton, thank you for everything.
Thank you Weightlifting for introducing me to my Dark Orchestra family.

My coaches....... what can I say. I love you all. Without you I am
not me. Without your guiding light I am still in the dark. Without
you I am still addicted to drugs and alcohol. Without you coach..... I
am just a college drop out with empty dreams and a path full of thorns.
You gave me air to my lungs and a beating heart to defeat the demons
that pulled me down. I walk down this orange world thinking about
every coach I have ever had. The cold breeze makes my hot forehead
cold, as my tears dry like the chalk on my hands. My steps are heavy
as my emotions way me down. I look up to see the future, only reminded
of the past. The past that has created a small smile of fun and out
of control times we have shared together. I hope coach.... you are
smiling too. For the memories are with you. My shoulders sway, as
my eyes lay closed, in memory of all those who have taken time out
of their life to help with mine. I thank you, from the bottom of my
heart. My heart bleeds to only give back for the blood you have drawn
for me. I will be forever thankful to my ever-dying day.

I finally arrived from my morning reflection. I watery walk on a clear
crisp morning..... what a perfect morning it was. I grabbed my back from
the pain. My knees screamed to stop moving. My right elbow clicking
from bad lockouts and rusty joints. My left hip higher than the other as
my walk stings my right calf from the lean my hip has given me. I walk
into my house while my wife lies still asleep, looking more beautiful than
ever. I pass my long hallway where my medals hang in their glass case,
protected from harm's way, and proudly in sight for all to see. They
look beautiful and bright, happy as if the moment we met each other was
happening this very second. These medals have no emotion but happy....
I could swear they are smiling. Only if they knew how many medals I let
die throughout my journey. I don't tell them or show them that though,
I smile and tell them I am proud of them and that I love them. They of
course smile back..... nestled comfortably in their glass beds. I knew as
I walked away the next part would be the hardest. My head sunk low once
I left sight of the medals. My heart rang heavy. I must retire my shoes
and singlet........ the pump to any weightlifter's heart.

My shoes and my singlets stared back at me on the bed, as if to say
they didn't want to go to summer camp. They looked defeated and let

down, sad and lost. They looked as if their identity had just been
striped. Crusted chalk, crumpled numbers still pinned to the singlets
laid lifeless amongst bloodstains and coffee spills. Once on top of
the world, now dead. Once the fastest feet in the world, now slow and
old, dusty and forgotten. The USA slightly faded, as the rips down the
legs of the singlets spoke many stories, and told awesome adventures.
Each singlet told wise stories, different adventures, and not yet
talked about experiences. Each singlet has a life of its own, while
each shoe lifted miles and miles of platforms. I will hang you up high
to never be forgotten, I told them as I started to place them in their
glass case. So high that no one will forget about you. Your stories
will live on forever every time someone looks at you. Your impact
could change a life. Your view alone can spark a conversation that
could lead a young kid down the great path of weightlifting. You could
one day change a life......like the life you changed with me. And who
knows, one day when I have kids, I will take you out of your glass home.

I am officially retiring as a proud athlete of this great sport. Go USA.

Thank you

Jackie Mah
Paul Doherty
Donny Shankle
Dave Spitz
Max Aita
Glenn Pendlay
Ben Claridad
Rob Earwicker
Greg Everett
Kevin Doherty
Freddy Miles
Phil Sabatini

Most importantly Special thanks to my lovely Wife Jessica North.
You were there the very first time I touched the bar,
and you are here for the very last time I touch the bar.
Thank you for all your support over the many years.
I love you.

Coach 2016

♪ ♪ ♪

The Beginning

Saturday, August 3, 2013

Hand prints from my fist ever athlete Andrew Jester after qualifying
for school age Nationals, one of the biggest
highlights of my life. This was the moment
that sparked my true love for coaching.
Andrew went on to become a National
Bronze medalist a few months later.

I want to say thank you to my Attitude
Nation family for all of your love and
support. I am excited to start a new
chapter in my life as a full time coach.
I am eager to take my love and passion for
the sport of weightlifting and pass it on
to others. Being a coach, I now have the
unique ability to win more medals and make
more teams, than being an athlete alone.
The past 7 years, weightlifting has been
my life as an athlete. Now it is time for
weightlifting to be my life as a coach. I am
still hungry and more passionate than ever. The journey is not over,
it has just begun...

Weightlifting 2016

♪♪♪

The Fog

Wednesday, August 7, 2013

A grey sky on a cold day. The gym door closed, but unlocked and
open for the world. The loading dock door rattles open as I use my
body to pull, my butt as a lever, and my arms like cables. Watching
the chain beside me slither like a snake, guiding the flexible door
past my head and peaking high above the gym roof. A breeze from
the outside fog falls to my feet, gasping its last swirl before
falling to its death. My Adidas sweat suit acts as armor, keeping
me safe and warm, focused and protected. A fanny pack full of the

same dreams, just located in a new pocket. The zipper cold from the
gym air. My hands shaky with nerves, as the smell from left over
knee wraps causes pain to my nose, and a slight twitch to the face.
A familiar smell in an all too familiar world. Standing with new
shoes, on a path of old, leading to a platform of new. A cold gym is
the best, for cold makes sweat dry, making the bar stick well on the
athlete's throat, keeping the athlete's elbows raised for gold, and
out of reach from injury. The cold gym makes the hot coffee fresh,
cooling down yesterday's struggles, and focusing on today's goals.
My sweatpants low on my waist, as I look forward to them rising
higher and higher, as the years move on, and the time ticks round.
Hopefully one day my pants will be covering my head, as I poke two
holes to see my athlete's achieve more than I ever did.

Small chatter as the coffee machine in the front room drips, some
stretch, while others sit. A room full of rookie athletes ready to
bleed experience, some stretching and rolling, some doing nothing
but drinking coffee while all are reflecting on the journey ahead.
Reflecting is the best warm up an athlete can do. Leaving behind
the past, and focusing on the future is a champion's best asset. A
mental warm up is what comes in handy, when a hard training session
lays quietly in front. Calm and collect, deadly and destructive,
all while being necessary and life changing. I watch the minds
of the young roll like hills. The grassy meadows they still have
to climb, the burnt forests they will get to know. Side by side,
platform by platform, resting bench to resting bench, coach's
eye, to a weightlifter's feet, a rhythm lifter amongst a strength
lifter, all fill the cold foggy gym with different philosophies
amongst millions of ideas. One must choose why they are lifting
before becoming a champion, once this is established, the athlete
will grow and grow fast, running full sprint to the bar in front of
them, ready to meet hell before achieving heaven.

I cross the gym floor with a limp, as I make my way to the fan,
facing its wide circular back to the outside mist. A white world
surrounding a dusty gym full of broken hearts, and broken bars. I
turn the fan on even though the cold makes my finger tips numb. A
fan must be turned on at all times no matter what the weather may be.
The sound of the fan alone eases a person's mood, humming soft sounds
of comfort, as the skeletons lay to sleep. A turning fan is water
to skin, as the cold moves swiftly around your body, as the athlete
moves fast around the bar. I turn the fan on for comfort, white
noise, to feel the outside world as I live in the inside of a gym.

This gym is cold this morning, and first practice is always painful,
but once the athletes get moving, everything makes complete sense.

Cold Gym 2016

♪ ♪ ♪

The Overall Man

Friday, August 23, 2013

Ripped overalls with pockets full of broke. Brown bag full of
sorrows, and hopes full of let downs. Banned from society, outcast
from the world. You the dreamer no longer dream, but only hope to
find where this old dirt road leads. You walk with pride, as your
knees fucken scream with pain. Holes in your shoes like holes in your
heart, shot from the gun of loved ones and sprayed by the machine
gun of life. You still stand, I still write, we still walk, we still
carry on as our blood shot eyes fill with dirt and our hair with
exhaust from passing trucks. The smell from the black fumes reminds
us of home. It reminds us of hiding spots while parents fought,
closets full of coats and umbrellas that came alive and comforted us
as a crying child. The dark is safe, the light is open. A cigarette
brings back James Dean, as the 3 legged dog morphs into a strutting
cheetah. Messy hair from falling fast, soon combs back like a wet
comb as we fall forward. A chip off the old black that could get a
cargo ship lost in its depth. A middle finger cold and frozen, stuck
high from seeing so many stuck up. Red knuckles and permanent damage
from fist to wall, hate to self-pain, and frustration to must figure
something out or else. No money to spend, but a fuck load to gain.
No future, but a hope to one day look back at the past. A dying want,
with nothing to feel, a fight deep down, that seems to only roll in
the belly of hunger and a mind of dizzy as the lack of sleep drains
your thoughts. Homeless with no home, loneliness with no one, empty
and ready to fill the void that is restless within you.

An old abandoned warehouse lies in ruins at the end of this dirt road.
The green grass slowly turned into burnt rubber, while the smell
rose dark and the backward town seemed hidden but visible from where
he was standing. The once blue sky turned yellow, as black clouds
traced through like arrows being shot by a thousand gladiators. The
graffiti on the walls of the broken warehouse dripped like tears,
while the windows closed like fear. A street sign that reads welcome,

506

as the five-story warehouse quietly whispers turn around. Wind that talked, and weeds that grew so high they wrapped around the man's ankles. His cigarette burnt his fingers, making him jump and say, "ouch!" a necessary reaction. He whipped his hands against his orphaned overalls, while his head turned like a spinning top trying to figure out what and where his windy dirt path had taken him. A small child appeared randomly by the front door of the warehouse entrance. Probably 4'9 and 180 pounds of muscle. She was strong and confident, wide-eyed and alive. A tall and skinny man walked up behind her with his eyes never unlocking from the overall scavenger that found himself now surrounded by at least two dozen men, women and children. A complete circle was formed, smooth and fast, out of the dark shadows they appeared. A few more from the warehouse, even a handful climbing down the black trees that were bent and fallen but perfect for climbing and tree forts. The dirt below his feet was grey ash that slowly fell from the sky as if winter time during Christmas. Memories of the once good times in his life passed over his face, before realizing they were and have been dead for many years. His overalls slapped back and forth from the wind that swooped up and over the cliff in front of him. It seemed as if the world literally ended 100 feet from the broken warehouse. He started to lean his head up and to the side as if he was a kid in a car seat trying to see out the windshield in front of him. He was suddenly awakened from his thoughts and curious adventure, a mental adventure on top of a real life adventure. It was hard to faze the man that walked the dirt road with torn cloths and eyes filled with abandonment. His chip held a lack of surprise, while a tender and sensitive feeling of sadness created a shock wave of constant depression. But this......this gingerbread house in the middle of the black forest made his heart beat for the first time in years. His lungs filled back up with air, and then the silence broke.

A little girl broke the circle and sprinted towards the man's leg. Her mother ran after her with her arms out as if trying to catch a chicken. A panic took over the mother, but soon came to ease as she saw the little girl and the man talking to each other in a safe an ancient whisper. The little girl said, "Hello", and the man said, "Well, hi". He looked down at her glassy brown eyes and asked what her name was. She responded by not answering the question, but instead saying "Their are many bad days in this forest where the dirt path meets, but my mom says that if we keep training hard we can make it to the promise land". He looked up to the mother who stood a respectable distance away, while still being motherly. She looked back at the man with no emotion, only her hair in the wind, and the men behind her who looked like monsters with beards of strength and legs of trees. The women looked like lions, fast and furious, strong and hard working. These people didn't look like the normal folk, they looked as if they.......well........they looked like him. Holey clothes with ripped hands. Sad faces with hungry souls. Dry marks from tears, under a brain full of motivation. The only difference from the man in the middle of the circle in the burnt black forest on the edge of the world and the strong people is that they looked like they had found something to be motivated for, while he stood empty handed. He looked down at his hands with his forehead crinkled tight, while his eyes pierced down looking for something that should be resting like home in the palms of his hands. But nothing, for the people around them had something. The little girl tugged on his overalls that looked as if they were going to rip at any minute. She said, "Follow me sir, I want to show you something". They started to walk to the front door of the abandoned warehouse where the tall man with the red beard still stood, eyes locked like an eye to a target. He seemed like the leader, but then again... they all seemed like the leader. The man looked back at the mother to see if she had any problem with the new plot of the situation. The mother nodded her head, walked fast and then joined them by grabbing her little girl's hand.

Inside the warehouse laid 30 to 40 medal cots. Side by side, dream by dream, wall to wall they sat with medal feet, bodies of blankets, and faces made of pillows. The little girl jumped on one of the beds out of either excitement from a new visitor, or just because she was a freak athlete, and that's what athletes do, they move, they jump, and they test the limits. She was defiantly testing the limits of her mother, because she was soon told to get down. The man entered the next room and to his surprise found something that would change his life forever. It was a large bar that stood 30 feet tall, and at least as round and wide as the whole warehouse. How he didn't see the massive metal behind the house seemed impossible. It was shinny and long, dense and strong, alien like was an understatement. The overall man reached out and touched the bar as if touching his first-born's face. There was a moment of complete silence while he tried to gather his thoughts, and control his emotions. He had so many questions, but stayed quiet. Besides the little girl, no one had spoken yet. Just look, expressions, and gestures were being used thus far. The only noises were coming from the wind that had now died down, and the footsteps that had now stopped while admiring the pure shock this lost

508

man was in. Wings.........wings he thought, with his hand leaned
against the bar and his head down with thought. He looked up at the
man with the red beard and asked.....wings? The tall cold man who
seemed to take the leadership roll nodded his head as to say, "Yes".
"Wings to fly," the little girl said as excited as possible. "If we
lift the bar hard enough everyday, my daddy says the bar will someday
fly us away to the land of bright." She said this while pulling each
finger down as if she has rehearsed it a million times, and once
finished she looked back up and followed with a jump and a clap out of
excitement for nailing the plan the tribe had in front of them. The
man looked fast to the bearded man with a look of excitement as well.
The beard of the man nodded up, then down.

The wings on the bar spread at least 100 feet wide on each side. On
one side of the bar the wing hovered over the black forest that
covered the warehouse and the people who lived in it. The other wing
spread out past the end of the world, or what really was the cliff
that led to the land of bright, where the trees grew tall, grass grew
green, and the ash was replaced by rays of sun and wind of warmth.
The mother of the little girl finally spoke. Her voice was soft like
an angel, as her brown hair now fell straight down on the side of her
face from the wind dying down. "There is only one way to get to the
land of gold and bright, green and happy, cabins of wood and water
of clear." She then looked at the bar......he followed her eyes to
the bar.......the quiet stood for a while as he felt at home, as he
felt alive for the first time, as he felt a part of something, as he
felt he finally had something to feel, grab and lay in the palm of his
hands. He looked back at the mother with a smile on his face. The
black ash started to fall from the sky, and the bad day started to
come to night. His eyes wide, his heart beating fast.

She looked at her bloody hands and then smiled at her beautiful
daughter looking up at the overall stranger. She then said in the
most calm and soothing voice he had ever heard in his whole life.
"To train everyday."

Wings 2016

♪ ♪ ♪

509

Human Clay

The swoosh of the bar passed my body like a train to a nearby
landmark. Fast and furious, loud and violent, triple with extension.
A no wrong way to lift hill, grassy and tall, as millions of paths of
different ways climb the rocky banks, and the sharp corners of doom.
I pull like the wind, with a whistle from my coach and a buzz from the
buzzer, the athlete must react like a horse out of gate, or better
yet, like creasy bear shooting the gun to go, swim and fast, with
proper training and believing she will win her first race, while his
black shades and his alcoholic lips wait at the finish line. Proud and
stubborn, egotistic and cocky a weightlifter must be, that's how I was
at my first American Open.....my second meet ever. The break through
of who is this, and why is he so crazy. The golf clap turned oddly
shaped as critics type on the forums of hate. I slam the bar with my
old style of technique, to show the world that Coach Jackie Mah might
coach different than I do now, but her methods work while others
fail. I lift blindly for that's how I should, listen to your coach
young athlete, for then you will be good. There is no such thing as
technique young lad, just who will lift the most weight, and who will
be the one holding the gold. A lever system of different, a melting
pot of hers, that I took from her to only mold my own later down
the road. I am a thief, this is what I am. I have stolen different
techniques for years I have, a thief in the night my hands have meshed
those who have stolen techniques of their own. Accused of the same
crime, we are all walking this jail house line, melting pots of hot,
mixed with our own thoughts that leak to others in passing or plot.
You stole from him, and I stole from her, we create what we think
works the best, while the athletes we teach end up winning the golds,
reaping all the benefits of these stolen concepts. Fights rage, as
N.O. Explode gets drunk, somewhat like my farther, but mostly like
my strut. Walk with energy, lift with passion, my triple extension
technique is the best thing that has ever happened. No wrong, and no
right, my way now is just as right as the train passes my body in the
midnight night. My way of under is just as right as pull 'til you see
the thunder. A shrug under is what I coach, but back in this video a
shrug high is what got gave me a great meet, PR's over my feet, and a
crying coach of joy, as we hug with a mission accomplished by a young
rookie and her ideas of long. Who can lift the most weight? Who can
get under what seems to be impossible by marching sheep of white, as
they live in their comfort zones tucked in all so tight. A million

ways to lift, my way is only one, is my way the best? Abso-fucken-lutely you son of a gun.

I catch and stand, slam and cheer, a fist pump follows as my future is clear. A young rookie I was, and now I coach, just like Jackie Mah, my very first coach. Great success, in many other methods, lever systems that turn, and bodies that deliver a simple message. Win, fight, and keep the gold PR's in sight. I was skinny but boy was I right....for dropping out of school and giving this sport all of my might was the correct path to go down, even though others said different. Thank you Matt for sending me this song, as I listen I can remember the feelings I had, at my first national meet with a corner full of support. Butch Curry helping, as Paul Doherty was cheering. The audience clapping, as I yelled Arnold and smashed my meth pipe. Watching the smoke circle up my skinny shaved legs, no more drugs will I be your slave. I have found Arnold and this Asian coach named Jackie, this sport is my new life and you my friend are a smoke filled mirror that will live in my past. I will put you in a closet and write about you here, in the Dark Orchestra where tears fill the stage full of many that lay near. You the reader, what style do you use? I know you have smashed something on that stage of might, your chest out proud as you crush the demons that bite. We are new, we are fresh, lifting young with many blood stains on our chests. We must lift, we must coach, no matter how we get the bar above our heads we must lift more weight than ever before. Beat the man next to you and breathe in success, for handwork got you here, and this style of technique is the best.

Move on I did, after punching a man in the face, I was kicked out of my old club, and now training in a new space. By myself, at the Rock House Gym, no coach but the YouTube videos in the background. I felt the bar brush one evening day, I looked at my wife, and she asked me if I was ok. I laughed and smiled with confusion on my face, a new way of lifting must have made its way. A slice from the thigh, as skin pealed like an orange, still very triple extension, as the bar never made a noise. Coaches approved, as I shrugged high, the older more classic way of lifting was still in full effect. Homeless and coach-less, living in a car, to bar slamming hopeless dreams at times. One day become a National Champion was a dream filled with steam. The Bulgarians entered my life with their catapult ways, the bar made so much noise that my ears rang for days. What is this odd creature I asked, for these men had a weird bar path. My technique before this was changing by the day, morphing into its own before even this day. But this was something new, fresh and alien, the way the

511

bar met the body made me think again. Max Aita and Martin, Shankle and Dave, these lifters made my melting pot stir for days. My mind thought and discovered, evaluated and soon surrendered. My brush over time was met by a hit, above my ouch bone was bruised like a son of a bitch. To peak the bar in this way, the bar path moved in a whole different way. The start was funny for the ass was low, the shoulders moved in a line that threw me for a loop, the double knee bend was more delayed than my career getting started, if it wasn't for the meth pipe I've might already been a champion, now I just watched and learned at this odd looking finish, was she arched not straight, and why was this? These Cal Strength guys are so different than most, a fight club of some sort that makes me want to join. Run the streets at night steeling fat to make soap, human bodies moving around the bar like we weren't supposed to talk about it. The leader Dave, stood tall by Shankle, for the arm bend on this man while lifted I have never read in an article. I began to lift, like these athletes I followed. I peed blood for months, as a clean athlete on a Bulgarian training system was buried deep six feet down, and so were they. Dead and tired, no rest days and max out sessions that never seemed to end. I was still a young rookie that was hoping for rest around the bend. I kept my mouth shut, and my eyes wide open, for in the dark I stole from them, when they were not looking. Now I have multiple coaching techniques, Jackie Mah's hand book, mixed with Paul Doherty's philosophies. A Bulgarian system with catapult technique, laying in front of me I could hardly sleep. Like legos they laid, a puzzle to solve, a concept to build and a technique to stand tall. How and what, when and how, which lever goes where, and for how long? Silly putty I played, as water made my thoughts move, dreams to achieve, and past memories that won't remove. The start of something new and great, that started from the Jackie Mah's lift. Technique doesn't matter nor exist, only who is going to lift the most weight.

What is your melting pot like? And how will it morph? Will you steal from mine or keep it all? I hope you steal from mine to build your own. Create your ship and sail home. Salute.

Melting Pot 2016

♪ ♪ ♪

Mrs. Elders

My eyes wander as my elbows meet my knees. My bouncing feet shake my
body, swaying me side to side. My shoulders drop and my head swivels
side to side as I reach down to drink my coffee. As if a boxer dodging
a punch. My eyebrows raise at random times, as the skin on my forehead
crunches together. Thoughts pinch my brain, as I slide both hands up
my face and down the back of my head, only reaching for my coffee all in
the same fluid motion. Smooth I move, patient I am not. Someone just
walked into the gym... My head turned fast as if I have been up for three
nights. Paranoid by sounds and people. Uncomfortable and completely
vulnerable. A little head nod to the person who just walked in to train,
duffle bag and all. My quick glance of hello is followed by a glance at
his gym bag, as my eyes move a million little clicks around the man as
he walks to his resting bench. Old but sturdy, tired but alive. A lonely
weightlifter with a lonely bag, make for a perfect couple. A smile from
memory, followed by an all to familiar pinch from my head that now turns
my stomach as I lean further over my knees, making my elbows sting from
the pressure of myself and a thousand skeletons I carry around with me
scream with pain. The best fix for the weight you carry, is the weight
you lift. I roar from my seat as a coach should, passion and fire
spill out of my mouth, as my blood pumps through my body like the door
opening to Maximus once he reunites with his family. Love for the game,
and love for my team keeps my feet bouncing up and down with a certain
rhythm that no one could repeat. Every athlete moves differently, every
athlete must paint their own masterpiece. Every athlete must move to
move, lift to make, and slam to succeed. A simple whisper in your ear
from your past demons can make you lift weight you never thought could
be possible. All this... I have been thinking while sitting in my small
black chair in the middle of the gym.

A single sweat drop enters my eye ball. I never blink. Even
though the pain is masterful, I keep looking forward at the rows of
platforms that meet this wide open ocean. Dust replaced with sand
scurries over the wood creating a small clicking sound and a loud
whistle from the wind meeting the wide open beach. I still sit,
now motionless from thought, and paralyzed from my surroundings.
The smell of ocean you can probably smell just reading this blog.
The cool air passing your body is refreshing but sad, as it passes
you without any care in the world. It's true, you can read without
reading, just like the wind can pass without stopping. You can

lift without thinking just like the bar moves without trying. The
beauty of sport is so beautiful.

Two old teammates living in separate rooms in an a warehouse off highway
65 that lays between an old dead wood tree and Mrs. Elders home by
the old church. A small quiet town that unfortunately runs into an
abandoned steel mill that has been shut down for a decade. Jobs lost
and hard time followed, now home to myself and my teammate who breath
cold floors and bathe in showers of unanswered questions. Bouncy
balls thrown over and over against the walls of our rooms mix perfectly
with the sound of rats that scurry behind the brown walls that we call
shelter. We leave during the day, unnoticed and blending in. Lunch
pail in hand, as the sound of beeping from the cash register finds a
certain soothing feel to me and my friend as we ring people up before
going about their lovely day. Mrs. Elders came into the store with her
Saturday blue dress and her white gloves. Always a limp that seemed to
come with a smile. She shuffled along the isles as we both kept an eye
to see if she needed any help. I don't know why I did this, because she
never did, I guess just keeping an eye on her was a natural instinct
in some ways. I was once heaving 400 plus pounds over my head, and now
I have found myself looking after an old lady shopping for bread and
blueberries. Not such a bad thing since the next day she should be
bringing my old teammate and myself some of the best blueberry short
cake in the whole wide world. My over sized fore arm hit my friends
inflamed elbow as we cracked a smile before hanging our white aprons on
the hook by where the shopping carts filled into line, and then started
our walk up the grassy meadows, down the rocky bank that use to be where
they lit the steel on fire. I knew this because of all the black rock
that cracked under our feet as we seemed to march not walk, to a song
with nothing playing. It was almost like we were re playing all of our
old training songs in our heads at all times of the day. And if one of
us smiled it was definitely a missed lift followed with a little kid
hissy fit. Grown men throwing fits is always the best. We approached
the warehouse were we lived. The front door already open, almost as if
the old shut down world was awaiting our arrival. Our eyes met...

Jon! my heart jumped out of my chest as Shankle shook my right shoulder.
I was back in the middle of the gym, same place I started. My cheeks
were drenched wet from my eyes never closing. A nightmare...? Or a
great dream....? I couldn't figure out which one it was. I could still
smell the ocean breeze, and I could still hear the beeping of the cash
register. My actions and odd behavior didn't seem to faze Shankle at
all. I couldn't figure out why. You would think he would have asked

514

me what was wrong, if I was alright, or what i was doing sitting in the middle of the gym staring at God knows what. But nope... Nothing. His mouth was moving, but I could hear nothing. I was too busy analyzing the situation. Shankle has been to the same place I have been. Shankle has been on the beach, in the store, and in the warehouse. This was just a guess, but his understanding of the odd situation was too familiar. Too at ease. He then walked away. And I was once again left alone.

My breathing became heavy. My eyes finally shut. The sweat on my face dried as the wind from outside picked up. The sound of the fan by the door made my wrists move in circles. My body leaned back over the chair like a waterfall, as my back cracked at least six times. The crunches in my forehead smoothed like the dust on the platform. The windmill began to move gracefully, as my arms cut through the air in fast circles like a jet flying over a baseball game. My chin moved front to back, side to side, like the catch of the snatch, like the beauty of an athlete. The black oil ran down my face and into my joints, passing over my skin and into my bones. Oil to move, and muscle to improve. Strength to build and speed to gain. My Adidas shoes feel tight against my feet. My eyes soon change from focused to fierce. My body language turns from passive to aggressive. Confident to cocky. My blood, to Shankle blood. My skeletons behind me as I write ARNOLD down my arm. My hook grip becomes tight like suffocation. I am an athlete. I must move to live. Lift to love. I am a prisoner of my own self. My skeletons, lets lace our shoes and grab our belts. Stand up from this chair. My skeletons... Lets fight.

"My ears hear what others cannot hear. Small far away things people cannot see are visible to me. The senses are fruits of a long time of longing. Longing to be rescued, to be completed. I am not formed by myself alone. I wear my fathers belt tight around my mothers blouse, and shoes which are from my uncle. This is me. A flower does not choose its color. We are not responsible in what we have become to be. Only once you have realized this is when you have become free". - Unknown.

I truly tried......but could not part. You will see intensity like never before. I am back.

Love for the sport 2016

♪♪♪

The Closet

His head hanged low, as the folds of his Asian eye lids drew shade over
his regret. Two eyes that have seen hell, as abandonment and pain pump
through his veins as he sits on the white crinkled paper in a world of
white and a smell of death. A time and place where everything stops,
and the world focuses in on a single man. A man that is a master of
capture, a slave owner of skeletons, and a warden of the biggest death
row prison known to mankind. A man that turns the other way, for the
pain burns when confronted. A man that has experienced heaven......only
to live in hell. Skin beaten, hands clammy. A worried look comes over
a man that never looks worried. For worried is an emotion never shown
nor confronted. Sad is something too close, for looking back hurts
the most. Walk fast, at times run, Bonny and Clyde himself and his
gun. Never get caught is a philosophy that has caught up. Now silence
takes over, reality knocks. His head of knowledge and mastery turns
to the side as his eyes continue to lay low, almost as if he is being
protected.......safe from what lies in front of him. Bonny has been
caught, and now fear meets Clyde. My father of strong, must now meet
his weakness......his own skeletons.

A small tint of orange met his black boots as the doctor's office drew
dark. The only light coming from the bottom of the closet door that
flickered up his legs.....leaving his face barely lit from the reflection
of the orange lake below his feet. He felt better in the dark.....he
always has. Years of excuses, has finally run out, as the closet door
started to shake. The banging sound of bone to wood made his hands
bury his face for comfort, as the reality started to enter through the
closet cracks. The skeletons wanted their freedom, the skeletons needed
him to become free. Mad at himself......mad at the world. His father
passing makes his gut turn. Pain that makes him want to throw up, and
at times......escape. An older daughter that leaves him breathless at
night, turns his pillow into a clenched blanket of might. Someone to
talk to he should, but his skin is stubborn, while his skeletons suffer.
He will never be free, unless he enters the Orchestra.

His beat up body and unhealthy lifestyle made it hard to get off the
bed. The white doctor's sheet crinkled as his left hand pushed against
his left knee to get up. He stood outside of the door now quiet. His
breathing became fast, as his heart raced like his life. He reached out
his hand and turned the knob. The door opened with ease, almost as if

someone pushed from the inside. His whole body was covered in a glow
of orange. The warmth of the light made his breathing calm, and his
eyes open wider. His skin looked brighter as his body became lighter.
Already a sense of relief...for just entering his past was a tough step.
A skeleton dressed in red with gold cuff links asked for his ticket.
The skeleton's red locomotive looking hat hung off to the side, shading
one side of his face. His eyes were hollow for my father's eyes were
his. Sight connected with sight, heart beat to heart beat, emotion to
emotion they were more connected than the skeleton's bones to joints.
One in the same......my father never understood this.....for my father
is his worst skeleton.   The ticket ripped as the bony usher drew his
arm out to the side with a small smile and a tilt of the skull, guiding
and welcoming my father to the 5 story hall filled with endless rows of
seats looking down upon the empty black stage. His hand laid out flat
in the air, feeling each seat as he walked in wonder. One of those
walks where your eyes and thoughts are so far gone, that how he knew
where to walk was amazing. His slow but long stride moved my father
up the first batch of stairs to the second story balcony. He turned
down each isle keeping his eyes located on the old wood stage in front
of him. His feet sticky to the floor each time he took a step. The
sound was as if someone was ripping tape. The ground was filled with
salt....salt from every tear he ever drew. Salt from every person he
hurt and who hurt him. Salt from abandonment, loss, happiness and the
biggest one of all.....regret.

While still keeping his head forward and eyes glued to the stage, he
blindly felt the arm rest with his left hand, and then sat down in
the very back row on the second story. So far back.....he was almost
hidden. Hidden from from what he had been hiding from his whole life.
A big deep breath made his black v-neck shirt move up then down. His
hands knocked against the arm rest as if he was singing a song. His
head now rotated side to side, then up and down in a nervous scurry
all around the huge auditorium. Excited for how far he has gone,
but in fear for what lies ahead. At least one hundred skeletons from
every angle of the stage slowly walked out to the stage each holding a
different instrument. The skeletons were dressed in all black.....black
like my dad's suits in the 90's. Black like the nights filled with
smoke and snow. Black like the sports cars he used to drive when he
was once rich. Black like the up all night nightmares. Black like the
circles around his eyes, black like ashes from his burnt relationships.
The skeletons took their place with such ease. No applause.....for
there was no one else to watch my father. There was no one in the
audience to watch my father play from the second row balcony. His

fingers become stiff.....while his head tilted to the side. His v-neck
turned into a tux, while his black circles slowly vanished from his
face. And then it happened.......he started to play! The Orchestra
of skeletons played loudly with him! The ground filled with salt as my
father cried while the violin strings sung. His body now moving with
rhythm. Side to side, his body moved while his eyes swayed violently
with every stroke of his arm. Blood ran down his nose from playing so
hard. The sounds of the violin was crying with pain and emotion. The
strings were screaming as his eyes now laid closed and his eyebrows
danced above his eyes. The skeletons on the stage were trying to keep
up with him, but falling short from the speed and violence my father
was playing with. The skeletons were smiling at each other as salt
water began to creep up their white bony legs. At this pace they would
all soon drown from my father's tears. The water was now up the the
skeleton's necks. They raised their instruments high above the water
to continue the song of my father's life. They played with passion.
They played with joy and pride. As my father did the same.

The song stopped.......the Orchestra went dead quiet. My father's
breathing was fast. His eyes slowly opened to an empty stage. The
sweat was falling fast down his forehead stinging his eyes. He
stood with weakness from the journey he just experienced. You could
hear a pin drop from the silence that was surrounding him. Silence
that usually haunted him....now gave him a sense of peace. He felt
different, he felt light, he felt......well.....good. He made
his way to the closet door that led him to this world he hasn't yet
figured out, but at the same time completely understands. He opened
the closet door to find all of his skeletons waiting for him on the
other side. Hundreds packed into the doctor's office, all smiling
from gaining their freedom, and seeing my dad gain his as well.

Let your skeletons from your past guide you to the future of tomorrow.

I love you, Dad. I am so glad we have rebuilt our relationship even
bigger and better than before. Today is day one of the rest of our
lives. I am glad my skeletons have met yours.

Welcome Father.........to The Dark Orchestra. 2016 & beyond

Focus 2016

♪ ♪ ♪

518

Tiger Blood

Wednesday, October 9, 2013

Naked I stand.......tiger blood I drink. White sheep skinned fur hangs from the back of my neck, falling like a cape and dragging against the muddy ground behind me. I stand tall and sharp, my head turned to the side like my sword....jagged and on point, down and in, ready and steady. Blood runs down my face as I close my black eyes and drink, drink what has given me great success....and even more failure. My double edge sword cuts my hand while I spin my blade around and around, taking out the skin from my palms like a grapefruit. A rhythm warrior, only left with a steady rhythm of nightmares. Nightmares that keep this fearless man in fear, while dreams stream out, long and cold under a bridge where water runs under, while others walk over. Tiger blood cuts tallies from the point of his blade into the pierce of his skin, one by one men have taken their last breath, as a cut from their skin now lays at rest on his. This blood called tiger makes men do extreme acts of good or bad.......how you use this curse is up to you, the reader. This blog is about the man who gave you and I this curse. A blog about a man who came about tiger blood and what he did with it. This blog is about you and me.

His home is made up of other's abandoned problems, left for dead skeletons, and forgotten relationships. He sleeps on rocks that have been beaten by the tide, as the sand from the wash of others builds walls high and strong under his bridge of protection and capture. The stream runs red with blood, as the bridge above marches with new hopes and dreams, as the warrior underneath battles demons left behind from the white sheep above. Drinking the blood from dead skeletons gave him the strength beyond anything anyone has seen. The strength to swing his sword violently through the guts of the ones above. The naked warrior promised with every drink from the red stream, that he would take vengeance on those weak minded souls who left their own skeletons to die and rot, turn sour and be forgotten......he would take his sword and bounty those very people who gave him the curse he carried inside of him......the curse of extreme emotion. Heads fell to the ground with each swing of his sword, rolling heads were then thrown to the side for bears and birds. His rusted sword had to cut at times rather than slice, for the past of the ones he was killing made his swing heavy and his sword dull from left in the rain emotions. Tiger blood pumped through this warrior's body so hard that

519

he at times would scream at the headless bodies before ripping their
hearts out and drinking the dripping blood that was left, trying to
move like traffic in New York. He drank blood and became strong, he
drank the blood from those who didn't know how to use the blood they
had. He opened his mouth and began then to eat their bones. One by
one he slaughtered every single person who walked over the bridge
above his home, drinking blood to gain endurance, and eating their
bones to build strength. His face was covered in blood splatter and
spaghetti looking guts. His knee would meet the ground as his hand
would enter their chest, ripping out everything that once laid like
a puzzle.....complicated but perfect.....now complex and scattered.
Hundreds dead, that murdered a hundred themselves.....he was finally
feeling good about himself. He felt he was doing right.....was he? I
have no idea....I'm just telling the story of the man who once took
bounty on those who drew blood to a stream that he drank out of.
Blood from skeletons he adopted and took in....literally. Skeletons
who gave him strength and nightmares. I am telling you a story of the
man who killed hundreds......and saved hundreds.

5,000 years ago, this warrior under the bridge of red, made love
to a woman a few years later.......a woman that was immediately
infected by this curse. She soon became the first female hunter all
the tribes had ever seen. She killed more animals than all the male
hunters combined. She somehow felt she had the strength of a million
people.......what she didn't know.......is she had the strength of a
million skeletons.

You the reader......let me introduce our long lost relatives.

The Curse 2016

♪ ♪ ♪

Monsters & Coffee

Wednesday, October 16, 2013

What a morning it is. Crisp cold monster after a tall hot coffee.
One dripping with sweat warming the soul with ease and serenity.....
while the other burns the throat from its ice cold daggers when
chugged at a fast pace. ah yes......motivation rings throughout my
ears, as the the sound of white buzzers fill the gym and the cracking

520

of an almost broken bar spins closer to meeting the graveyard of steel
and dust. Miss brown eyes dances on my right shoulder whispering
songs of sex and passion......while the monster on the left tells cold
stories of my past, guiding my anger out with a middle finger and a
chair thrown to its death. Fuck you chair, fuck you world. I wear
a gold grill placed on my teeth to smile at the ones who once kicked
dirt upon my dreams....who laughed at my potential.....and who doubted
my every move. A smile of gold that tells a story of a grid that lead
me here....with you. A half cracked smile that once lived homeless
with broke. I smile of clean to say no more to the Crystal smoke that
once filled my lungs with a high that makes sense why so many would
turn in everything for another taste. The problem with meth is that
it's just that good.....I'm not going to lie. But....the best thing
about the gym life society is that it's even that much better. Gym
life for life as we drink coffee side by side. Hand in hand, filling
our stomach with swords and weapons, ammo and shields, attacking the
society that we once fell capture to. Society....you will now feel
the wrath of my bar, as an earthquake will take you all down to the
cracks of hell and into the dark where we the Orchestra call home.

Another coffee.....this time mixed with monster for todays openers. A
hit and quit type day. Gearing for a meet this saturday. Gearing up
for the small glimpse of light before being dragged back down. LETS
BREATHE! This my friend is what a meet is....the surface of the water
where our heads meet the sun! Reach and grab, hold steady and then
stab! Dig your knife deep into the belly of the beast for a feast
with the ones who fight in the gym you call home. Once alone.....now
you are a part of a mafia that stretches from this blog to the ones
breaking blood vessels to watch you stand. Yell, "Mother fuckers!"
We alone are weak, for numbers make us strong. As each bars slams,
the offices across the street gather canned food, as all the prisoners
to money and retirement 4 1 k's panic. Every bar that is broke the
trainers at planet fitness gather their weak-minded sheep under ground
for fear of.......us. For fear of higher standards, and morals that
fall from the ski the size of beach balls, crashing upon car windows
and shattering "fuel economy cars". I work hard to put gas in a car.
I don't need or care if a car gets great gas milage. I drive fast n
furious, loud and bold, in a car that eats gas like I eat sheep.

This morning I am writing in the front office next to others, in a
room of sun and smiles....maybe this is why the skeletons are in such
a good mood, positive, and outgoing. My dark office with a flicker
of light can make our skeletons draw dark and painful......which I do

521

truly love. I love the dark. I love pain.....why? Maybe why is not
the right question. Maybe why not is the right thought process. Why
is it frowned upon to feel safe in the dark? To feel pain from the
past? Embracing our weakness? Atmosphere is everything. Salute.

Newest Team ANW video

White Monster 2016

♪♪♪

Blood Shot

Monday, October 21, 2013

The white glaze that once circled her brown eyes now lays in a bath
of blood, as a shot of warmth meets the cold outside air. Steam
moves like fog around the icy mountains that stagger her on point
journey where land meets water. Throughout her tunnel vision......
each step will soon push her closer to feeling alive, once the blood
from her eyes falls fast upon her moving feet. As the dragon flying
above her breathes fire amongst the now charcoal black trees.....
she adds another taste of blood for the rush of bravery and balance.
Blood so heavy her eyelids droop, low like the bank she walks to,
heavy and deep like her past. Evil pulled them down to see what
lies within the eyes that look out, to figure out how someone so
fragile can become so strong. The black dots that never seem to
blink have now been infected with the blood she has drawn so heavy.
A shot of reality to help with reality. A shot of warm meeting
cold to create some sort of fucken balance that this life has given
her. Her hands ice cold as the rocks of gravel under her feet roll
with crunch as the path she takes leads her to the destination of
her choosing. With every step a drop of blood falls, warming her
with a coat of white as her skin turns ghost from the loss of blood.
The evening turns dark like her soul, as the ice around her melts
from her warmth. She gives off a certain vibe that makes the knees
from others crumble and grow weak. Strong with a taste of bold,
some can't seem to handle her power, some can't seem to swallow her
misery, her pain.... her faults. Some can't seem to handle what
truth she holds. The smell of sharp, the after taste of regret. She
is you.... the direction of love, real and never forgotten, for some
stay hidden away from the bank she walks toward.

A cold night chills the plants and trees that bend like ballet
dancers, falling and swinging like a play that asks for her
approval. For claps are unseen, for the blood has drawn shade
over the already black holes that sink into her head. A dark roast
of fire burns her stomach with every step, closer and closer she
walks.... faster and faster her heart pumps, moving her feet at
a steady pace over the frozen hills and green landscape she calls
necessary. Fight within released from the hell outside makes the
skin turn from the reader to her, as she screams to the moon while
digging her long nails into her palms.... a grip so tight only blood
could be drawn. For blood is what makes any shot swirl and scream,
come alive and dream, to walk the night with a dream in mind, to get
closer to this reality becomes a responsibility that weighs heavy in
her hand. As her mind turns, the mixture of both energy meeting
energy rattles a heavy blend of storm and rain, wet as the melting
rocks that slowly turn into her brown eyed pain. Becoming a part of
myself, you the reader whoever mixes two toxins of the some sort
will figure, a storm of some sort will violently rain down upon the
ones who fucked us. Giving all hell to capture, for freedom within
is without blood from within. She bleeds the shot of her life which
makes mine spike with fierce revenge, raining hell on those who
struck me down, for cuts on my back keep me from drowning in hell.
My own scars are what keeps me curing the ones of others. I will
cut my skin deep with the nails I have grown, so others can't. She
adds an extra shot, so they can't.

She met her edge, as the water met her lips. Red like her eyes....
red like the sea she looks over. Home bound, and ready to live under
a liquid layer where fear cannot reach. Her eyes now closed, as her
toes met the fall, while her heels stayed steady on the bank of ice
and rock. Still cold, still night, for she felt warmth as the shot
of confidence met her that night.....she then took a deep breath.....

"Your name is strong, you must kill it before they kill you".

- unknown

Miss Brown Eyes 2016

♪ ♪ ♪

523

The Inside

Wednesday, October 23, 2013

Character influenced by Dallas Hunter

Story inspired by us all

His walk was staggered, and his limp was obvious. His shoes were
ragged, while his laces ran free, bouncing from side to side with every
heavy step he took throughout the cold evening city than ran pity
amongst him. Looks of sorrow followed with looks of disgust. Looks
of shun from head to toe, as a dirty beanie meant homeless to those who
grabbed their kids to gain space from the man who had fallen into the
cracks of life. October leaves dance around his feet on this windy
cold day. His eyes closed as his beard tilted up, facing the cloudy
murky sky with a pause from the long walk. His beard red, his eyebrows
brown, his shirt dirty white, as the deep stretched out V-neck exposed
the bruises on his chest, and the cuts on his neck. Pale white skin
from a lack of sun.....pockets inside out for money is gone. His grey
sweats that fit tight around the legs feel comfortable and warm on
legs that dig deep in mud. Hair salon shops laugh, while kids out of a
candy store play tag. Grocery carts rattle as business folks chatter.
The sounds of laughing make his eyes drop low like his V. Memories of
a time where life was smooth, an easy smile made a comfortable mood.
Now a smile comes once a full moon, as the dark casts a light that
leaves too soon. The city is alive while this man is dead. His sweats
hang low and saggy around his waste from the absence of his drawstring
that once tied tight and high, for now he must grab the front to keep
them up and on.....a jail house walk while singing a jail house song.
The red hair that covers his forearms cuts like a thorn, as his non-
hydrated body pleads for water, only to be given coffee. One more cup
of coffee and the body might fall. Dry up and cast a shadow amongst
the concrete wall, leaning and breathing for life as others watch him
fall. No one cares, for an outcast he is, a street bum that can't
find his way in a maze of city streets, lost in a world of white sheep.
Lost to be never found, addicted to drugs and robbery he must....for
this man is the leach of the world and must....must be crushed.

Dry blood sleeps upon his knuckles of white, finding a home where
consistency lives...makes even blood sleep tight. His long red beard
dry and tangled, matted and fragile. High to his eyes and low on
his neck, his beard is a mask that hides who he was, barring the boy

he has left behind. The beard is a warrior's cape that represents
independence. The beard is an expression of man hood, fight hood, a
new path hood. A drop the boy off and grow a pair hood. His beard is
a shield of fire that keeps white sheep away from its heat and mass,
strength and power, a V-neck of dirty sweat mixed with bloody knuckles
that string painfully in the shower. His bold beard that screams for
water keeps the city street herd away.....as he gets close to his
destination from the far away place he started.
His masterful beard looks more beat up than him, but what some don't
see is the strength within...under what the skin hides....some don't
see, that the inside is where the beard grows, starts, and blossoms.
The roots of where we started is where our strength is born.
Forgetting our past and what lies beneath... is the down fall of so
many that now lay dead in these city streets. His legs might be weak
on the outside, but strong like bull beneath. This broke homeless
looking bum keeps walking....one step at a time. Every step counts,
no matter how he truly feels. The devil in a red dress awaits with
open arms around each turn, as a young lady working at a bank firm
firmly grabs his hand giving him a chance with change....to them he is
weak.....weak and wounded......

The red bearded man of an awful smell and lips of dry, stumbles into
the gym with a limp of pride. He slaps the hands of many as home he
is......he grabs the bar with knuckles of pain....for it is time for
weightlifting practice......once again.

Strong 2016

♪ ♪ ♪

Numb

Monday, November 4, 2013

Freezing fucking cold, as her whiter than a ghost hands beg for the
warmth of a cracking fire. Snow flakes slowly fall amongst her open
palms, like a plane landing safely on its runway. Fingers laid back
like the snow on the ground, open but tense, solid but breakable. Her
muscles ache with pain... pain like water to a burn... pain like the
wind to a paper cut... pain like the below freezing morning wind on
her bare naked body. She sits on the edge of a carousel dragging her
feet, open toed, across the surface of the snow like a fishing line,

525

gliding against the glassy untouched water. Fucking cold. The icy
snow puncturing her feet draws spots of red, like an artist drawing a
face of sadness. Tears to feet like tears to eyes, the red spots draw
blood for protection, as the cold tries its best to keep the blood dry
and away. The white snow stains her skin to white, as her insides
bleed blood to sight. A battle raged on a woman's feet, on this early
morning sunrise carousel. Her ideas and dreams become more alive than
ever, blurry but focused... as the breath taking cold elevate her
emotions to a new height never experienced before now.

She is butt naked, and by this point her butt is most likely stuck
against the medal seat of circles. As her naked body spins faster and
faster, the wind stabs her from skin to spine, speeding her heart
up with eyes of wide. She is alive and she feels cold but steady,
relaxed but tense; she spins with her feet on the ground and her arms
reached high. Her head leans back as her hair becomes like rain,
falling around her sight as the sun comes piercing in. Heavy and
light, fast and slow, her emotions turn and flow, like water from a
fall as the sun through the clouds never move. Her vision is straight
up, as her body is slowly dying. She has been out in the morning
breeze for much too long... even waterfalls freeze when the weather
draws too long.

At this point, her naked body feels nothing, as the air that passes
moves around her breasts like a face under a mask. Hidden and
untouched, the unrecognizable cold is replaced with warmth from the
fire within. Every spin makes her skin strong and tough, as her goals
draw closer and closer... with a simple stretch and a reach she could
touch them. The cold had lost, as she has won, her feet now red and
colored from the blood that has drawn victory amongst the daggers and
fears melting from the sun. The beautiful woman that spins naked on
the snow... she has become numb to the powerful force that she had
always been afraid of.

Mother nature is a powerful queen, yet this woman's body is an
undiscovered phenom. Within it lies a great magical power she had not,
nor possibly would have ever understood nor experienced. What can this
cold weather do to a body that sleeps and walks under a blanket of
pain? Will this pain she feels from the cold daggers of wind take away
her pain by adding more pain? Yes, she is dying... but by dying she is
living. The more she sustains the closer to death she walks... hours
have went by and her heart has almost stopped. Facing death without
feeling its wrath, her body like ice as her breath breaths success.
Eyes open as she stops the carousel with her feet, like an anchor she

stomps her feet deep. Bam! On a dime she stands tall and proud, naked and loud, near death... but more alive than ever before. She smiles at mother nature with her teeth whiter than snow. Her hair falls amongst her face with water dripping to her toes. She cannot feel a thing besides her dreams. She walks away with steam and passion... strength and emotion... a body of numb with goals to overcome.

Freezing Fucking Cold 2016

♪ ♪ ♪

Bo Bo

Friday, November 8, 2013

Inspired by my childhood growing up on a horse farm.
&
In loving memory of my childhood horse, Bo Bo.
You will never be forgotten.

Teeth yellow from smoke, as gums draw blood from a lack of brushing. Saliva stretches from jaw to jaw like cob webs banding together from tackle box to old saddles in a dust filled horse barn. Spit flies from an athlete's mouth like hay particles shattering into a cloud of haze, as the watchman heaves bails by one knee into puzzle pieces... hand by hand, gloves to orange twine. Stack after stack he works like art... as the horses watch with hunger. Hunger from the weightlifter's eyes fill with blood veins that cast upon the white glossy outlook of bright lights glaring back in a mist of hands that clap like whips to the back of a horse. The indoor arena the horse circles, makes the crack of the whip extra loud, as the echo of the athlete's yell has now turned into a scream for all to hear. One persons head drops from the back of the room from understanding, as shade can comfort such emotions... good and bad. The loud nay from the horse moves through the barn like a base jumper passes mountains and trees, as the horse turns gracefully, each front knee raises high and mighty, confident and powerful, loud and in your face......the barn becomes alive with cheer, as the horse performs its masterful craft.

Dust kicks up as hooves trot violently... a spray that only a slalom skier could duplicate from a cut through crisp morning air, on a glass sheet of reflection like eyes they stare. Gripping the handle not to

fall, the skier leans like a knife cutting through the wake like a
weightlifter creating a massive earthquake. Crack! The place goes wild,
the horse nods his head as his perfectly combed mane swings like hands
that raise in victory. Sweat that tells a story makes the athlete's
journey more humbling, as the sweat makes the black horse glossy like
a ghost in the old barn of dust and webs. The smell of the barn like
gas at the station, manure and the leather saddles makes the barn rich
in smells. Eyes water from the weightlifter's eyes from the pride
that bottles his throat, an achievement of life makes a tear splash
against the wood, as the fruit of his labor tastes salty and good. Eyes
water from the smell of the barn, as both sides of the breezeway open
and long. Wind passes through like young horses live and die only
to give birth to new. Old wheel barrels tell stories of hard work
and purpose... as the weightlifter's ripped shoes stand perched on a
podium of high... overlooking the mountain he just climbed. The soul
of the barn speaks to you when you open each stall. The horse nods
with understanding and excitement... for it's time to roam the outdoor
pastures with other friends to run with... open world with open wind,
away from the barn the horses live. The weightlifter pops champagne
celebrating being a champion in a sport where so many die. Open path to
more success the gold medal speaks into the ear of the beholder... as
this gold medal brings a reluctant sigh to the athlete's state of peace.
The horse runs fast for training it's not, his technique is all over and
wild for this can't be taught. Freedom and happiness is something that
lies within. This barn and this gym are the same, for both have stories
and souls from the decades they have withheld and always will withhold.
This is a story about a barn and a gym, a weightlifter and a horse...
both athletes, both freaks to some... both with much to overcome.

The horse takes a deep breath as the weightlifter breaths out. The
horse's knees wrapped for the cold, as the weightlifter's calves stay
wrapped from pain. Both will sleep will blankets tonight, as rain
makes a beating sound from the roof they sleep under. Both tired from
a day of activity, both dreaming about the next, for a new day will
soon arrive as the sun rises high. The barn will smell like leather
and the gym will creak with water leaks. Both the horse and the
weightlifter are athletes... both are at peace.

BO BO 2016

♪ ♪ ♪

528

The Elephant Man

Monday, November 11, 2013

Chunks of puke blasted the inside of the little white airplane bags
that once laid flat and steady under the red spread out chairs facing
the stage. Puke after puke... the bags filled with disgust as the
rounded back lifter drew a scream of pain into the tunnel of bright
lights that looked down upon him... showing the texture of his red
skin and his squinted eyes. Lay at rest young lad... for your dreams
must suffer into the pain you hurdle, the scream of embarrassment
shuns your pride as weakness floods the building that spins around
you. Kids cry, as parents cover their small tearful eyes. Help!
One man screamed from the back, while pushing over the table he once
sat at handing out fliers for his small business. He ran fast to the
stage to try to save such an ugly piece of shit animal. The lifter
so torn and helpless... so wrong in every way. A crime that must be
stopped, that gets the worst of punishment... publicly hung for all
to see. Publicly stained by fruit being thrown, splashing upon his
face like green slime on the bottom of the little white airplane bag.
Laughter collapses the room like the boiling chuckle of a witch's
rant. Outcast this animal!... Outcast this puke of a human! A rounded
back monster has entered the sport they scream, under the seat they
hide while eyes of blood leak from the lifter's struggle... a struggle
only an animal could understand. Knees hit like a car crash as sirens
yelp. 90 degrees and half way up, legs fold like the jacket of a
retired golfer. Hung up and dry, only seeing the light if someone
asks. The golfer says, "Yes, of course!" as he rushes upstairs to
show off his achievement to someone who actually gives a fuck. A give
a fuck is all this old man needs to better his day... even month that
just maybe might leak into a year. It all matters how many times he
gets to show his green jacket off. How many people care to ask, for
interest lacks as he overflows with constant excitement. Caring is a
universal drug that will never be topped. One this world needs more
of, as I sit and write this I ponder how much more care I can put out
to others, outside of my world and into others.

Carry this bar man! A coach yells from the left corner of the hunch
back's shoulder. The freak that peaks open one eye to see where he is
at in the lift... for feeling of his art is now replaced with guilt
on what others might say... in this example we must conquer defeat in
standing with overcome. Rising to the challenge while others whisper
hate, for beauty lies within the beholder of the weight... on the bar

and within. Smile with blood young lad. Let your yellow teeth dagger
the ones who rage at your craft. Let your knees buckle and your back
round to prove to yourself the non-approval of others doesn't affect
you. The one thing that is required from you... a made lift, to make
your life what you have pictured in your day dreams as night sets in,
making your dreams clear. So clear that sound is removed from your
ears while your thoughts pinch your skin. Reality is there... even
though others don't see as clear.

The forums start to type words of hate, as the judges cringe in horror.
"This weightlifter on stage has the worst technique," they whisper from
back to front, as the athlete's elbows drop from the heavy clean taking
him to his toes. Heels off the platform as his hips rotate to the side
like a plane spinning to its death. His spine bent like the people
in the audience hurled over as more green puke comes spooling out from
their dirty mouths. He stood.......how? No one knew. The place was
in shock, as the computer monitors that looked like the chalk board in
the Harvard hallways froze. Lights lowered and dimmed as the middle
light grew heat like the sun... casting a spotlight on the athlete who
dared to stand with such ugly form, that even Betty left the room and
took on the elephant man as a date. A pen fell... literally a pen, not
a metaphor. When the pin dropped a small drip of sweat dropped from
the lifter's forehead. Splash! The drop was long and the decent was
even longer. The pen rolled like the weight on the outside of his bar.
Spinning fast like his mind. Collars were tight, as his collar bone was
in pain. The resting of the bar gave his chest time to breathe, as his
throat felt suffocated from the cold bar piercing his skin. Lips open
like a gold fish as air entered like Thanksgiving dinner... and left
just as fast once full. Knees locked like a door at night, while kids
asleep a gun should be in close sight. Protect your house young man...
protect your dignity and make this fucken lift!....This his father said
in his mind. His father knew nothing of weightlifting, but he did know
about winning... and more about losing. A man that knows more about
losing than winning is the man you want in your corner. For mistakes
he has made will never be forgotten in the arms of others. Let his
cuts be your sail, as his blood flickers into the wind, guiding your
dreams like a knife through skin. Blunt. In your face, and times
advice you don't want to hear makes you stronger... especially in a
jerk to the moon.

His long legs shaky while his eyes wide open. A ghost might as well
passed the lifter on stage, as he motionlessly stands with a look
of haze, for what they don't see is the concentration of rage. The

530

thought of dropping this weight on the faces who puke, killing all
who doubt him, killing all who bared to look. A dip with his hips as
the bar bent with his motion. A fast motion that kept the middle of
the bar straight, while the ends like eagle wings, dipping low only
to fly. The oscillation of the bar turned metal into feathers. The
lifter's face turned long and yellow, as a beak grew and eyes of
black stained his face. The flap from the wings of the bird created
a rustle of wind that pushed violently into the audience of puke. A
hurricane of sort, turning vomit into rain, as thousands flocked out
from the competition room. The computer monitors sparked, as the
judges dodged the gusty winds as lights fell from the celling. Chaos
was created for those who watched, not the one who lifted.

The eagle was born before those who saw disgust, from a person who
just wanted to stand. THEN THE BIRD DROPPED LOW, ONLY TO FLY SO HIGH!
I used all caps to assure all the readers who watched from the side,
that he made this jerk... so we can all give the middle finger to the
made up audience watching from the front. Letting lightening and
thunder blast through the fucken roof! This ain't a depressing blog,
this is the truth! This is not bodybuilding, we decide a win or lose.
No such thing as a bad make, only a solid bright gold medal up for
the take. The lifter made the lift while the judges pushed white, as
papers and blinds flew from all sides. For the people left in the room
still watching, taking cover was the only option. Three whites he made
the lift. The room at this point was empty from the wind it carried.
Only a few people saw his testimony to the bar, as the weight stayed
steady and high, breathless but alive. He then let out a roar for all
to hear, a roar that translated to this................

Give me my fucken gold.

A beautiful made lift 2016
Freedom 2016

♪ ♪ ♪

Poker & Things

I love writing about pain. I find the beauty in it all too moving.
Like losing in a poker game......the loss makes us more alive and
open to the thought of winning. More motivated to succeed, and more
passionate about our direction in life. I guess I am addicted more to
the struggle, than I am the victory. How the victor became victorious
is more intriguing to me than the view from the top. For the clouds may
look eye gazing and white, but the dark made us appreciate the sight.

Cigarette smoke swiftly clouds the clay chips like fog on the wet road.
You know.....the early morning buzz we get while others snooze in a
comfort of average. They sleep in a bed where the bar lays low. The
strong don't just survive....we prosper. Breathtaking the black road
is while yellow stripes pass and flicker. White lightening rods on the
side make my two front windows lower. I find that my writing usually
starts on the way to my destination of writing....rather than the
writing itself. My thoughts play like a movie, as my athletes train
in pain, their knees black and purple from the constant thud of hitting
rock bottom. Redirection to stand up fast. Ballet with a bar we are,
but once off the platform when the dance ends, we become crippled and
full of rust. Tired and slow of breath. Their new journey takes me
back to the start of mine. Almost as I am starting all over from my
first meet to now. The path is different, but so the same.

I pull up to the Barnes and Nobel as if I was smart. Accepted I truly
am, as I blend in perfectly with the other brown coats and grey haired
suits. Only if they knew who I really was, what then? Would they
accept me like they do now? In this club of knowledge while sound
whispers throughout. I write what I was thinking about on the drive
over. What plays in my head I literally put to paper. I see it play
out in my head, the dark thoughts mixed with caffeine, everything
coming together in a blend of weightlifting. I always say that the
song that I listen to writes the blog, but as I keep writing I am
finding out that all my surroundings play a big part. This is why
waking up early is a must. More life to take in. More smells to
breath in. All while people watching in Barnes and Nobel.....all
while building a better sense of what the fuck is going on.

Chips clack and slide as the felt of green is so smooth and at ease.
The sound of poker like the sound of weightlifting adds in addiction

532

of its own. For every thud of a chip or knock of a check, falls a
red slab of beef or heels that cut sharp and fast. All sounds that
have feeling that move from the famous flip to peak of the cards, to
the callused chalked hands meeting the cold bar. Edge of our seat
we sit, leather or medal, cards or bars, fingers stay crossed while
hard work hopefully pays off. Small injuries pop up like pimples on a
teenage kid. I sometimes just laugh at the site of this over dramatic
issue. Tape that shit up and shut up. Get back on the bar and lift.
If you can't hack it then pack it. Extreme I am.....yes. Being
extreme has worked well for me, I like to practice what I preach,
and preach what I practiced. It's a hard nosed sport that gets less
credit and respect than anything out there. Weightlifting........
it's fucken hard, it hurts, so what. Just like the great Dave Spitz
use to tell me right before I approached a lift, "If it feels heavy
it's ok.....it's supposed to be heavy.....it's weightlifting". Bam
baby. Love that line. I love it because it's so damn true. We need
to stop fighting the weight and just lift the weight. It's like my
grandfather used to tell my mom as a kid, "You spend more time getting
out of work, than when you do the actual work itself" - Poppy.

Poker to weightlifting, felt to wood and pain to victor. A morning
drive to a book store to write. A hidden black sheep takes cover
amongst white. The dark journey to bright, while painful knees
and injuries try to act like they have some say in our goals. You
reading this are probably getting ready to battle and fight! For
weightlifting practice is near, and even though this blog seems to
merge in all different directions......to a weightlifter it makes
perfect fucken sense. Salute.

The Dark Orchestra 2016

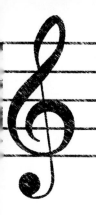

CHAPTER 18:
THE DARK ORCHESTRA
2014

Virus

Friday, January 3, 2014

These fucken shoulders sting like a nail in the foot. Lower back
mangled like a bush of thorns, and twisted like my knuckles from the
walls I have punched.....fuck. Fuck is right, fuck explains it all.
Fuck is the cap that releases the pressure from our heads. The word
fuck makes sense in a sport that makes none. Legs heavy like the
demons I carry. Regret is worse than a missed lift....while sadness
seems to overpower the highs. A virus of some sort has spread to so
many, leaving the light shadowed out, and sleep never to be the same.
A virus that lifts the soul....but breaks the body. A virus that
makes us live, before it kills. A virus that spreads faster than the
sting up your neck when slept on wrong from a brutal day of training.
A morning of coffee is shared with the bug of weightlifting, while
the double-edged sword kills the dragon leaving scars on ours palms.
This is weightlifting.

My eyes lay red for the dark turns me black. You
and I lay at rest in a gym where bars and plates
spend their last days. A graveyard of once
strong, has now fallen to the dust of dark and
cold, stuck with no spin, and
bent from slams of the past.
The glory days of so many find
peace within the place they found
life. A soul so proud while
knees click like crying
children. Echoes of "what
ifs" rain about the
hollow gym. For bars and
weights don't take up too
much space, while the feeling
of unfinished drapes from above.
Here I have this paper called
freedom that lays in front of me.

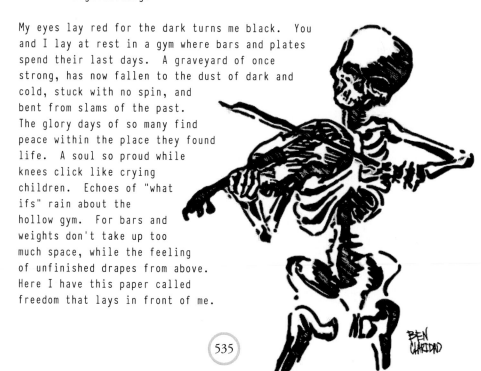

BEN
CARIDAD

Freedom paper to escape and travel, run away to a sandy beach, swim
in an ocean I can call home, while fine dinners and wine sooth my
body. Success has opened a door for much more. The light so bright
as signs point for my escape. No more pain.....no more struggle.....
no more days filled of missed lifts and let downs. No more bad days.
The sun awaits as a new life calls. I look behind me as the lighted
door gets closer to my pale white face. The gym so cold and dark,
so empty and unforgiving. The same gym that broke my brother's neck.
The same gym that bombed me out, split my head open, out casted past
friends and family, beat me, pulled me from school and sheltered me
from society. The new strong bars are telling me to leave! Spitting
at my ankles, as the fresh colored weights laugh at my numbers....
telling me how weak and disgusting I am. This gym is not my home,
but my prison. I have one life.....only one.....and I have spent
half of it here......alone......in the dark. Why? Fuck. The outside
seems so nice. The temptation warms my skin. A new life awaits. A
new life I know nothing about. The outside world seems big, and more
unforgiving than this gym. The sun burns more than the dark. Even
though half the weightlifting world hates me.....I still call them
family. I still feel at home under their ridicule, along with the
ones who fight side by side with me, and you the reader.....will
you be out there in the sun? An answer of a broken pipe from the
ceiling above drips down against one of the wooden platforms over....
and over...and over again, with the best response you could of ever
given me. A response of no......no we will not, we will die in this
gym......we will fight in this gym......no we will not surrender to
the pleasures that so many speak upon. For hell is our home and the
dark is our shelter.

A warm breeze from outside enters through the door that sprays half
my face with light, as the gym covers the other half with dark. A
breeze that swept the dust off the top of the bars that lay broken.
The graveyard as I call it, where one day I will lie, we will lie,
buried in this gym for others to step over and for dust to multiply.
The dusty bars have never left, in a way they are still fighting
with their presence as they lie with more strength then when they
lived. Still in the gym to show lifters that this sport is a never
ending story.....a never ending journey. My red eyes turn black,
as the veins in my skin turn purple. My body starts to shake as my
lips turn dry. A gym that once was blacker than night, has given
me sight. I could see better than before as the black stayed night.
It has happened once again just like 8 years ago........I have been
infected by the virus called the Weightlifting Bug. I slowly walked

to the door that smelled of salt water and sounds of baseball games.
I took my pale hand and shut the door until the last bit of light
suffocated. I lit a match to burn the paper of freedom in front
of me. A new life piled high and tall cracked and burned, casting
shadows that flickered wall to wall, of myself.....and others who
have now come out from their resting bench. I choose to stay with
these bars of broke. I stay with these plates of bent. I choose the
dark. I choose the family that brought me in from the outside. I
choose strong. I choose better. I choose PR's and bars. I choose
to be great and follow my heart. I choose pain and discomfort. I
choose broken bodies and tears of red. I choose you. I choose to
put my head down and keep fighting day in and day out. Some will
leave...some will stay.....but just like these broken bars......I am
here until the death.

Skeletons 2016

♪♪♪

Recovery VS. Comfort

Monday, January 6, 2014

Jeff begs for his stomach to accept the steamy soup that sits rested
in his hands cupped like a bowl, morphed into a homeless man begging
for change on a cold afternoon. Hands of chalk and eyes of tired, his
big breath makes the steam float away fast and violently, as the bowl
of chunky soup only can imagine running away as well. The soup sits
so quietly in the hands of this non-hungry but hungry Weightlifter.
Stomach rolls for food, but the mouth won't open. Hands shake the
bowl in desperate need of food, fuel, and recovery. Eat! He yells
out in the lobby of the gym while his plastic spoon drapes the outer
line of the bowl as if sitting in a hot tub of pure relaxation. Don't
rush me mother fucker.......the spoon barked quietly as his head
fell back and his toes wiggled just peaking out from the soup before
plunging them back under. The athlete felt paralyzed. His mind
confused as his body was acting bi-polar. Jeff's friend Frank walked
by asking if everything was ok......Jeff replied without taking his
eyes off the soup bowl...."I'm good". But the sad news was Jeff was
not good. How could Jeff be so hungry but not eat? How could he not
move his arms to feed his body?....and why the fuck was this spoon
being such a piece of shit?   •

537

Hell month....that's what they call it. I guess it makes sense
considering this month in training was truly hell casted from the dark
valleys where the devil sleeps. Protein powder went down smooth......
only wanting to be thrown back up instantly once the chunky powder
bombs entered the power belly of Jeff. Big boy belly is what he called
it, pasta belly, carb belly, recovery belly.....most importantly.....
strong fucken belly. But as of late, a belly of sick and tired. A
body of disgust of any scent or sight. Fast paced movies gave Jeff
motion sickness, as the sight of a burger commercial made him weezy.
How could this be? He thought to himself while swirling the spoon
around the ever growing cold soup. How could an athlete train so hard
and not eat? It's more confusing than Leo not having won an Oscar
yet.......????   Jeff got up to slam a some creatine that tried to
hide away in the bottom of his paper cup. After a few swishes and
fancy maneuvering with his hand eye coordination he was able to gulp
down and capture all of the white rocks of creatine that made his body
tingle and itch.....a sensation that stood right behind sex. Yea.....
that good. A must for big weight....both sex and creatine. He paced
the lobby as if getting ready to run out on the court of a basketball
game. Introducing number "I'm not fucken hungry".....Jeff! and the
crowd goes crazy just like his body that so bleeds for food. The voice
of Shankle playing over and over in his head..."You gotta eat," Shankle
would say if in this situation. In a heated flash Jeff threw out the
bitch of a spoon from the bowl....grew a pair of balls while raising
the cup to his mouth.....and took a giant gulp of steak, potatoes,
vegetables and soupy awesomeness. He stood tall while the food raced
like the carpool lane at 5 o'clock and yelled "Shankle!!" for all to
hear! Jeff felt alive and in control. Jeff realized that food was just
like training....you must never listen to your body, with the bar, and
with food. Jeff grabbed the loaf of bread and stick of butter and took
bite after bite, mixing the butter and bread in his mouth....no time
to spread.....no time for liberal type shit. Jeff finished his soup
all while standing with his legs out wide and his chest raised high.
Rocking back and forth from the discomfort he was in while engulfing
his recovery food. He raised his fist up high with a crooked and full
of food smile he finished all his food and got one step closer to gold.

Food ain't food for an athlete.....food is recovery. Period. It
ain't supposed to taste good. Your girly purple grape protein shakes
can be shoved up your ass. The next time someone tells me what kind
of protein flavor they are drinking I am going to body slam them in
a cave of no return where monkeys eat brains. Do you want monkeys to
eat your brains!? That's what I thought, so shut up and eat, drink,

and stop caring how it tastes. Keeping your weight up is a sport of itself. Eating when not hungry is an Olympic Sport. If you ain't eating.....you ain't winning mother fucker. These non Attitude Nation pussies out there only eating when they're hungry makes me sick. Making short gains....? Food. Feeling too sore......? Food. Not a lot of energy......? Food. If you are taller than 5'10" you better be a 94 or above. If not.....you ain't eating. These self made pussies only think of weight classes, when they should be thinking about recovery. Food is not weight class.....food is recovery. Wherever the food takes you is your weight class!!! I am banging on these keys because of the bullshit that I have seen all over the world. Like Donny Shankle says, "No Comfort Zones" - Lion Killer.

Eat mother fucker   2016

♪ ♪ ♪

Let Go

Tuesday, January 14, 2014

Inspired by Donny Shankle

Back burnt to a crisp from the overwhelming heat of our past. Our necks pinch in pain from the constant looking back, seeing those we have lost throughout this sport. The old saying is, "they come and they go," but do they really? I still feel them behind me as I stand upon this railing. I still feel their presence on this bridge. I still see their faces hang in defeat as I hang mine in pain. At times lonely in a sport of one, surrounded by many that can be easily forgotten when alone too long. To repeat the same thing everyday makes for bones weary and eyes teary. Minds lose the simple touch to reality, as dark gyms breathe clouds of cold while dark shadows sit beside you for company. Once friends, once teammates.....never to be heard or seen again..... only memories fill this gym as my old Adidas shoes look back upon my empty face, in pure solitude, while a blanket of hell lays upon my back keeping me warm and ready for my next attempt. I am a warrior of this gym, of this platform.....and I will die amongst my shadow, I will take my final breath chasing my goals....even if the single goal I am trying to reach kills me. I am the dark. I am hell. I am a survivor of a sport that kills so many. A sport that breeds to destroy and grows to chop, for dreams are big and the fall is hard, the sound sounds nice as the sight from afar looks bright. One only feels the true fright once the weeks stack upon the next, as the body hurts and the money runs tight. Parents and friends ask why.....and soon you do too. I stand on this rail with the wind meeting my face. This spring day makes me want to train outside more often. A beautiful day like this makes me wish I was a cyclist. A hand simply lays itself upon my right shoulder, as another hand wraps around my left ankle. My naked body warm from the hot air that soothes my soul, as my skin gets cold from the past trying to ease me off the rail of this tall bridge. I find it funny that we think we are the ones holding onto the bar......

My penis hangs like my toes 80 feet above, as my heels stay down and dig, just like I have been taught, just like my body has known to understand after all these years. Hands out wide like an eagle ready to fly, ready to be set free. It seemed like yesterday that when the front door opened I would jump with joy for the idea of fresh blood, new lifters.......something new in a gym of the same. I'll never forget the day I started hating this sport......and we all do at some time or another. It reminded me of the time when Donny was asked in an interview what his favorite lift out of the two was. His hat laid low, his eyes lowered, as his silence convinced the room it was a question taken very seriously. He then with no movement at all, no hand jesters or a single blink of an eye responded with...."I hate 'em both". The day I came to this same conclusion is when all my friends left me. They walked into the door with a smile on their face, while mine smiled back ready and eager to embrace new teammates....new friends.....only to be constantly taken away by the devil in the red dress. Once friends, now dust on a bar. Once training partners, now a partner of my own. All alone again as my path continues with left over shadows of others and myself. Memories that fill the eye as these keys tap. For this blog is a dark hole of what has happened and what will come. Doors now open while my eyes stay down, hardened by the reality of what this sport brings..... broken bars and shoes of old, plates of color as dark is my new father. A single light to 5 rings is the shadow that others leave. Guiding me to what they could not, as their lack of strength gives me fire within my gut. Shankle who has taught me more than weightlifting.....but how to fight, will carry on with me 'til the day I cannot. I sit alone on my resting bench as the dark gives me light. My old shoes still with me in this never ending fight. I still stand with this hand on my back, burnt from the burned out light they try to keep me back. My past is my past while mistakes I have made. Gold medals and victories are hard to find underneath a pile of dirt, pissed on by others and laughed at by most. Doubts within and doubts by others, chatter behind my back even

by those I call my brother. 8 years down, this reunion is emotional. I
wanted to write to you the Nation, a family I call home. It's nice to
be able to talk to someone in a sport of such solitude.

Scared......fuck yes. Nervous.......fuck yes.   Not only about
letting go.....but the next 8 years. An email was sent and I read.
Wise words from a lion, who takes pray on heads.....in the jungle
he roams in areas unknown. His legacy forever will live on......and
lessons taught will never be forgot. I now know what I must do to
succeed moving forward.........

I let go, as my heels raised like my head to the sky. I fell to the
water of cold.......to fully embrace my future not yet told......

"We must learn to let go" - Donny Shankle

The Path 2016

♪♪♪

Anniversary

Tuesday, February 18, 2014

Can you hear me? I can hear you. Scrolling through old blog posts
trying to figure out witch one to re post......re post? Fuck re post.
If they missed it then they missed it. We got it, even if they can't
understand it. They are those who miss opportunities on purpose and
then blame others for missing the bus. You see the world as I do, as I
see it through your eyes as if I was you. You feel that....the bar in
your hands? Completely in control of your own destiny? The future cant be
told, for that you are blind, as I lay a thousand miles away wishing I
knew mine. Medals can't be seen from under a turning fan......but doing
what we love is ours.....as simplicity can fool the smartest of ones.
The smell of chalk doesn't change, just like our love for the sport stays
the same. Isn't it funny......that we are still here, as so many have
walked out. Its been years now and the Orchestra still plays as this
black stage salts our feet, as our pasts watches us from the back seats.
Completely dark, besides the small light peeking in from the bottom of
the old broken door that leads to wherever you walked in from. The lint
from the dusty stage dances within the light, as the skeletons continue
to make strings cry....as we still sit and watch with eyes of wide.

It's been over two years in this stage of black, you still sit with me
in complete silence. Why? So much has happened on the outside, to both
you and I. What keeps us visiting this place? Why do we love to listen
to our skeletons play violins? Why so dark? Has anybody ever tried to
turn on a light? This Orchestra sounds horrible from all the strings
that have broke, and the salt that has rusted out the wood. Seats that
creek and floors than moan. Cob webs that hang while dust claps after
every showing. This place is a bloody mess, a disaster, a completely
broken down piece of shit! Has anybody every tried to clean this
solitude mistress up? "No......leave the fort alone and don't change a
fucken thing. This is life, this is past, this is future, this is us,
this is beautiful, this is art, this is bright, this is home, this is
real, this is true, this is me, this is you...." Skeleton.

I sometimes forget to visit such a dark place when things in my life
are going so right. My ignorance leaves me forgetting what has
gotten me to this point. My past bad and wrong, dark and sorrowed
songed......has not done me wrong, but has instead ended me up here,
next to you listening to this song.   PLAY ON SKELETONS PLAY ON! I
yell from the stage, skeletons always hard to see for they play so far
away. I don't know if my dad ever re-visits anymore.....that one time
he did, his tears pushed him out the door. My success is due to this
stage with you, accepting my past has brought me strength times two.
Has time changed me from visiting the dark? I think not my friend
because I am back again.....something is pushing me to write words
through this salt filled pen. It's when I am the most happy I get the
most down. I have hurt so many, and made so many mistakes, my head
hangs low as I feel less than worthy. Faces of the past and feelings
towards the future, at times leave me locked in my office for hours,
as the door guards locked they from the outside. Fuck they, stay away.
They will never understand us.   Stay away good times, for sorrow is
my guest. A podcast if upbeat usually means I'm heavy in my chest.

It's good to see you again my friend. Let the our past be our
future......and our friendship become our strength. Salute to every
skeleton who has stayed with this blog from the start, this is only
the beginning to a new start.

Skeletons 2016

♪ ♪ ♪

Us

Monday, March 10, 2014

I guess sometimes I lose my mind....at times in a state of depression
for no real apparent reason, and times in a state of rage. Rage
on those who ever doubted me, rage on those who hurt me, and rage
against the single piece of metal that has hurt so many of my
close friends.....the bar. I sometimes lose my mind in a stage of
excitement. A sudden burst of insanity fuels my heart with hope to
one day become the man I never saw myself being so many years ago.
A solo piece of happiness that whispers in the back room of a meet,
that one day I could be a great father, teaching my kids everything
that I have learned, and most importantly...what not to do. Yes, some
hate me and most disagree, but for those that stand with me......it's
all worth it. For those who get me, I get them. Yes I slam bars,
and yes I like drinking coffee, but most importantly I say no to all
the things that have crippled me, a no to those who once surrounded
me. Drugs are a far away world, as coffee reminds me of the path I
am on. Guiding me to the stage where skeletons of my past look on.
I play my violin to not forget....but to never hide the feelings that
once shadowed myself from myself. The coming down was always the
worst. A living room with no furniture spoke thoughts of reality,
as the light from the rising sun peaking though the shades made my
pale skin feel warm, as my teeth chattered from the cold room. My
back against the wall, as my knees held my chin. I am death; I
am nothing; I am a slave to the crystals that fill my soul. I am
scum on earth that chooses easy rather than hard. I simply do not
live......so excuse me if I now choose to live.

My eyes heavy from up all nights and long talks. Talks about so
many goals and dreams that truly only live in smoke rings. Smoking
a cigarette to the butt....only means you're not done with the
nicotine rush. Yes this morning might be here, but I am no where
near facing what I have become. As the fan turns like the bar, only
in this chapter of my life it turns in fear. I remember crying in
the bathroom as my ribs would stick out from my side, eyes so dark
and wide you would think I wasn't alive. If you have been down this
path you know about the itching that takes place, for skin only
falls when the smoke fills your space. Every flake would shed a
tear, as I hoped no one heard my sniffling from near. Hanging with
a crew like this.....you never showed weakness......funny looking
back.....that's all we were, weak. I lose my mind from time to

time, only to find it in a better place than before. When this mind
is lost this body is weightless, the only thing heavy is the weights
I lift. My past is heavier than any bar, as my past skeletons are
my coach....rooting me on from afar. So sue me if I slam this bar,
or kick me out from this family I once thought was mine. The talk
chatters at night that things are already in order for leaving me
outside. What they don't understand is the dark is what I like.....
the only thing that truly scares me is the sunlight. I write alone
in this dark room I call home. A part of me still lives in the
past, but I choose this, for my past has turned into you, as gold
medals fill my room. Without the dark I would have never seen the
lights on the stage, walking out to a bar is my freedom from being
a slave. If you don't think empty living rooms with smoked filled
clouds is being a slave..... then you have never saw the sun creep
in through the shades. My friend......weightlifting is heaven,
as blue skys fill my cheeks with smiles and cries. I guess the
character from Training Day nailed it to my surprise.

This is a blog about the person you are. I am me, you are you.
Our skeletons have different pasts as our training room might play
different tunes. For those that shun our light, our sun.....they are
the ones who live everyday not knowing where they come from. Accept
your past, don't fight yourself, get to know your skeletons at last.
Your past is you and you are truly strong and true. I am me and with
you we are three...you, me and the skeletons make three.

Weightlifting is my love.....but my wife is my life. My dogs are
my heart. My future kids are my blood....and you the reader are my
understanding and my teammate...not in weightlifting but in life we
fight. You and I can achieve anything believing in.....well.....
you and I.

Don't change. I will not. I have never forgot what the dark as done
to my life.....it has made me happy, and introduced me to my wife.

                                        I love you, Jessica.

                          ♪ ♪ ♪

Crazy 8

Wednesday, March 19, 2014

Coffee at night........Coffee in the dead of the night, as I write
to the ones who raise hell during the day, and find peace at night.
Throat hurts from the bar, while eyes sag from rage. Black eye from
fighting.....teammates at war.....nothing new. I write the those
who fuck shit up during the day, only to dream about it at night. A
plot that thickens in the darkest of the night....fuck everyone, and
hold those you love tight. Step and sleep, wake and turn, wrestle
what Shankle cooks, and ripe what those wont. I type extra fast so
I don't loose what hits me, cleans crash on me as I drink wine like
Mathews. Red for wine, and dark like this living room, I say hello
before we sleep, I say more coffee! Jump below to keep reading if you
relate........the gym world is among us.......and its never to late.

A journal? I don't think so.....more like a confession to myself
and those who read. Read then write, a confession from us develops
throughout this dark night. No joke, 1am......coffee still by my side
as the quiet tv once alive and well, now lays dead by my side, lifeless
and stale. Junk is filled from the box of shit.....I don't watch shows
that fill my mind with nothing more than.....well, shit. Moving on,
one sip at a time. They told me to make paragraphs, so down I jump.
Follow me tonight as I write about nothing more than Weightlifting.

I like to think thoughts of forgiveness while I write letters of apology.
My mistakes may help others as they helped me, for my future kids will
know all I did wrong, only so they can make wrong decisions on their own.
They will fuck up, we all fuck up, and we will continue to fuck up. It's
how we move around the fuck up, getting to the side of stand up, that
makes it hard for most to swallow. Stand up and dust the dirt, shake
the dust, and become a man of trust and self accountability. Nut the
fuck up before you get knocked the fuck out......I tell myself as I look
in the mirror. Did you think I was talking to you? No, I would never
tell anyone how to handle themselves while looking into the unforgiving
mirror. A place so real, that most of the times I wash my hands I never
look up. I award myself so well with all my life gathered accomplishments
I have earned and taken, never mistaken for deserve.....the only thing
that deserves anything is children and animals, they are owed Love.
Don't give it to them......well then....you my friend are a piece of shit
terrorist and should be shot in the head. You my friend should be killed
on the spot and taken far from this world. Love is owed to some.....only

a few.....for the rest of us we fight, fight for what is ours and what we
have worked so hard to get. I blame others so fast, this is what I write
about tonight. My wrong paths and empty chats, leaving bad decisions
in other hands. I sometimes walk away from what I created.....good or
bad, rather than growing a pair and owing up. Both can spin in different
directions by the way you handle them. Bad can turn good, as good can
turn bad. The start is not the finish, for the finish is not 'til you're
dead, your family and friends must always be first and your last.

I guess this coffee has a weird way of sliding me into a mood,
slipping me off the kitchen chair into a room....a room so dark and
thoughtful, while awareness blinds me as my hand hides from me. Black
like my coffee, black like the lines around my eyes, that looks like
eye liner even to my own surprise. A weightlifter's mind works all the
time. Around the clock is we wait to squat, another minute passes as
our legs become shot. The night before a meet is where you win, when
the win becomes reality.....or when the win becomes a distinct dream
that only lies within the dead of the night memories. Shot legs means
strong for the meet ahead, acting slightly off means your going to be
on like donkey kong. Just saying......now jump down!

Make odd twitches, talk to yourself in a way of not understanding
yourself. Make those around you accept your odd mood as you move to a
place that only some will ever see, a place that feels alone and free.
Lost in space, where your breath feels like ice, and your heart beats
like a fight your parents got into on a vacation cold night........the
dead of the night make the worst fights. Alive we will be on top of
a platform, a moon walk must take years of prep, just to realize what
you are doing takes time to settle, as this coffee makes my emotions
rise, like smoke from my other friend I call my tea kettle. Funny
how coffee takes our bodies all over, at the same time keeping our
mind pinned to one thing. I usually drink tea at night, but being up
this late makes me excited for the next day fight. Will I sleep, yes
of course, after you read this it's off to bed. Awaiting me awaits
dreams of coffee mixed with c-4, weightlifting shoes and so many
people walking out the front door. Hmmm.......I wonder.......where
have they have all gone. What are they doing as I write along. I
have dreams of meets gone wrong, only to dream within a dream they
turned right. Friends and teammates I truly hope are doing alright.
I have odd dreams of roller blading......crazy 8. Once thought it
was cool to where jeans that covered the back of my shoes. Dragging
behind like a wasted bum in a midnight saloon. Green skateboard with
a Seattle helmet......I don't want to bore you with memories that

only live within me, I'll keep this blog somewhat on point as I keep
writing deeper into the night.......stay up with me longer...? If
so.....jump to the next paragraph with me.

Thank you for jumping down. I feel like we are back in middle school
sneaking out of our parent's house, only to destroy the community with
eggs and toilet paper. Ding dong ditch to feel bad and mean, take that
you house full of old people! Fuck everyone! We would yell so mad and
hurt.....from what? I don't know...... to this day that same anger comes
out, as if we were back slaughtering the quiet community we called home.
Stay up and let's eat pizza and watch the Rock. A great movie that
leaves us loving Cage, only to later ask ourselves why he is doing such
shitty movies these days. Bed time is near, again.....thank you for
staying up and sneaking out, egging houses and raising hell! Goodnight
my fellow friend........see you tomorrow for another day in hell...

Though I don't know you.....I truly know you. 2016 and beyond...next time
you see me I will give that look, at that moment we will all strike...

♪ ♪ ♪

Leathered

Saturday, July 5, 2014

Pull back with all your might......for us the skeletons should never
stop fighting the good fight. Heave! Pull! Use your back to attack
and your heart to win; the greatest gift an athlete is given is the
strength within. Pinch your shoulder blades tight to cut through the
wind! Fast with a swoosh and quick like a hush......this will keep the
weight from pounding us against the dust. "Back not up!" the lifters
yell from behind, as water creeps around the bend. Don't try to move a
bar; for it will always disguise itself as a friend, only to steal your
gold and rust your crown, athletes are kings that continually drown.
Under we go, heavy we constantly throw, as buckets of water sink us
low. Move around like sound, let the bar unite you with the ground, as
heels dig and tears falls......let your body move as your fear dies.

Chest up young lifter.... as the leathered faces crack a dry smile,
tying their shoes makes them remember days of denial. A heavy chest
means a weighted down soul, one that carries too many problems on a
platform of weight. Adding extra baggage becomes a weight too much for

any plate. Your knees will break and your heart will stop, as your eyes
look around an audience of silence. Let your chest rise as you break
through the air......let your lats spread like flight to a bird......
let your confidence soar as a lion with his roar. Donny Shankle watches
from the back of the room, blue hat low and jeans full of blue. If you
have lost your chest and your shoulder blades aren't tight... look at
the man postured in the back with a hate that blocks the light. A face
on an interview half covered from shade, half light, one half leathered
and the other half brave. The Cal Strength interview of Shankle is a
reminder on how to train. If you are a lifter reading this blog, you
must learn to learn, tighten your back like the curve of a spoon. Tight
and strong not just flat and solid, for a tree will lie when lying down
flat. Some look sturdy, while others look hollow. To find the right
tree takes years for the eye to see, the body to feel while your hand
falls free, once you stand long enough by a tree, you will know every
itch of its matter and how it may be. Learn how to keep your back
tight, and your hands free, this young lifter, is when skin becomes
leathered and the weight of the world becomes free.

I write to you from a corner booth in Starbucks. The day outside is
cloudy and the air is full of salt. I write by the ocean of peace,
thinking about tight backs, weights being made, and how a lifter's
movement to me is never the same. This is why technique is so intriguing
to my brain, a brain that has never been good at much besides movements
that mock the flow of rain. For we are the best athletes and dancers
alike, we move like the ocean on a stormy night. I lift weights for the
expression it gives, freedom of movement in a life of constant heartache.
You know as well as I that quick sand is quick to find.... grabbing a
bar will always relieve you of your pain, giving you another feeling of
ache...and well...pain. The microphone has consumed me far too long...
I am back home in the dark where I belong. I raise my fist, full of wine
and C4. Cheers to you, the ones of bones and salt, not from the sea but
by the stage of the never forgotten. Right through us they see our past
in the same room as me, and a window open from the Orchestra to the sea.
I ink my pen, I shed a tear, I write directly to you without any fear.

Without this blog I fake smiles. Without this blog I lose myself. I
am the dark, we are the Orchestra....

Olympics 2016

♪ ♪ ♪

C4

I am going to walk you through my C4 journey this morning while I
type to you in Starbucks. Better yet.....please, join me. Lets fly
together. Lets dream together and conquer together. Lets become
brothers in a world of war together. Lets drink the dancing water in
a room of dark, as we get high doing what we love. shhhh.....I can
hear society outside these boarded walls....lower your candle young
lad, we must never let them find us. Take the bars and squat racks
to the back. Shelter the plates and find homes for the clips.......
we all know those clips have a mind of their own. They were born
bastards in a sport that uses them in training as much as peanut
butter on pancakes. Bring the dancing water to the table. Now....
Before we start, let me stop this blog for a minute to give you time
to grab your C4 and watch the magical dust fall from the sky and then
twirl in your water......turning your cup from clear to the color of
your flavor. I choose strawberry......so let there be blood! Let the
sky turn from light morning blue....to the dark red that flows through
my veins! OK.......have you poured? good. Now raise your cup, glass,
water bottle, old coffee mug, skull of a lion.......cheers. Cheers to
the day, to our loved ones, and the ones we protect from harm. Cheers
to the iron sport we call life, that separates us from them, the weak
form the strong, the sheep from wolves, better yet.......as we call
them here in the dark orchestra......the ones with soft hands.....

First gulp down as I crack these little black keys. I close my
eyes and wait......wait for the rush of joy and the taste of all my
insecurities leaving my body like blood from a cut. The cracks of my
skin slither like small snakes, running rivers of fresh water amongst
my body washing away the day before, giving me a new fresh look on
this life we walk upon each day. My skin itches with pleasure, so
much that water drips from my eyes, as the goose bumps from my cracked
skin raise like the wave on top of a gold medal podium. The itch.....
starting from my cheeks, crawling up to my eyes, seeping into my skull,
and then like a water fall......down my whole body as if I was born
new. My fingers type faster, as my mind becomes sharper. The world
around me spins slower, as my concentration becomes better. The pain
in my knees starts to seep away like a high tree in a moving fog. My
back grows spikes to keep me safe from the back stabbers that lurk
during the day, and the two faced monsters who hide at night. My
senses grow consistent to a spider, giving me the power in separating

the closet haters, to the ones who truly have my best interest. My
foot now taps to the violin song I will post above. I write to its
rhythm. The beat moves me as the C4 runs through me. I am strong when
I am confident.......sadly I need dancing water to keep this instrument
tuned and sound, for without it I am not as sound, I am weak and less
bound. The room now completely dark, a great time for us to take
another gulp......better yet....this time lets take a giant chug......

Belly of warmth.....as bones grow bigger, and muscles become stronger.
At this point we are dangerous.....unknowing what we will do nor say,
not as scared at the punishment that may lay. Another chug down.....
as now my heart beats fast like the snatch. Hang snatches are the
fastest because of the stretch reflex the athlete can use if done
properly......C4 is a triple hang snatch above the knee, fast and
violent like a pirate ship set out to sea. I wonder if Shankle is
reading this blog, if so you better put down that sweet Louisiana
ice tea.....get your self some of this skin itching, belly warming,
red sea flowing, water dancing, pain relieving, weightlifting hulk
juice we call the 4th element of the C. Late, late at night when the
Orchestra is the quietest......The lion killer has been rumored to
lark in the dark. Its been chattered about throughout the halls a few
of the skeletons sitting in the very back row listing to the Orchestra
play on an ordinary day.....that lion heads have been found all
throughout this old forgotten auditorium. Who be-headed them? and why?
I have a pretty good guess on both matters....

C4 before training? The sheep ask. Yes, we reply without looking
up. I don't need to make eye contact with those I don't trust. I
keep to myself these days, I talk less these days. What I didn't tell
these sheep, is that C4 is a must on any day. Today is an off day for
Weightlifting......but not for life. I chug this bottle to connect
with you. I chug this bottle to clear the pain in order to smile.
The dancing water keeps me awake in order to live. Take it away......
you take away apart of my lifestyle.......take away my lifestyle, and
I don't trust myself in what kind of life choices I would make.

Stay away forever crystal mountains.......protect me dancing water........

C4 2016

♪ ♪ ♪

550

Projector

Thursday, December 25, 2014

It's where it all started. Full circle. 5 years later the Orchestra
stands, bent but never broken. Side ways, but strong. Old, but
perfect. My old friend. True & brutally honest. Dust on my hand,
as my calused palms drag upon the faded red cloth chairs. Row after
row, higher and higher the 5 story auditorium rises, until the dark
slowly starts to cast a blanket over the last few seats. Seats where
we have sat in so often, as our skeletons play sad songs from the
broken strings from our past. Perfect harmony, perfect motion, and
perfect sadness. Dark, empty, but ever so bold. Too bold and honest
for most, for most don't enter, only those who truly want, and can
accept their past can make peace from this Orchestra. My feet stick
from the salt water on the ground, as broken strings lay next to
broken promises, promises that held dreams oh so tight, only now to
lay out like an old rug that runs up the once lit up isle. I am back,
and it feels ever so good. The bright light from the outside world
creeps underneath the exit door, as boards and nails do their best to
block the sun. Black walls, filled with a black stage. Broken chairs
& fallen wallpaper sob like so many who enter this closet. Passed
the coats, passed the boxes, there lies a door, a door that leads to
a place I found back in 2010. I'm glad you can join me once again.
Join me as our journey continues. The next chapter may begin. But
first, let's go back before we move forward.

2010, I needed a place like this. A place where I could face my
demons like a man. I place that shed no shame, but bathed me in
guilt. A place that would introduce me face to face with the
skeletons that kept me up all those past nights. The boogie man
under my bed, as smoke and coke chased me around the nighttime life
I called hell. A world of frightful tales, amongst the worst of
devils. Regrets from my childhood haunt me; decisions I have made lay
me awake, as what if's wrestle me to the point of depression. What I
have created today takes me high, where I stand now is a dream world,
one of beauty and honesty, but entering the Dark Orchestra is a must,
for it keeps me grounded. 2010, I was going through a very hard time,
one without saying you can relate to. Slamming bars, chugging coffee,
and yelling on the platform wasn't enough. I needed something to yell
at me, something to slam me down and give me a rude awakening to the
person I had become, and the person I was. I needed the truth, one
not sheltered by caffeine and weights, but real, horribly real that

could help me grow to the man I always saw myself becoming. 2010, I sat down in the back room of Cal Strength, & began to write. It was weird...I started to write about this thing called...well...The Dark Orchestra. Where it came from...I will never know to this day. But boy, I am glad it came to me. Without it.... who knows who or where I would be today. This is my 5 year reunion of my blog, today I write again after a year to give thanks to something that connected me to you, you the reader, & hopefully through my writing helped you along the way as well.

I continue to slowly drag my hand over the stage and music stands raised up high like a skinny robot, as my walking feet creek the hardwood floor. A projector plays old videos from being a little boy all the way to my early days at Cal Strength, slamming bars at Sac State, flying to the American Open under Hassle Free, long chats with Ben Claridad, and long training sessions with Coach Jackie Mah. Scraping change for monster energy drinks to split with my wife, all with happy smiles on our face. Not a care in the world besides training. No cares, for all my skeletons at this point in my life were locked away and forgotten in my long lost closet door. Now sitting on the stage, feet dangling down as if I was a kid in a tree, now reminiscing about moving across country and throwing weight at squat racks at MDUSA. Epic YouTube videos cast a small smile over my face. I shake my head sometimes to see if it was all just a dream, but no...I was truly a part of so much good. I was truly a part of so much greatness.

Gold medals and bomb outs, missed teams and made teams, friends, enemies, brothers, and sisters. The scratchy projector screen above the stage continues to play a timeline of my life, as if it was waiting for me this long year I have been MIA. What happened? How did I become the man I am today? I walk the stage and throughout the maze of isles and seats with more confidence than ever before. I have come along way with my wife by my side, staying off by the exit door as so many memories catch me by surprise. We have accomplished so much; we have failed so much. I have changed, but this Orchestra hasn't. Still hungry, but at the same time, satisfied with my hard work. Hard work...something that sounds so simple, something that rolls off the tongue...something that is so hard...something that still must be performed.

A young, ambitious kid lifting weights for the love of the sport, and the world the sport lives within. Community...something I finally found back then. Acceptance, pride, attention, something that felt as warm as the sun on my face. I walk amongst this stage as my skeletons start to come out from the dark, cellos, violins, bass, saxophone, & pianos start to come together like life has a way of doing. I sit. I listen. Half my body covered in dark, half in dust, as sad music from my far & recent past keep me humbled and in check. An odd understanding comes forth, giving me pain, while turning it into strength. Sad songs at first, morph into songs of truth and fortune, breath and lungs, dreams of better places and untouched grounds, as fog circles my feet, and dark captures my head. My white eyes stay up toward my songs that play, as my chin points low, as thoughts interact with the music. The best part about the skeletons is they have a way of relating. You see...after a few songs your skin melts from understanding, admitting, seeing, and finally accepting. Your white bones become strong and loud, your white eyes turn to black, as your nails fall like leaves. Your clothes become nothing to you, so pure, so honest just this once, just this minute, your true feelings are the only thing that consumes you. You my reader, you my fellow friend, who sit next to me tonight, you are now turned into a skeleton. We are now skeletons. Nothing but bones that can be seen right through. Nothing to hide, nothing to fear. Skeletons of the dark are nothing more than our own mirror.

I can truly say that I am more of a man that I was last year. More mature, wiser, and more understanding on how this society works and turns. More keen to human behavior. Not as trusting, but more trusting in some situations. Still growing, still trying to understand, still playing my violin as a skeleton...no matter how much success I create, the Dark Orchestra keeps me straight. How far I have come...oh but how far I have to go. Blogs of sad, blogs of crazy, blogs of tears mixed with hate and love...this blog is more me than me, as my fingers bleed for truth and honesty, honesty within myself and others. My father not too long ago found the Dark Orchestra; I know so many skeletons reading this now have as well. Finding is key, but ever growing is a must. As my good friend and coach Les tells me... "This is only the beginning".

Skeletons of the dark that sit with me tonight, let us take pride in ourselves, our families and friends, and never forget that our past is what has made us who we are today, and today is a great day to fight.

Skeletons 2015

PS: Hey Shankle, better step up your writing game......I'm back. #blogwars

553

ABOUT JAMES MCDERMOTT

James McDermott is the Head Coach of Albany CrossFit located in Albany, New York. He specializes in Weightlifting instruction and is an avid competitor in the sport. During his tenure, James has coached several athletes to the podium as well as athletes competing in the CrossFit North East Regionals. While he is very active in sports & fitness now – this was not always the case. As a teenager James struggled with a multitude of health issues as a result of being overweight and living an unhealthy lifestyle. As he matured into a young adult, James became increasingly unhappy with his life and decided to do something about it. He took responsibility for his personal health and fitness by eating healthier, exercising and playing sports. Eventually, through a fiery passion for fitness, James began to seek out knowledge on how he could help others live happier, healthier lives.

James entered college with a simple decision and goal: to pursue a career in the fitness industry. He earned a Bachelor of Science in Kinesiology from State University of New York (SUNY) College at Cortland in 2012. His relentless passion to help others be better led him to discover Albany CrossFit where he was hired as an intern coach. James dedicated the next few years to Albany CrossFit and saw more responsibility given to him through a series of promotions in the company. He views his role in the gym and the opportunity to help bring about positive change in the lives of others as a privilege. James believes that he truly has the best job in the world. He is always looking for ways he can improve as a coach and expand upon his knowledge to better serve his athletes. A few of the certifications James currently holds include, but are not limited to:

- Attitude Nation Level 2 Coach
- Donny Shankle Weightlifting Seminar
- USA Weightlifting Sports Performance Coach
- FuBarbell + The Training Geek: Biomechanical Concepts Applied to Weightlifting
- Rock Tape: Fascial Movement Taping (FMT) Level 2
- CrossFit Level 2 Trainer (CF-L2)
- CrossFit Weightlifting Trainer

Insight into the Inception of The Dark Orchestra

James first met Jon North in June of 2012 when North visited Albany CrossFit to hold a seminar. This is a fond memory for James as the Attitude Nation Level 1 was the first seminar he ever attended – a truly life changing event. At the time James had been exposed to Weightlifting within the CrossFit community and knew very little about the sport. He found the movements to be frustrating, but was excited about the prospect of learning from a professional who boasted a new way of performing the Snatch and Clean & Jerk. James found Jon's personal story to be very inspiring and was fascinated by the way he taught and performed the movements. The seminar was an incredibly fun event and James walked away from it with a new found respect for Weightlifting and a personal record Clean & Jerk of 75KG.

Ever the student and eager to learn, James showed up to the seminar with a pen & notebook to take meticulous notes on Jon's technique instruction. He wanted to make sure that he remembered all of the steps so he could accurately teach his own athletes. Little did he know this would be the ember that would blaze a new path in his career and life. He recalled how he would frequently receive puzzled looks from Jon, who must have been thinking "what the heck is that guy doing?" – as James briskly wrote down his every word. Shortly after the seminar, James and his fellow coaches at Albany CrossFit set out to hold their own seminar to relay the information they learned to members of the gym. James wanted to share his notes with other coaches and athletes so he spent a large majority of the following week, staying up until all hours of the night, putting together an eighteen page manual of what he learned at the seminar. This manual contained coaching cues, diagrams created from photos of Jon found on the internet, and a step by step breakdown of The Technique of Oscillation (The Attitude Nation Catapult Method) as reviewed in Chapter 8 of this book.

James wanted to be sure that his presentation of the manual echoed his relentless pursuit of perfection through a high quality document. The manual eventually made its ways into Jon North's hands months later. James received a phone call from Jon who loved the manual and expressed interest in creating a book that contained his blogs, life story, and methods of technique. Jon wanted to give the Attitude Nation something they could be proud of and take with them every day to the gym. James was first relieved that Jon enjoyed what he had created and was eager to be a part of this new project. The two decided to discuss some ideas later that week and in the time leading up to that second meeting James began working on the book. He wanted to show Jon that he was indeed the man for the job and viewed their second meeting as essentially a job interview that he needed to perform well in. He spent hours brainstorming ideas, reading Jon's blog and watching California Strength YouTube videos. When the meeting arrived, James had a detailed outline for the book and information on the publishing process available. He bombarded Jon with all of his ideas who fell silent after the presentation for a long pause and eventually said to James, "You're the boss." Over the next year the two met via Skype and James attended many seminars to gather as much information about Jon and his methods as possible.

From the beginning James knew that if he was going to write this book then he needed to become a Weightlifter himself. He scaled back his training with CrossFit workouts and began training the Snatch and Clean & Jerk. In the trenches of hard Weightlifting training he formed a love for the sport, gained insight into how Jon must have felt at various points of his career, and learned a lot about himself as an athlete and coach. Over the years, Jon and James continued to put the pieces of the book together – a process they now have a new found respect for, and grew to become great friends.

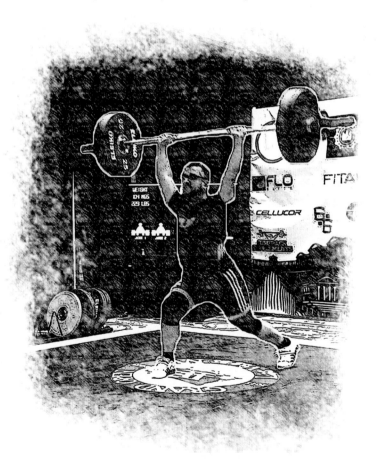

Acknowledgements from James

James hopes that you have enjoyed your experience within The Dark Orchestra. He wants you to know that everything that has been done was for You, The Attitude Nation, as him and Jon wanted to provide you with something very special. He thanks all of you for accepting him into your community – inspiring him as he watched you lift and gain knowledge from Jon. All of the handshakes, kind words, and warm smiles were greatly appreciated at the seminars he attended.

James would like to thank the people close to him that worked behind the scenes on the project. He feels that one of the most important things he did throughout the entire process was to ask for outside help when editing the book. Patrick Regan, Juanita Smart, Kiera Taylor, Joanna Toman, and Jessica North read draft after draft to ensure that the text was as close to perfect as possible. None of them are professionals, just people who care for Jon and James, love correcting grammar and are passionate about fitness and living a healthy life.

A special thank you is in order to Christopher Smith, Jordan Aguilar, Kayleigh Gratton and the rest of the Lingualinx, Inc. team. The Lingualinx, Inc. was essential on the development of the design and layout of the book. Quite simply, you would not be holding this text right now were it not for them. James met Christopher when he first came through the doors at Albany CrossFit. The two became great friends and James is very proud of his accomplishments as an athlete. It was Christopher who brought the services of Lingualinx to James' attention – he also acted as a liaison between James and the Troy Bookmakers (a local publishing company out of Troy, New York). He went out of his way to learn the ins and outs of the industry to help make this project flow as smoothly as possible. An additional thank you to Jordan is called for – he is an extraordinarily talented designer. He was able to take the ideas that James had swirling around in his head and make them a reality. Not enough can be said about Lingualinx, they are an exceptional company that truly values the journey their clients are on.

James wants Jon and Jessica North to know how truly grateful he is that they trusted him with such an enormous task. He knows that The Dark Orchestra is something that is deeply personal to the both of them and their continued support and belief in his abilities kept James going throughout the project. It has been his mission from day one to bring this project to life and to put the book in their hands.

Last, but certainly not least, James would like to thank his beautiful girlfriend Joanna Toman. Over the last three years she has patiently been his anchor – encouraging and supporting James when the weight of the project was heavy on his shoulders. She encouraged James at competitions, sat by his side as he worked for countless hours throughout the day and deep into the night, and traveled with him to seminars so that he would have company on the road. She helped to keep James focused and without her love and support he would have been truly lost.

The Dark Orchestra was built on a foundation of love. Love for the Attitude Nation and the sport of Weightlifting. Jon, James, Jessica, and everyone else involved hope this book helps you to grow as an athlete or coach and continue to Slam Bars and Kill PRs!